GIS in Healthcare

GIS in Healthcare

Editor

Fazlay S. Faruque

MDPI • Basel • Beijing • Wuhan • Barcelona • Belgrade • Manchester • Tokyo • Cluj • Tianjin

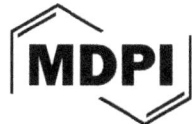

Editor
Fazlay S. Faruque
University of Mississippi Medical Center
USA

Editorial Office
MDPI
St. Alban-Anlage 66
4052 Basel, Switzerland

This is a reprint of articles from the Special Issue published online in the open access journal *ISPRS International Journal of Geo-Information* (ISSN 2220-9964) (available at: https://www.mdpi.com/journal/ijgi/special_issues/gis_health).

For citation purposes, cite each article independently as indicated on the article page online and as indicated below:

LastName, A.A.; LastName, B.B.; LastName, C.C. Article Title. *Journal Name* **Year**, *Volume Number*, Page Range.

ISBN 978-3-0365-3423-7 (Hbk)
ISBN 978-3-0365-3424-4 (PDF)

© 2022 by the authors. Articles in this book are Open Access and distributed under the Creative Commons Attribution (CC BY) license, which allows users to download, copy and build upon published articles, as long as the author and publisher are properly credited, which ensures maximum dissemination and a wider impact of our publications.

The book as a whole is distributed by MDPI under the terms and conditions of the Creative Commons license CC BY-NC-ND.

Contents

About the Editor vii

Abrar Almalki, Balakrishna Gokaraju, Nikhil Mehta and Daniel Adrian Doss
Geospatial and Machine Learning Regression Techniques for Analyzing Food Access Impact on Health Issues in Sustainable Communities
Reprinted from: *ISPRS Int. J. Geo-Inf.* **2021**, *10*, 745, doi:10.3390/ijgi10110745 1

José Manuel Naranjo Gómez, Rui Alexandre Castanho, José Cabezas Fernández and Luís Loures
Assessing Health Resources Equipped with Hemodynamic Rooms in the Portuguese-Spanish Borderland: Cross-Border Cooperation Strategies as a Possible Solution
Reprinted from: *ISPRS Int. J. Geo-Inf.* **2021**, *10*, 514, doi:10.3390/ijgi10080514 21

Maohua Liu, Siqi Luo and Xishihui Du
Exploring Equity in Healthcare Services: Spatial Accessibility Changes during Subway Expansion
Reprinted from: *ISPRS Int. J. Geo-Inf.* **2021**, *10*, 439, doi:10.3390/ijgi10070439 39

Nathaniel R. Geyer, Fritz C. Kessler and Eugene J. Lengerich
LionVu 2.0 Usability Assessment for Pennsylvania, United States
Reprinted from: *ISPRS Int. J. Geo-Inf.* **2020**, *9*, 619, doi:10.3390/ijgi9110619 57

Claudia Costa, José António Tenedório and Paula Santana
Disparities in Geographical Access to Hospitals in Portugal
Reprinted from: *ISPRS Int. J. Geo-Inf.* **2020**, *9*, 567, doi:10.3390/ijgi9100567 75

Gianquintieri Lorenzo, Brovelli Maria Antonia, Brambilla Piero Maria, Pagliosa Andrea, Villa Guido Francesco and Caiani Enrico Gianluca
Development of a Novel Framework to Propose New Strategies for Automated External Defibrillators Deployment Targeting Residential Out-Of-Hospital Cardiac Arrests: Application to the City of Milan
Reprinted from: *ISPRS Int. J. Geo-Inf.* **2020**, *9*, 491, doi:10.3390/ijgi9080491 103

Zhenghong Peng, Ru Wang, Lingbo Liu and Hao Wu
Exploring Urban Spatial Features of COVID-19 Transmission in Wuhan Based on Social Media Data
Reprinted from: *ISPRS Int. J. Geo-Inf.* **2020**, *9*, 402, doi:10.3390/ijgi9060402 121

Nivedita Nukavarapu and Surya Durbha
Interdependent Healthcare Critical Infrastructure Analysis in a Spatiotemporal Environment: A Case Study
Reprinted from: *ISPRS Int. J. Geo-Inf.* **2020**, *9*, 387, doi:10.3390/ijgi9060387 135

Liang Zhou, Shaohua Wang and Zhibang Xu
A Multi-factor Spatial Optimization Approach for Emergency Medical Facilities in Beijing
Reprinted from: *ISPRS Int. J. Geo-Inf.* **2020**, *9*, 361, doi:10.3390/ijgi9060361 165

Abdulkader Murad and Bandar Fuad Khashoggi
Using GIS for Disease Mapping and Clustering in Jeddah, Saudi Arabia
Reprinted from: *ISPRS Int. J. Geo-Inf.* **2020**, *9*, 328, doi:10.3390/ijgi9050328 181

Bandar Fuad Khashoggi and Abdulkader Murad
Issues of Healthcare Planning and GIS: A Review
Reprinted from: *ISPRS Int. J. Geo-Inf.* **2020**, *9*, 352, doi:10.3390/ijgi9060352 . . . . **203**

About the Editor

Fazlay S. Faruque is a Professor of Preventive Medicine at the University of Mississippi Medical Center (UMMC), USA. He joined UMMC in 2000 as the founding Director of GIS and Remote Sensing program. For the last thirty years, Dr. Faruque has been teaching and conducting research in the area of environmental health, utilizing a variety of geospatial technologies. As a principal investigator, he has managed extramural grants, including projects from NIH and NASA. His research projects are mainly within the areas of environmental health and the application of spatial methods in epidemiological and healthcare delivery-related studies. Since 2012, he has been serving as the Chair of the ISPRS Working Group on Environment and Health. Through his academic training, Dr. Faruque is a geological engineer.

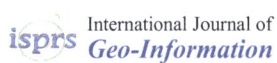

Article

Geospatial and Machine Learning Regression Techniques for Analyzing Food Access Impact on Health Issues in Sustainable Communities

Abrar Almalki [1,*], Balakrishna Gokaraju [1], Nikhil Mehta [2] and Daniel Adrian Doss [3]

1. AI&VI Lab from NCAT and Visualizations and Computing Advanced Research Center (ViCAR) North Carolina Agriculture and Technical State University, 1601 East Market Street, Greensboro, NC 27411, USA; bgokaraju@ncat.edu
2. Department of Information Systems and Supply Chain Management, University of North Carolina at Greensboro, Greensboro, NC 27402, USA; n_mehta@uncg.edu
3. Interim Chair of Johnston Division of Business and Associate Professor of Cybersecurity, University of Tennessee, Pulaski, TN 37478, USA; ddoss@tulane.edu
* Correspondence: aaalmalki@aggies.ncat.edu

Citation: Almalki, A.; Gokaraju, B.; Mehta, N.; Doss, D.A. Geospatial and Machine Learning Regression Techniques for Analyzing Food Access Impact on Health Issues in Sustainable Communities. ISPRS Int. J. Geo-Inf. **2021**, 10, 745. https://doi.org/10.3390/ijgi10110745

Academic Editors: Wolfgang Kainz and Fazlay S. Faruque

Received: 28 July 2021
Accepted: 27 October 2021
Published: 3 November 2021

Publisher's Note: MDPI stays neutral with regard to jurisdictional claims in published maps and institutional affiliations.

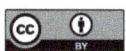

Copyright: © 2021 by the authors. Licensee MDPI, Basel, Switzerland. This article is an open access article distributed under the terms and conditions of the Creative Commons Attribution (CC BY) license (https://creativecommons.org/licenses/by/4.0/).

Abstract: Food access is a major key component in food security, as it is every individual's right to proper access to a nutritious and affordable food supply. Low access to healthy food sources influences people's diet and activity habits. Guilford County in North Carolina has a high ranking in low food security and a high rate of health issues such as high blood pressure, high cholesterol, and obesity. Therefore, the primary objective of this study was to investigate the geospatial correlation between health issues and food access areas. The secondary objective was to quantitatively compare food access areas and heath issues' descriptive statistics. The tertiary objective was to compare several machine learning techniques and find the best model that fit health issues against various food access variables with the highest performance accuracy. In this study, we adopted a food-access perspective to show that communities that have residents who have equitable access to healthy food options are typically less vulnerable to health-related disasters. We propose a methodology to help policymakers lower the number of health issues in Guilford County by analyzing such issues via correlation with respect to food access. Specifically, we conducted a geographic information system mapping methodology to examine how access to healthy food options influenced health and mortality outcomes in one of the largest counties in the state of North Carolina. We created geospatial maps representing food deserts—areas with scarce access to nutritious food; food swamps—areas with more availability of unhealthy food options compared to healthy food options; and food oases—areas with a relatively higher availability of healthy food options than unhealthy options. Our results presented a positive correlation coefficient of $R^2 = 0.819$ among obesity and the independent variables of transportation access, and population. The correlation coefficient matrix analysis helped to identify a strong negative correlation between obesity and median income. Overall, this study offers valuable insights that can help health authorities develop preemptive preparedness for healthcare disasters.

Keywords: disaster preparedness; smart cities; sustainable cities; food desert; regression analysis

1. Introduction

City planning for sustainable communities requires equitable distribution of and access to healthy food options for inhabitants. This study examined the statistical association between food access on people's health and its connection to income and mobility access. The unbalanced distribution of food may have consequences concerning health and other factors. In this study, we examined these issues in Guilford County, North Carolina. Guilford County was ranked as the highest in food scarcity in North Carolina by the Food Research and Action Center in 2020 [1]. Since then, the county has worked to analyze the factors associated with food scarcity, studying the area's income, education, and poverty rates. To advance Guilford County from a scarcity condition to sustainable equal distribution condition, an estimate of the scarcity situation and an analysis of the geographic areas for improvements in food access were needed. A key objective of sustainable communities is to effectively manage the health issues of their inhabitants. The process included gauging food access distribution by spatial methods, analyzing potential factors, and finding areas with remarkable numbers to start development. Recent studies have examined the distribution of food outlets and peoples' buying habits and their food options. However, there are several studies that have presented the investigation of food outlets' distribution geographically by integrating the health issues correlations to people's habits or food distribution. This study focused on the density of food outlets, the health issues regarding the food outlets' distribution, food access areas, and its correlation in terms of income, vehicle access, and health issues. Ultimately, we also simulated an improvement to provide suggestions and strategies for enabling Guilford County to become a smart, sustainable community in terms of food access.

Planning future cities requires scientists' and planners' points of views in solving current issues and prioritizing the service sectors according to the areas' needs. As a result, concepts, such as smart cities, intelligent cities, sustainable cities, and creative cities, were invented. The definitions of these concepts vary from one author to another based on the planning priorities. Several models have been applied to investigate health-related issues. A socio-ecological model (SEM) is an approach that investigates health as influenced by environment, social, policy, and physical factors [2]. SEM investigates levels of influence at the interpersonal, institutional, community, and public policy levels [2]. This model investigated factors at each layer to understand their relationships [3]. Nevertheless, this model estimated prediction [4]. For instance, a study presented the application of the SEM model to investigate obesity-related variables such as vesical activities [3]. The layers that presented the strongest on predicting childhood obesity were neighborhood characteristics, parent demographics, and parent participation in their community [3].

According to [5], more advanced management technology can be used to manage a city's resources and provide security [5]. In city planning, food access is primarily analyzed by scientists and decision makers to show its influence on the health of people living in these areas [6]. Food security and access were measured using several methods. Several techniques and methods were applied to measure food distribution and security. Measuring the geographical location of food outlets was performed based on applying GIS methods and tools. GIS is a software manager that analyzes data based on their geographical location [7]. GIS is applied to a wide range of problems such as natural hazards and public health [8]. GIS methods were used in different food analyses such as buffering, kernel density estimation, and spatial clustering [7]. More methods were applied depending on surveys and statistical data. For instance, an example method was based on the retail food environment index (RFEI) [9]. However, some methods have limitations concerning the application and presentation of results. The RFEI method has the limitation of not covering all tracts because of the need of calculating all food outlets categories such as supermarkets [9]. A study performed in California showed that data maples covered only 3719 out of 7049 based on the RFEI method [9].

Techniques, such as machine learning, are now used for research related to food security, as they are highly data-driven models. Machine learning (ML) is a programming technique that is used to solve nonlinear problems efficiently. It has models and algorithms, where the algorithm executes on the data to create the model [10]. It has serval different models to investigate relationships and compare results. The ML techniques were used to solve major problems such as classification, regression, reinforcement, and clustering [11]. The regression analysis was applied to detect continuous metric output [12]. Regression problems were investigated by several models, for instance, linear and non-linear regression. These models also worked in hyper feature space for illustrating the relationship and were applied to different scientific fields [13]. A further example is the K-nearest neighbors regression model, which presents appealing results for small data [14].

Random forest regression models, as part of tree multioutput regression, were used to predict the variables [12]. More than one regression analysis can be used in comparison to find the best-suited model for higher performance. A study investigated food security using machine learning models (extreme gradient boosting, random forest, and CatBoost) to predict monthly variations [15]. This study investigated data involving food choices, income, geographical location, and climate [15]. It showed Xgboost was the best model and better results were presented when fewer changes in time and place accrued [15]. A further study in food security discussed the application of machine learning techniques to predict the modified retail food environment index (mRFEI) and found that a food desert differs from a food swamp thereby necessitating the application of different policies [16].

Furthermore, sustainable communities give priority to people's health [5]. However, currently, it is recommended to use smart and sustainable terms as one concept, which converges the application of data-driven technologies of smart cities with the key goal of creating sustainable communities to provide an equal right to the benefits and an equal access to healthy food [17].

Studying the distribution of food outlets involves studying the distribution of groceries, restaurants, and residents' density. Food access can be analyzed by studying the two key elements known as a *food desert* and a *food swamp*. Food swamps are areas with more unhealthy food options than healthy food options [18]. On the other hand, food deserts represent areas with low access to healthy food, and the expected distance was 500 meters, 0.3 miles, or 5–7 minutes of walking [19]. The characteristics of food deserts include availability of inexpensive food, poor nutrition, and limited healthy items in small stores [18]. Food insecurity is not only the critical area to be investigated. The availability of food sources is also very important. Food oases represent areas where people have an abundance of healthy food options rather than unhealthy food options [20]. In another study, the difference between food item prices was investigated with respect to food access areas, food deserts, food swamps, and food oases, and it was determined that there were no remarkable differences in the process [20].

Several studies investigated the influence between food distribution and other variables such as location, transportation, time, and behavior. A study of 36 counties of a suburban area showed that these areas suffered because residents needed to travel up to 30 miles for healthy food access [21]. Another study analyzed food access in the suburban areas and rural areas of Louisiana and determined that suburban areas near urbanization had greater access to healthy food [22]. Time could be analyzed by two dimensions including the time of events (such as weather events) and the time of source existence (such as food trucks and farmers' markets) [6]. For example, the accessibility of food by walking was found to be different in summer than in winter, as the time of the year and day were different. As a result, in the case of a health disaster, socially isolated communities with food scarcity were most severely affected [23]. A study applied GIS and analyzed people's access to transportation where the results indicated the importance of transportation access to improve people's food choices [24]. Another study analyzed people's behavior using data from an application designed for people to donate food [25]. The results showed a correlation between a higher number of donations points and more bus stops as a means of access to transportation [25].

Analyzing food access is a complex process that includes observing the current distribution of food outlets and analyzing the residents using different methods, factors, and scenarios. These factors were transportation access to supermarkets, the ethnic group of population distribution in food deserts, economic status, and chain and non-chain stores [26]. A study by Eckert and Shetty (2011) used block methods in geographic information systems (GIS), which applied network analysis to determine the distance between each resident and the grocery store (considering the residents' ethnic group and income) [27]. The result showed that there was no connection between income and ethnic group in relation to food access [27]. Regarding chain and non-chain stores, a report by the Economic Research Service (ERS) explained that smaller stores sold smaller packages at a higher cost compared to supermarkets and non-chain stores [26]. Moreover, they were typically situated in poorer areas [26]. Another study showed that more options for greater food items were available with lower prices in supermarkets compared to small stores [28].

One study on food access and its consequences examined the relationship between fast-food restaurants and obesity in the surrounding areas [29]. The study considered two miles as the accessibility distance to analyze the health records but found no connection between obesity and fast-food accessibility [29]. Another study in Philadelphia, which was considered the second lowest in food access among major cities nationally, concluded that many low-income and food access neighborhoods had a high number of health challenges such as diabetes, heart diseases, and cancer [26]. An additional study also found a connection between food deserts, low income, lack of transportation, and diabetes [30].

There have been several studies on the consequences of inadequate food distribution, and they included the number of diseases spreading. Healthy food access was a key factor in the obesity epidemic, and the high consumption of unhealthy food was a critical factor in diabetes, hypertension, cancer, high mortality rates, and life loss [18]. There were some studies on the health risks and mortality rates regarding food access, and some of these suggested looking into the factors of these rates after mapping them. A study by Cossman and others (2003) mapped the mortality rates in every county in the United States for 30 years and determined the highest and lowest mortality rates [31]. The study suggested looking into the continuous high mortality in a county and analyzing it to determine the involved factors [31]. Another study looked into mapping health issues, such as tuberculosis, and the correlation with human development such as food access, income, education, and health [32]. The study concluded that there was a connection between human development and tuberculosis [32], where neighborhoods with less than the average income and education had higher tuberculosis rates [32]. A further study illustrated the investigation of type 2 diabetes per county level by machine learning [33]. Its results illustrated no correlation between the health issue and the variables of physical activities, access to exercise, and food environment [33].

Several limitations on food access were presented in recent studies. A large percentage of studies focused on only one to two outlets or categories, and only a few investigated the effect of all types of food outlets [34]. Another method's limitation involved hypothesizing that people's health was only influenced by the stores located closed to their residential location [34]. A further limitation involved using separate methods concerning food, where nutrition studies were separated from food environment research (combining them with the support of more methods and techniques would present a comprehensive overview of food access and health consequences) [34].

The reviewed literature illustrated that several studies focused on a few parts or variables of the overall problem regarding food access, health issues, and regional distribution. We studied all food access areas together with their influence on three health issues as a holistic case and to help local authorities in decision making for future planning. According to the literature review, food scarcity was studied in the form of a food desert and food swamp but lacked their influence on health conditions and the comparison to food abundance. The research questions in this study were:

Using GIS spatial mapping, can we find possible correlations between food access distribution and health risk issues?

Do health issues depend solely on univariate food access distribution or multivariate analysis of transportation access, income, population, and food access?

Can the linear or nonlinear ML regression models be developed for dependent variable health risks with better determinant coefficient?

This study addressed the gap by finding the correlations of food desert factors, food swamps, and food oases impacting on health issues and mortality using geospatial information analysis, surveys, and machine learning techniques. Our contributions in this study included reporting the results of:

Investigating the geospatial correlation between food distribution and health issues;

Comparing the number of health issues between food access areas;
Estimating the statistical correlation between health issues and several variables;
Comparing the results of the regression analysis models regarding health issues related to several variables.

2. Materials and Methods

We examined Guilford County in North Carolina as our study area (Figure 1) including tabular attribute data. Data were obtained from the Health Department in Greensboro based on a crude survey, USDA Environmental Atlas, and the American Community Survey. Health records were collected by the North Carolina Department of Public Health. These data were geolocated by tracts. The data included income, food outlets, health records, low transportation aces, and mortality rates. Health records included (i) high cholesterol, where cholesterol was higher than 240 mg/dL and higher than 18% lipoprotein density; (ii) high blood pressure, where the systolic was 140 mm and diastolic was 90 mm or higher; (iii) obesity as defined by the World Health Organization, when an individual's body mass was greater than 30 [35–37]. At the time of this study, Guilford County aimed to become a smart, sustainable community. With a population of 533,670 within 645.70 square miles, it was the third most populated county in North Carolina and was also among the top five most densely populated counties in the state of North Carolina [20]. It was also the largest county in terms of acreage [38,39]. Guilford County had 118 census tracts, and it covered the cities of Greensboro and Highpoint and eight towns consisting of Gibsonville, Jamestown, Oak Ridge, Pleasant Garden, Sedalia, Stokesdale, Summerfield, and Whitsett. The county was identified primarily as a food desert in 2014 [1]. The median household income in this county was $51,072 [39]. Methods (see Figure 2) included applying GIS and regression analysis. The GIS method was selected to investigate the geographical correlation, and the regression analysis was conducted to combine it with statistical association. Regression analysis is a machine learning technique that can be applied to forecast prediction or investigate relationships [40]. Regression models were applied (as multioutput regression and multiple linear regression) to present relationship and compare their results. The mathematical foundation lies in deriving the nonlinear relationship of the dependent variable against the multivariate independent variables. We based our nonlinear multivariate regression model with a polynomial of the order 3 and 3 independent variables giving up to $2^n - 1$ coefficients. We compared this model against the other ML models and found that the random forest regression model performed better next to the nonlinear multivariate regression model. The hyper dimensional feature space transformation in the random forest technique yielded a better performance.

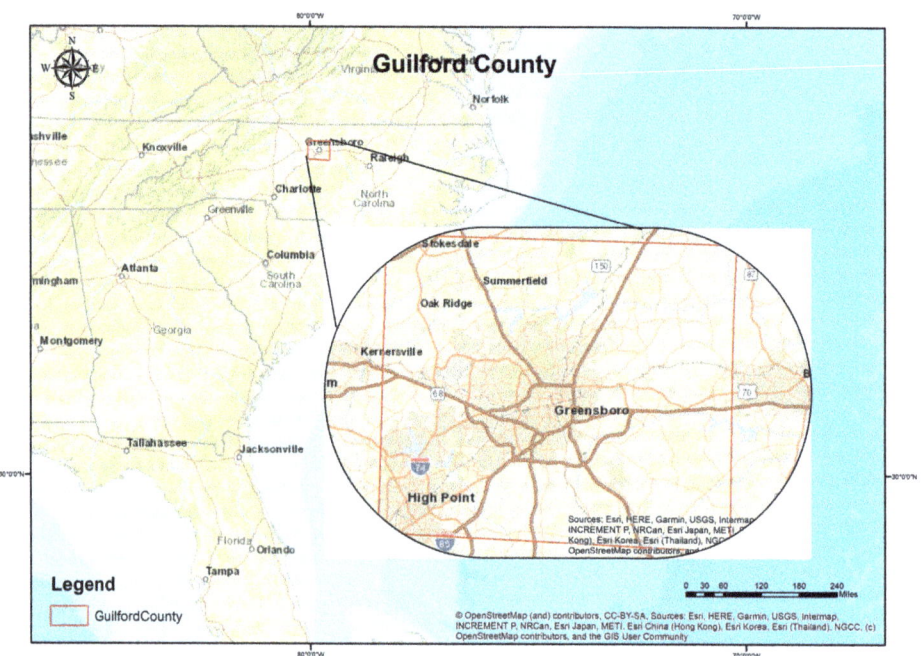

Figure 1. Study Area: Guilford County, North Carolina.

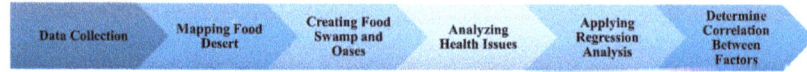

Figure 2. Methods.

2.1. GIS Method

First, we developed the geospatial maps of health (Figure 3) and mortality outcomes for Guilford County. Figure 4 llustrates the geospatial map of heart disease-related mortality rates in Guilford County by percent in each census tract. The descriptive statistics of these health issues are presented in Table 1.

The mortality rate due to the fact of heart diseases ranged between 0.002% and 0.008% per census tract. Figure 3 shows that there was a high density of obesity and high blood pressure in central Greensboro, Downtown, and Highpoint (outlined in the bounding box). It also coincided with the high density of high cholesterol issues. Notice that the density markers of high cholesterol had higher percentages than hypertension markers. These density maps were developed using the point density tool in ArcGIS software and were overlayed against the obesity density map. Interestingly, the west part of Guilford County showed low obesity numbers. However, high cholesterol and high blood pressure numbers were shown in few census tracts. The distribution of high blood pressure and high cholesterol showed a higher density around Greensboro and Highpoint, too. Figure 5 shows the mean household income distribution of Guilford County with obesity distribution. A low income was from USD 0 to 30,604, a middle income was between USD 30,604 and 91,812, and a high income was more than USD 91,819 per year [41]. The overall mortality rate map shows a similar pattern in the downtown Greensboro and High Point cities.

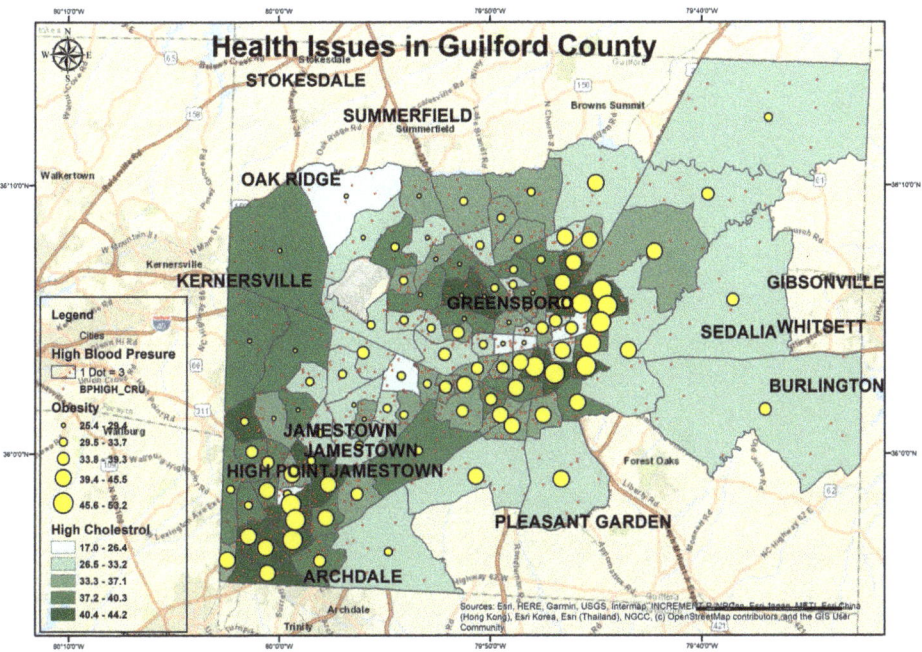

Figure 3. The distribution of health issues (i.e., high cholesterol, hypertension, and obesity) in Guilford County.

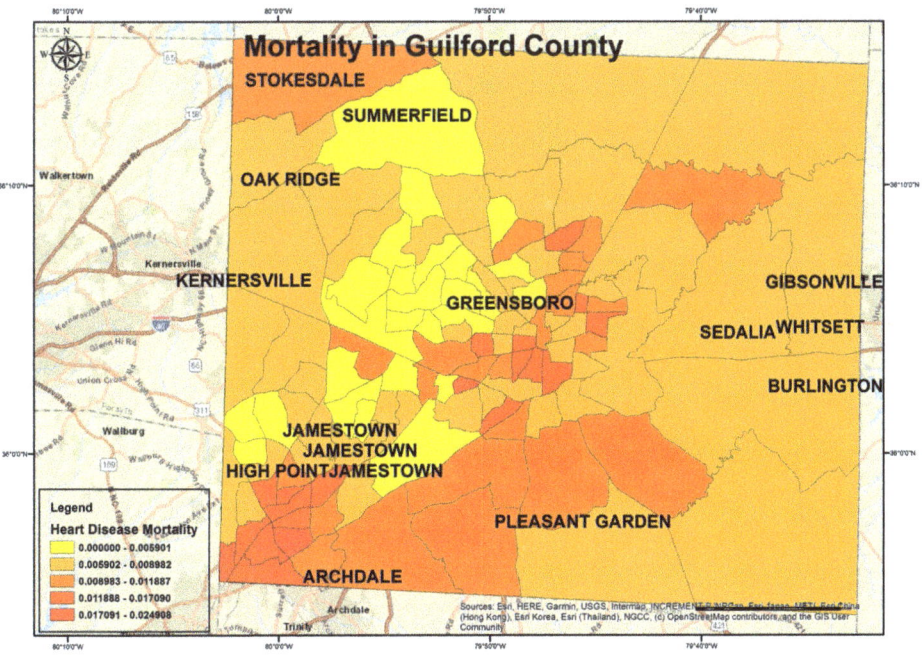

Figure 4. Heart disease mortality rates in Guilford County.

Table 1. Descriptive statistics.

Statistics	Median Income (USD)	Population	High Blood Pressure	High Cholesterol	Obesity
Mean	51,440.06	3979.78	34.10%	35.70%	35.87%
SD	25,725.97	1498.57	7.59%	5.01%	7.13%
Minimum	14,695.00	1300.00	13.30%	17.00%	25.40%
25% Quartile	33,889.00	2862.00	28.80%	32.80%	29.90%
50% Quartile	47,500.00	3903.00	33.10%	36.20%	34.20%
75% Quartile	60,653.00	5063.00	38.00%	39.60%	53.20%
Maximum	170,625.00	7791.00	55.00%	44.20%	53.20%

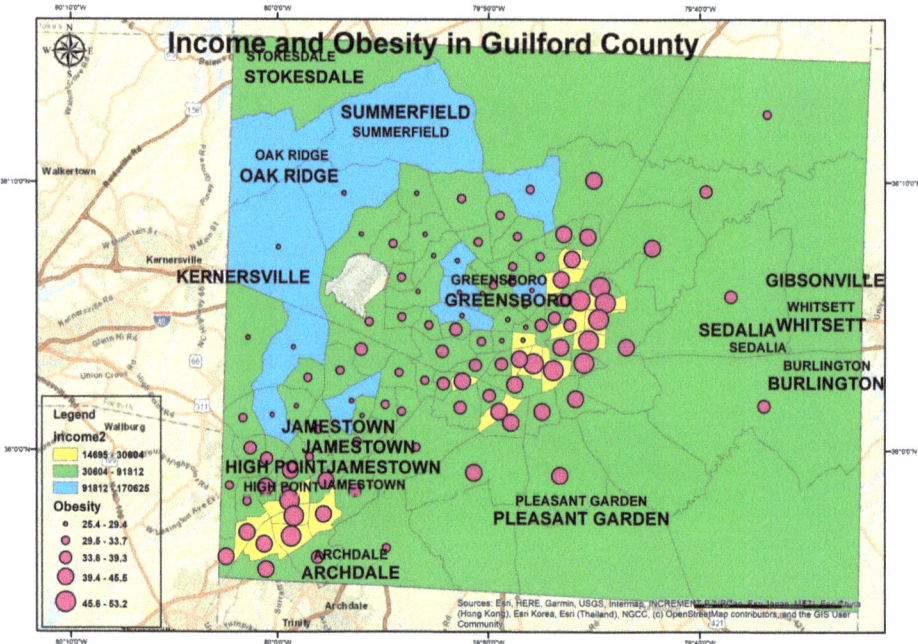

Figure 5. Income and obesity in Guilford County.

Later, we calculated the total number of healthy and unhealthy food outlets per census tract using the tabulate intersect method, which gave the result in a tabular format. Afterward, the resultant table was joined to the study area using the "Mathematical Join" option. The census tract shapefile was used to find the areas with higher unhealthy food from the intersection of healthy and unhealthy outlet maps in Figures 6 and 7. We then performed spatial analysis using the clip tool in the ArcGIS software to find the number of health issues and the mortality rates in all three food access areas (see Table 2).

Table 2. The statistics (mean and standard deviation) of health issues, density, income, and mortality rates in each food access area.

	Income (USD)	Population; Acreage	High Cholesterol (Mean, SD)	Obesity (Mean, SD)	Hypertension (Mean, SD)	Mortality (SD)
Food Deserts	41,369.35	105,695, 1418 acres	36.5%, 5.34%	42%, 6.52%	38.8%, 8.38%	0.01%
Food Swamps	51,783.43	189,166, 6485 acres	35%, 4.39%	34%, 6.63%	32%, 6.75%	0.0085%
Food Jungle	60,595.80	13,847, 27,584 acres	37%, 5.58%	35%, 7.84%	36.25%, 7.00%	0.0079%

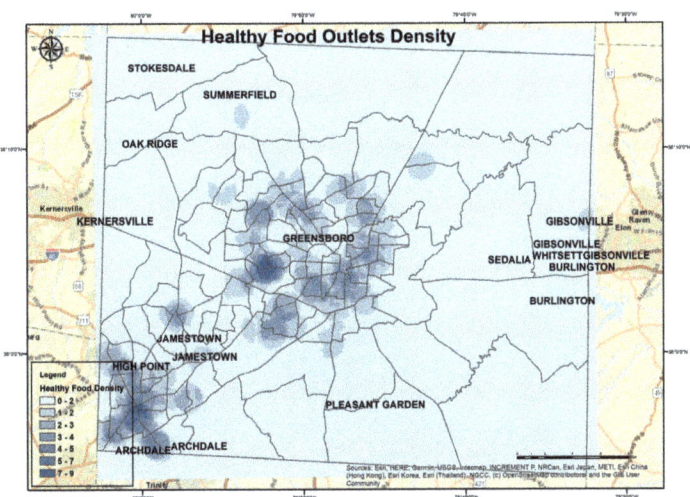

Figure 6. Geospatial map showing the density of healthy food options.

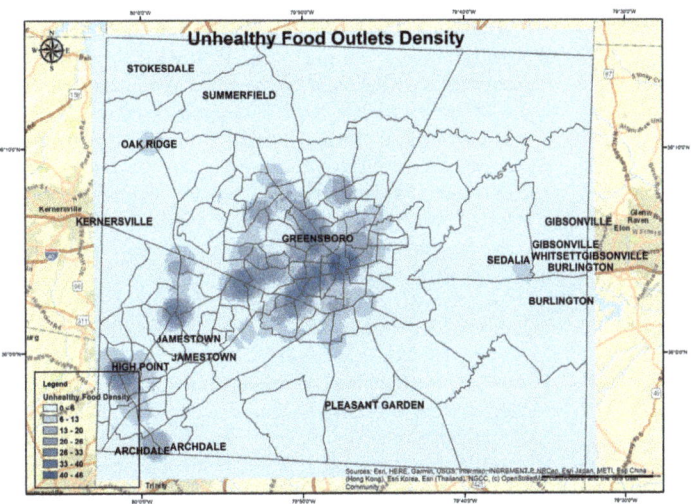

Figure 7. Geospatial map showing the density of unhealthy food options.

Next, we developed geospatial maps of the three food access areas. Based on healthy food access, Guilford County was divided into three food geographies: food deserts, food swamps, and food oases (Figure 8). Food deserts were measured based on the USDA Economic Research Service definition as the census that had a poverty rate defined as more than 20–30% of its people living more than 1 mile away from a full-service supermarket [42]. In addition, we included where the minority rate was higher, i.e., more than 30% of the total population [43,44]. A food desert is presented in the equation below:

Food desert = low access to supermarkets (the tracts with more than 30% of its people in more than one mile from supermarket) + low car access (households with no personal transportation) + high poverty rate + low income (<USD 30,000 p.a.).

The food desert method started by buffering 1 mile around supermarkets and applying the symmetric differences tool to find the tracts with 30% of the population living one mile away from supermarkets. After that, we applied the intersect tool to the previous layer with the layers of low income, low car access, and high poverty.

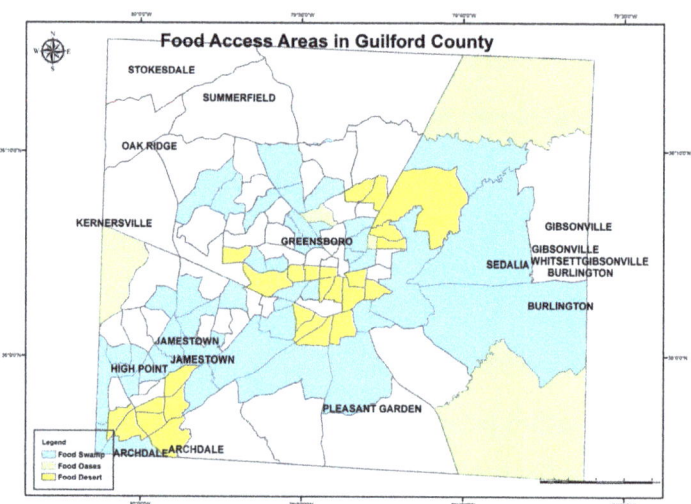

Figure 8. Geospatial map of food access in Guilford County.

The method started by buffering 1 mile around supermarkets and applying the symmetric differences tool to find the 30% of the population that was more than one mile to supermarkets. Afterward, we applied the intersect tool to the previous layer with the layers of income and poverty. Then food deserts showed areas where residents had scarce access to nutritious food. Geospatial mapping of food deserts in Guilford County was developed by identifying areas with the following overlapping characteristics: (i) healthy and unhealthy food density (Figures 6 and 7); (ii) high population density; (iii) high poverty and low income (Figure 5); (iv) low access to transportation. A food desert is a census tract that has less than a 20% poverty rate and at least 30% of its population lives more than one mile from supermarkets.

Afterward, we identified food swamps and food oases. A food swamp had more unhealthy food outlets than healthy outlets, but a food oasis had more healthy than unhealthy food options. Food outlets were categorized as healthy based on fresh food availability such as supermarkets and farmers' markets. Unhealthy food outlets were packed, and fast food was sold in various places such as restaurants and convenience stores. To develop the food oases and swamp geo-maps, we categorized healthy and unhealthy food outlets (Figures 6 and 7). The healthy outlets were where fresh vegetables, fruit, and meat were available. This category contained supermarkets, grocery stores, meat markets, farmers' markets, community gardens, farm road stands, and food parties. Although the second category represented relatively unhealthy food, it comprised convenience stores, dollar stores, and restaurants. We computed the density maps for healthy and unhealthy food outlet stores (Figures 6 and 7) using the region growing density tool. These density maps present the volume of stores for each category. For healthy food outlets, the highest number of stores ranged between 5 and 6 (dark spots in Figure 6), and the lowest was 0–2. For unhealthy food outlets, the highest number of outlets ranged between 40 and 46 stores (dark sports in Figure 7), and the lowest was 0–6.

We computed the descriptive statistics (i.e., mean values and standard deviation) of each health issue in these food access areas for correlation analysis. We used the clip tool additionally to merge the income layer by each food access area to compute the mean household income for Table 2. After developing the overall map showing the three food access areas' geographies (Figure 8), we compared the health records in each area to determine if there was an effect of healthy food access on health and mortality outcomes. The spatial analysis method showed positive correlations among food outlets and health issues, mortality rates, and income. The results are corroborated in Table 2.

In Table 2, the percentage of the population in food access areas may not provide a clear illustration of the number of people impacted by health issues. For instance, the quantity of 36.5% of the population in food deserts having high blood pressure was 38,578.674, which was higher than 37% of the population in the food jungle (consisting of 5123.39).

2.2. Multioutput Regression and Multiple Linear Regression

We used machine learning techniques to examine the quantitative analytics of population and median income on health issues by specifically applying multioutput regression and multiple linear regressions. Multioutput regressions are regression problems that involve predicting two or more numerical values given several independent variables. The multioutput algorithm is more efficient than the single-output algorithm, because the relations among outputs can be estimated simultaneously by the proposed prediction model. Moreover, application of more than one regression was necessary to compare their results. In this work, we predicted high blood pressure rates, high cholesterol rates, and obesity rates based on the inputs (independent variables) of population, income, and low car access.

The data set was divided into 80% training and 20% testing for multioutput model development. The training set contained eighty-seven (87) observations and twenty-two (22) observations in the testing set, and two different metrics: root mean square (RMS) and R-Squared (R^2) which were used to evaluate the models developed. The implementation of multioutput and multiple linear regression models was conducted with the Sklearn package in Python and MATLAB 2020a, respectively. The default parameters for the multioutput regression models are shown in Table 3.

Table 3. Regression models' parameters.

Model	Parameters
Linear Regression Model	copy_X=True, fit_intercept=True, n_jobs=None, normalize=False.
Decision Tress Regression Model	'ccp_alpha': 0.0, 'criterion': 'mse', 'max_depth': None,'max_features': None, 'max_leaf_nodes': None,'min_impurity_decrease': 0.0, 'min_impurity_split': None, 'min_samples_leaf': 1,'min_samples_split': 2, 'min_weight_fraction_leaf': 0.0, 'presort': 'deprecated', 'random_state': None, 'splitter': 'best'
Random Forest Regression Model	bootstrap=True, ccp_alpha=0.0, critrion='mse', max_depth=None, max_features='ato', max_leaf_nodes=None, max_saples=None, min_impurity_decrease=0.0, min_imprity_split=None, min_samples_leaf=1, min_samples_split=2, min_weight_fraction_leaf=0.0, n_estimtors=100, n_jobs=None, oob_score=False, random_state=None, verbose=0, warm_start=False
K-Nearest Neighbor Regression Model	lgorithm': 'auto', 'leaf_size': 30,'metric': 'minkowski', 'metric_params': None, 'n_jobs': None, 'n_neighbors': 5, 'p': 2, 'weights': 'uniform'

The below equation, based on multivariate linear regression, was applied to predict and investigate the relationship between variables, where 49.855 and 0.00029 were the coefficient for the median income variable, 13.233 was the coefficient for car access, and 0.00025 was the coefficient for the interaction between median income and low car access.

$$y = 49.855 - 0.00029 * MedIncome + 13.236 * Low\ Car\ Access - 0.00025 * MedIncome * Low\ Car\ Access.$$

3. Results and Discussion

3.1. Geospaital Correlation

Figures 5 and 6 show geospatial maps of the density of healthy and unhealthy food outlets in Guilford County. In Figure 6, the highest density cluster represents nine healthy and fresh food stores. They were located in the southwest of the county central and the south of the county. In Figure 7, the unhealthy density shows that 42 was the highest number of unhealthy food outlets in a square mile. These clusters were in central Greensboro

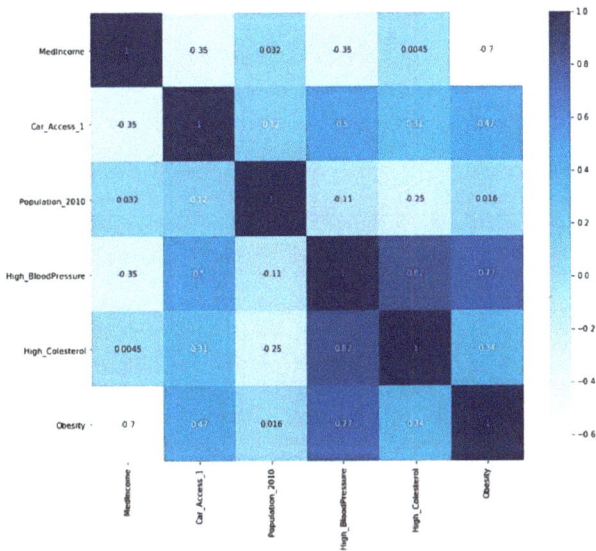

Figure 9. Correlation matrix with heatmap.

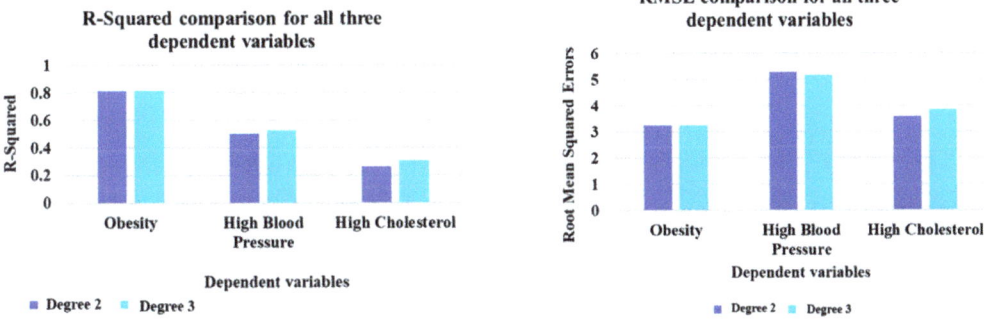

Figure 10. R-Squared and RMSE comparison of multivariate polynomial regression of second and third degrees.

3.2.1. Multioutput Regression Models

Multioutput regressions are regression problems that involve predicting two or more numerical values given several independent variables. The multioutput algorithm is more efficient than the single-output algorithm because multiple outputs can be estimated simultaneously by the proposed prediction model.

Based on the R-Squared values in Tables 4 and 5 below, none of the multioutput regression models can be recommended. Nevertheless, the R-Squared values of all four models with obesity as a dependent variable consistently achieved a higher score, with the highest being approximately 79%. The independent variables, namely, median income, low car access, and population, had a significant influence on obesity rate and a negative correlation with high cholesterol.

Table 4. R-Squared values of the k-nearest neighbors, random forest, and decision tree for multioutput regression.

Models	R-Squared		
	High Blood Pressure	High Cholesterol	Obesity
Linear regression for multioutput Regression	0.375	0.236	0.600
K-nearest neighbors for multioutput regression	0.349	0.045	0.771
Random forest for multioutput regression	0.350	0.054	0.797
Decision tree for multioutput regression	−0.261	−0.806	0.586

Table 5. Root mean square error (RMSE) values of k-nearest neighbors, random forest, and decision tree for multioutput regression.

Models	Root Mean Square Error		
	High Blood Pressure	High Cholesterol	Obesity
Linear regression for multioutput regression	5.348	3.921	4.417
K-nearest neighbors for multioutput regression	5.50	4.385	3.347
Random forest for multioutput regression	5.457	4.363	3.149
Decision tree for multioutput regression	6.733	5.682	3.792

3.2.2. Multiple Linear Regression Models

Implementation of the multiple linear regression models on the data set was evaluated considering the three dependent variables separately. The value of the coefficient of determination (r-squared) when high blood pressure and high cholesterol were used separately as dependent variables remained significantly low with or without interaction terms. The R-Squared value obtained from these models was below 40%. However, promising results were achieved when "obesity" was used in the multiple linear regression model as a dependent variable. Table 6 presents the independent variables and dependent variables for the multiple regression model. The predictors or features were transformed to give interaction terms to improve the model (as presented in Table 7). This means approximately 81% of the variability in the obesity rate (dependent variable) was explained by the independent variables (high blood pressure rate, high cholesterol rate, and obesity) in the multiple linear regression model. There existed a significant interaction between the variables median income and low car and transportation access.

Table 6. Variables for multiple linear regression model development.

Inputs	Output
Population	Obesity Rate (Figure 2)
Median Income (Figure 6)	
Low Car Access	

Table 7. Results for the multiple linear regression using obesity as a regressor.

Interaction Terms	Normalization	Outlier Removal	Root Mean Square Error	p-Value	R-Squared
No	No	No	4.870	6.10×10^{-18}	0.546
Yes	No	No	4.280	7.94×10^{-22}	0.660
Yes	Yes	No	0.516	7.48×10^{-25}	0.733
Yes	Yes	Yes	0.449	1.78×10^{-28}	0.809
Yes	No	Yes	3.110	1.93×10^{-28}	0.816

3.2.3. Multivariate Polynomial Regression Models

Implemented on all three variables (i.e., high blood pressure, high cholesterol, and obesity) separately as dependent variables yielded the results. The multivariate polynomial model of the second degree, with "obesity" as the dependent variable, again attained the highest accuracy score of approximately 81%. This was followed by the multivariate polynomial model of the second degree with "high blood pressure" as the dependent, scoring a slightly above 50%. The accuracy for the multivariate polynomial model of the second degree, with "high blood pressure" as the dependent variable, was better than the accuracy obtained for the same variable modeled with multiple linear regression (which fell below 40%). Figure 11 shows the predicted trend versus the test data. The peaks and troughs were very well in sync, using the multivariate polynomial regression for the obesity rate model. In addition, Figure 10 shows the R-Squared and RMSE comparison of multivariate polynomial regression based on second- and third-order polynomial functions. The performance of the model was quite similar in comparison.

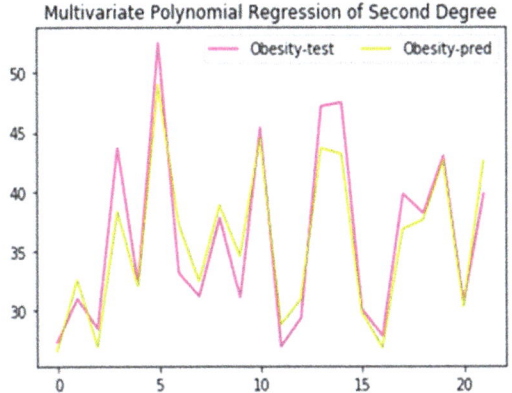

Figure 11. Multivariate polynomial regression of second degree.

4. Conclusions and Future Research

This research investigated the possibility of the geographic correlation of three health issues (i.e., high blood pressure, high cholesterol, and obesity) with food distribution and the statistical correlation with income and car access. These health issues were investigated together to provide a thorough analysis of the chronic health conditions in Guilford County. This study used geospatial technologies and machine learning techniques to provide insights into developing sustainable and healthy communities by examining the presence of food deserts, food swamps, and food oases. We demonstrated how access to healthy food options influenced health and mortality outcomes in one of the largest counties in the state of North Carolina, USA. Specifically, we co-intersected county-level data on representing food access, income distribution, and access to personal and public transportation with data on health or issues and mortality rates.

We started by showing the food outlets' density and health records in the county. The density measuring technique was an alternative method to creating food access maps. The RFEI measure showed only the quantitative index value and may not have covered all tracts based on the equation's requirements. Then, we analyzed the health records in the food desert, where people had limited access to healthy food options due to the low income and low transportation access. We also created geospatial maps of food swamps and food oases. Geospatial data presented the distribution of food deserts in Greensboro and Highpoint downtowns; high income distributes in the northwest of Greensboro, in Summerfield, Oakridge, and Kernersville; high density of food outlets, both healthy and unhealthy, in Greensboro and highpoint. The results clearly showed that food swamps had a higher density of unhealthy food outlets than healthy outlets, while a food oasis had a higher density of healthier than unhealthy food options. We then compared the health records in each of these food geographies to examine any influence of healthy food access on health issues.

This study was limited to the study area of Guilford County. The county-level was practical for showing the current stage and helping local decision makers. Involving more counties for comparison would have supported the study's hypothesis that health issues had a positive correlation with food distribution.

The results of the GIS analysis demonstrated that food deserts with low income, high population density, and low access to transportation were less sustainable, as they showed a high correlation with severe health issues and mortality. Food swamps and oases showed lower health issues and mortality rates compared to food deserts due to the availability of transportation access and income higher than poverty in these areas. The food swamp was a better option than food desert because, nonetheless, the unhealthy food options were accessible. The study's results presented the correlation of food environment with three health issues, unlike other studies. For instance, a study analyzed the numbers of healthy and unhealthy foods and the rate of obesity and found a correlation with unhealthy food options [45]. However, our study investigated more variables, such as income and car access, which were parts of food access areas.

Food deserts showed greater health issues. This could be related to one of the area's characteristics: the availability of unhealthy food outlets, high poverty rates, and low access to transportation. Regarding the availability of unhealthy food, some studies showed no association between unhealthy food and health issues such as obesity and hypertension. A study applied statistical analysis to investigate the correlation between unhealthy food options and obesity and hypertension in children but found no significant correlation [46].

Regression models were used to detect relationships and predict results. The application of several regression models was objective in comparing their results. It illustrated the most correlated variables regarding health issues for inclusion in the development plan. Moreover, illustrating these strong variables would benefit stakeholders in directing new plans and investments. Multi-output regression and multiple linear regression analyses were used to examine the correlation between independent and dependent variables in the study area. Multi-output regression is a series of independent linear regressions. There are three outputs and three inputs. The linear regression for the multioutput model coefficients and intercepts is given in the table below (Table 8) and the parameters in Table 3. We included different regression models for comparison and evaluated the model with the highest performance. In machine learning, it is not always straightforward that a better model will consistently give higher performances across all distributions of a data set.

Table 8. Models' coefficients.

Models	Coefficients			Intercept
	MedIncome	Car_Access	Population	
High blood pressure	-4.04×10^{-5}	7.72	-4.18×10^{-4}	35.64
High cholesterol	3.79×10^{-5}	4.31	-7.89×10^{-4}	35.37
Obesity	-1.47	4.05	2.65×10^{-4}	41.44

The obesity and high-cholesterol output variables showed high positive and negative correlations (R^2 = 0.79 and -0.81), respectively, based on the independent variables of low car access, population, and median income. The obesity and high cholesterol variables were modeled using random forest and decision trees for the above performance. In contrast, the linear and nonlinear regression models could only help to predict the dependent variable obesity with an R^2 value greater than 0.80.

The correlation matrix results illustrated a strong, negative relationship between income and obesity and a positive relationship between independent variables, high blood pressure, and high cholesterol. In addition, it presented the correlation between obesity and income. There was more of a correlation of the independent variable with obesity than between high blood pressure and high cholesterol.

Overall, our results suggested that when compared to food swamps and food oases, food deserts would be the most vulnerable and would probably experience the highest mortality rates in the case of health-related disasters. The presence of such food deserts challenges the sustainable community goals of city and county administrators and directs the need for development in these areas for better future planning.

Future studies may examine the long-term statistical association of food with respect to commercial and governmental policies implemented and its impact on people's health and conditions. More specific future studies may investigate the low rate of health issues in food swamp areas. Moreover, future research may investigate the increase in health issues and potential cause(s) in various areas over time and recommend possible solutions.

Author Contributions: Conceptualization, Abrar Almalki and Balakrishna Gokaraju; methodology; Abrar Almalki, Ba-lakrishna Gokaraju and Nikhil Mehta; validation, Abrar Almalki and Balakrishna Gokaraju; formal analysis, Abrar Almalki, Nikhil Mehta, and Balakrishna Gokaraju; resources, Balakrishna Gokaraju, Nikhil Mehta, and Abrar Almalki; data curation, Abrar Almalki; writing—original draft preparation, Abrar Almalki; writing—review and editing, Nikhil Mehta and Balakrishna Gokaraju; supervision, Balakrishna Gokaraju; funding acquisition; Abrar Almalki. Daniel Adrian Doss, emergency management subject expert; homeland security subject expert; draft manuscript preparation; English language; editing and revision; content advising. All authors have read and agreed to the published version of the manuscript.

Funding: This research is sponsored by the partial funding from North Carolina Department of Environmental Quality (NCDEQ) and NC CARES Act. 2020-21.

Data Availability Statement: Data, such as income and food access, were downloaded from the USDA Food Desert Locator Map website at https://www.ers.usda.gov/data-products/food-access-research-atlas/go-to-the-atlas.aspx (accessed on 18 November 2020).

Acknowledgments: We thank Mark Smith from the Health Department in Guilford County, Greensboro, NC, for providing the preliminary data sets on health statistical records and other data. The authors also sincerely acknowledge the Health Surveillance and Analysis Unit of the Guilford County Department of Health and Human Services, Division of Public Health, as a source as well as the NC Electronic Disease Surveillance System (NC EDSS) of NC DHHS for providing data sets. The authors would like to thank Marwan Bikdash, Chair of Dept. of Computational Data Science and Engineering in NCAT for supporting the publication cost of this manuscript.

Conflicts of Interest: The authors declare no conflict of interest.

References

1. Greensboro, High Point Top Nationwide Hunger List. News & Record. 2021. Available online: https://www.greensboro.com/news/local_news/greensboro-high-point-top-nationwide-hunger-list/article_88828c52-e568-11e4-9b5b-db55afd7f635.html (accessed on 15 April 2021).
2. Neufeld, H.T.; Richmond, C.; Southwest Ontario Aboriginal Health Access Centre. Exploring First Nation Elder Women's Relationships with Food from Social, Ecological, and Historical Perspectives. *Curr. Dev. Nutr.* **2020**, *4*, nzaa011. [CrossRef]
3. Ohri-Vachaspati, P.; DeLia, D.; DeWeese, R.S.; Crespo, N.C.; Todd, M.; Yedidia, M.J. The relative contribution of layers of the Social Ecological Model to childhood obesity. *Public Health Nutr.* **2015**, *18*, 2055–2066. [CrossRef]
4. Dammhahn, M.; Kappeler, P.M. Females go where the food is: Does the socio-ecological model explain variation in social organisation of solitary foragers? *Behav. Ecol. Sociobiol.* **2009**, *63*, 939–952. [CrossRef]
5. Letaifa, S.B. How to strategize smart cities: Revealing the SMART model. *J. Bus. Res.* **2015**, *68*, 1414–1419. [CrossRef]
6. Widener, M.J.; Shannon, J. When are food deserts? Integrating time into research on food accessibility. *Health Place* **2014**, *30*, 1–3. [CrossRef]
7. Charreire, H.; Casey, R.; Salze, P.; Simon, C.; Chaix, B.; Banos, A.; Badariotti, D.; Weber, C.; Oppert, J.-M. Measuring the food environment using geographical information systems: A methodological review. *Public Health Nutr.* **2010**, *13*, 1773–1785. [CrossRef]
8. Chang, K.-T. Geographic information system. *Int. Encycl. Geogr. People Earth Environ. Technol. People Earth Environ. Technol.* **2016**, 1–9. [CrossRef]
9. Truong, K.; Fernandes, M.; An, R.; Shier, V.; Sturm, R. Measuring the physical food environment and its relationship with obesity: Evidence from California. *Public Health* **2010**, *124*, 115. [CrossRef]

10. Brownlee, J. Difference between Algorithm and Model in Machine Learning. Machine Learning Mastery. 2021. Available online: https://machinelearningmastery.com/difference-between-algorithm-and-model-in-machine-learning/ (accessed on 22 September 2021).
11. Alzubi, J.; Nayyar, A.; Kumar, A. Machine learning from theory to algorithms: An overview. *J. Phys. Conf. Ser.* **2018**, *1142*, 012012. [CrossRef]
12. Segal, M.R. Machine Learning Benchmarks and Random Forest Regression. 2004. Available online: https://escholarship.org/uc/item/35x3v9t4 (accessed on 22 September 2021).
13. Mahmoudi, M.R. On comparing two dependent linear and nonlinear regression models. *J. Test. Eval.* **2018**, *47*, 449–458. [CrossRef]
14. Teixeira-Pinto, A. 2 K-Nearest Neighbours Regression | Machine Learning for Biostatistics. Bookdown.Org. 2021. Available online: https://bookdown.org/tpinto_home/Regression-and-Classification/k-nearest-neighbours-regression.html (accessed on 22 September 2021).
15. Westerveld, J.J.L.; van den Homberg, M.J.C.; Nobre, G.G.; van den Berg, D.L.J.; Teklesadik, A.D.; Stuit, S.M. Forecasting transitions in the state of food security with machine learning using transferable features. *Sci. Total Environ.* **2021**, *786*, 147366. [CrossRef]
16. Amin, M.D.; Badruddoza, S.; McCluskey, J.J. Predicting access to healthful food retailers with machine learning. *Food Policy* **2021**, *99*, 101985. [CrossRef]
17. Ahvenniemi, H.; Huovila, A.; Pinto-Seppä, I.; Airaksinen, M. What are the differences between sustainable and smart cities? *Cities* **2017**, *60*, 234–245. [CrossRef]
18. Statement of Policy, Healthy Food Access. NACCHO: Washington, DC, USA. Available online: https://www.naccho.org/uploads/downloadable-resources/13-04-Healthy-Food-Access.pdf (accessed on 15 April 2021).
19. Hodgson, K. Planning for Food Access and Community-Based Food System. 2012. Available online: http://citeseerx.ist.psu.edu/viewdoc/download?doi=10.1.1.593.1056&rep=rep1&type=pdf (accessed on 22 September 2021).
20. Jin, H.; Lu, Y. Evaluating Consumer Nutrition Environment in Food Deserts and Food Swamps. *Int. J. Environ. Res. Public Health* **2021**, *18*, 2675. [CrossRef]
21. Kaufman, P.R. Rural poor have less access to supermarkets, large grocery stores. *Rural Am. Rural Dev. Perspect.* **1998**, *13*, 19–26.
22. Kuai, X.; Zhao, Q. Examining healthy food accessibility and disparity in Baton Rouge, Louisiana. *Ann. GIS* **2017**, *23*, 103–116. [CrossRef]
23. Frankel, L.K. The Relation of Life Insurance to Public Hygiene. *Am. J. Public Hyg.* **1910**, *20*, 258.
24. Abel, K.C.; Faust, K.M. Modeling complex human systems: An adaptable framework of urban food deserts. *Sustain. Cities Soc.* **2020**, *52*, 101795. [CrossRef]
25. Nica-Avram, G.; Harvey, J.; Smith, G.; Smith, A.; Goulding, J. Identifying food insecurity in food sharing networks via machine learning. *J. Bus. Res.* **2021**, *131*, 469–484. [CrossRef]
26. Walker, R.E.; Keane, C.R.; Burke, J.G. Disparities and access to healthy food in the United States: A review of food deserts literature. *Health Place* **2010**, *16*, 876–884. [CrossRef]
27. Stucker, H.; Parmenter, B. Multi–level Food Retail Opportunities: Improving food access in Boston's most underserved neighborhoods through grocery store development, small food market improvements, and mobile produce market stop expansion. *Appl. Geogr.* **2013**, *31*, 1216–1223.
28. Guy, C.M.; David, G. Measuring physical access to 'healthy foods' in areas of social deprivation: A case study in Cardiff. *Int. J. Consum. Stud.* **2004**, *28*, 222–234. [CrossRef]
29. Jeffery, R.W.; Baxter, J.; McGuire, M.; Linde, J. Are fast food restaurants an environmental risk factor for obesity? *Int. J. Behav. Nutr. Phys. Act.* **2006**, *3*, 1–6. [CrossRef]
30. Sisiopiku, V.P.; Barbour, N. Use of gis spatial analysis to identify food deserts in the state of alabama. *Athens J. Health* **2014**, *1*, 91–103. [CrossRef]
31. Cossman, R.E.; Cossman, J.S.; Jackson, R.; Cosby, A. Mapping high or low mortality places across time in the United States: A research note on a health visualization and analysis project. *Health Place* **2003**, *9*, 361–369. [CrossRef]
32. Gehlen, M.; Nicola, M.R.C.; Costa, E.R.D.; Cabral, V.K.; de Quadros, E.L.L.; Chaves, C.O.; Lahm, R.A.; Nicolella, A.D.R.; Rossetti, M.L.R.; Silva, D.R. Geospatial intelligence and health analitycs: Its application and utility in a city with high tuberculosis incidence in Brazil. *J. Infect. Public Health* **2019**, *12*, 681–689. [CrossRef]
33. Quiñones, S.; Goyal, A.; Ahmed, Z.U. Geographically weighted machine learning model for untangling spatial heterogeneity of type 2 diabetes mellitus (T2D) prevalence in the USA. *Sci. Rep.* **2021**, *11*, 1–13.
34. Black, C.; Moon, G.; Baird, J. Dietary inequalities: What is the evidence for the effect of the neighbourhood food environment? *Health Place* **2014**, *27*, 229–242. [CrossRef] [PubMed]
35. Obesity. 2021. Available online: https://www.who.int/westernpacific/health-topics/obesity (accessed on 21 September 2021).
36. High Cholesterol Facts. Centers for Disease Control and Prevention. 2021. Available online: https://www.cdc.gov/cholesterol/facts.htm (accessed on 21 September 2021).
37. High Blood Pressure Symptoms, Causes, and Problems Cdc. Gov. Centers for Disease Control and Prevention. 2021. Available online: https://www.cdc.gov/bloodpressure/about.htm (accessed on 22 September 2021).
38. The Demographic Statistical Atlas of the United States-Statistical Atlas. Statisticalatlas. Com. 2021. Available online: https://statisticalatlas.com/county/North-Carolina/Guilford-County/Population (accessed on 10 May 2021).

39. U.S. Census Bureau Quickfacts: Guilford County, North Carolina. Census Bureau Quickfacts. 2021. Available online: https://www.census.gov/quickfacts/guilfordcountynorthcarolina (accessed on 10 May 2021).
40. Maulud, D.; Abdulazeez, A.M. A Review on Linear Regression Comprehensive in Machine Learning. *J. Appl. Sci. Technol. Trends* **2020**, *1*, 140–147. [CrossRef]
41. How Much You Have to Earn to Be Considered Middle Class in Every US State. Business Insider. 2021. Available online: https://www.businessinsider.com/middle-class-in-every-us-state-2015-4 (accessed on 15 April 2021).
42. Dutko, P.; Ver Ploeg, M.; Farrigan, T. Characteristics and Influential Factors of Food Deserts. Economic Research Report Number 140. Washington D.C. USA. United States Department of Agriculture. 2012. Available online: https://www.ers.usda.gov/webdocs/publications/45014/30940_err140.pdf (accessed on 21 September 2021).
43. Access to Healthy Food. Health Concern. Guilford County Department of Public Health Community Health Assessment. 2013. Available online: https://www.guilfordcountync.gov/home/showdocument?id=268#:~{}:text=Food%20deserts%20are%20defined%20as%20areas%20where%20at,high-poverty%2C%20high-minority%20areas%20of%20Greensboro%20and%20High%20Point (accessed on 23 September 2021).
44. Green, D. Your Census Tract May Get You Lower Mortgage Rates. Mortgage Rates, Mortgage News and Strategy: The Mortgage Reports. 2021. Available online: https://themortgagereports.com/18912/census-tract-low-income-high-minority-mortgage-rates-homeready (accessed on 23 September 2021).
45. Morland, K.B.; Evenson, K.R. Obesity prevalence and the local food environment. *Health Place* **2009**, *15*, 491–495. [CrossRef]
46. Cummins, S.C.J. The local food environment and health: Some reflections from the United Kingdom. *Am. J. Public Health* **2003**, *93*, 521. [CrossRef] [PubMed]

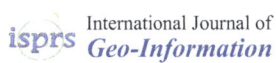

Article

Assessing Health Resources Equipped with Hemodynamic Rooms in the Portuguese-Spanish Borderland: Cross-Border Cooperation Strategies as a Possible Solution

José Manuel Naranjo Gómez [1,2], Rui Alexandre Castanho [2,3,4,*], José Cabezas Fernández [2,5] and Luís Loures [2,6]

1. Agricultural School, University of Extremadura, 06007 Badajoz, Spain; jnaranjo@unex.es
2. VALORIZA—Research Centre for Endogenous Resource Valorization, 7300 Portalegre, Portugal; jocafer@unex.es (J.C.F.); lcloures@ipportalegre.pt (L.L.)
3. College of Business and Economics, University of Johannesburg, Auckland Park P.O. Box 524, South Africa
4. Faculty of Applied Sciences, WSB University, 41-300 Dabrowa Górnicza, Poland
5. Environmental Resources Analysis Research Group (ARAM), University of Extremadura, 06009 Badajoz, Spain
6. Research Centre for Tourism, Sustainability and Well-Being (CinTurs), University of Algarve, 8005-139 Faro, Portugal
* Correspondence: acastanho@wsb.edu.pl

Abstract: Portugal and Spain share one of the greatest European borderland areas. This fact has direct impacts on a large territory and consequently on the communities' living in it. Still, even if the border areas represent an essential fraction of the territory, planning policies have not resulted in specific cooperation programs that could enable sharing general leisure and recreation assets and infrastructures and collaboration in critical domains—i.e., the case of the health sector. The present study aims to assess the territorial accessibility to the hemodynamic rooms by the potential population of the Spanish-Portuguese transition areas that may suffer an acute myocardial infarction. Contextually, this study employed a spatial interaction model based on the three-step floating catchment area method (method-3SFCA). By applying these methods, it was possible to develop a map of accessibility to health infrastructures equipped with hemodynamics rooms on both sides of the border that may answer the Spanish-Portuguese border populations' needs. Besides, while granting valuable information for decision-makers regarding the need to develop new infrastructures to guarantee that even considering cross border cooperation, everyone gets access to a hemodynamics room within the critical intervention period.

Keywords: cross-border cooperation; geographic information systems; Iberian borderland; strategic planning; sustainable planning

1. Introduction

Providing adequate essential services is an increasingly important issue in livelihoods, sustainability, and public policy [1]. Equality of access to these services must be achieved between different population groups regardless of social, economic, demographic, or geographical differences that in many cases lead to inequalities in the provision of these services [2–4]. Mainly it must be achieved in those services that are vital, such as the health service [5,6].

Nevertheless, in many cases, the provision of health services is not distributed equally in one region and among different population groups due to a variety of spatial and non-spatial factors [7,8]. As for non-spatial factors, these mainly significantly affect the quality of the health service offered [7,9]. However, spatial aspects can become a physical barrier that hinders adequate access to health services, depending on the separation distance where the patient needs medical assistance to the nearest hospital where he or she can be assisted [10,11]. For this reason, health service planning must make it accessible and

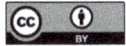

effective for the whole of the served population [12–14]. For this reason, the location of health infrastructures has a social impact among residents of cities and towns [15,16]. In fact, a country's health care capacity affects others due to the interconnection between economic, social, technological, and political systems [17].

In this regard, considering the different political systems of Spain and Portugal, each country depends on its criterion of self-sufficiency to provide health infra-structures, producing unequal technological development. These differences are more prominent in high-tech sanitary technology equipment, mainly because it is more expensive and requires more skilled human resources. In fact, the non-existence of prior collaboration agreements or previously established protocols causes the patient to be treated primarily in the same country where he or she requires healthcare. Likewise, if the population's access to health services may in some cases be inadequate and unequal [18], this is aggravated concerning high-tech health care [19], like hemodynamic rooms that are considered representative precisely of high health care technology for three fundamental reasons. Firstly, access time to these rooms is a vital factor for the patient. Secondly, they offer urgent health benefits by treating myocardial infarction through percutaneous coronary angioplasty (PCA) which is a treatment potentially usable in the vast majority of patients with acute myocardial infarction, achieves the recanalization of the coronary artery in more than 90% of cases, with better perfusion of the infarcted area and a lower incidence of re-inclusion when compared with thrombolytic treatment [20]. Thirdly, these rooms must be integrated into a hospital [10].

The assessment and optimization of cardiovascular and hemodynamic variables is a mainstay of patient management in critically ill patients in the intensive care unit (ICU) or the operating room (OR). Therefore, it is of outstanding importance to meticulously validate technologies for hemodynamic monitoring and to study their applicability in clinical practice and, finally, their impact on treatment decisions and patient outcome [21]. Indeed, hemodynamic monitoring provides the basis for optimizing cardiovascular dynamics in intensive care medicine and anaesthesiology [22]. The hemodynamic room has the most advanced technology for the diagnosis and treatment of coronary diseases. On the one hand, the virtual histology offers differentiated and percentage information of the four components of the atheroma plaque: the fibrotic, lipid, calcium, and chorionic content. On the other hand, intracoronary ultrasound consists of a 1 mm catheter incorporating a small ultrasound emission system (transducer) at the distal end connected to a console that generates images in real-time.

The use of indicators makes it possible to assess the geographical distribution of the applicant population of these services, the transport infrastructures that allow access to them, and the provision of services offered by health infrastructures. In this sense, the proliferation of spatially disaggregated data and the increasing use of Geographic Information Systems (GIS) has led to a plethora of spatial accessibility analysis to health services, combined with criteria for quality and efficiency of the service provided [10]. In the bibliography on accessibility, a great variety of indicators that evaluate them is observed (see, for example, [23–27]). Moreover, all of them offer a measure to close the existing separation between human settlements and activities depending on the transport network made available to defining a single indicator of accessibility that includes all the approaches is nearly impossible to realize since each indicator measures this variable from a concrete point of view, to evaluate the quality of the access to the transport infrastructures and to determine strategic locations or as tools for the planning in the decision-making process [26]. However, these indicators can complement each other to provide a clearer picture about the benefits that the analyzed infrastructure will facilitate the territories affected by it [28]. Therefore, it makes it possible to analyze whether societies are inclusive [29], that all their members have access to high-tech healthcare services and impartial, and whether they have the same healthcare opportunities [30–32]. This kind of analysis has produced different approximations [18,33], including the regional availability model [34–37], kernel density models [29–31], and gravity models [38–43]. Among the latter models the two-step floating catchment area method (2FSCA) stands out [44,45]. However, the adoption of an equal catchment size was criticized for the lack of nuances in interpreting the effect of decreasing distance [43] and to adapt to the different travel environments where health search behaviors take place, the enhanced two-step floating capture model (ESFCA) was proposed [46]. Nonetheless, in these latter two methods, there is the oversight of regional competition [7]. In fact, it is also known as "intervention opportunities" in the language of spatial interaction models [47], as they limit search behaviors, as in many cases, the patient can be treated outside a particular administrative unit [48,49], to minimize this defect the three-step floating catchment area method (3SFCA) was developed [50–52]. Regarding the choice of 2FSCA versus 3FSCA, it is a necessary combination of both a distance-decay function and variable catchment size function for the 2SFCA to appropriately measure healthcare access across all geographical regions [53,54]. The 3SFCA method is based on a more reasonable assumption of healthcare demand for medical services [51]. Suppose it is considered the chance that a patient could be treated in two neighboring countries. In this scenario, the boundary line would be considered non-existent to serve the population regardless of the country in which it resided. To seek collaboration between both countries to seek a better health service to the population. 3FSCA assumes that a population's healthcare demand for a medical site is influenced by the availability of other nearby medical sites. Indeed, it assigns a travel-time-based competition weight for each pair of population-medical sites in addition to the E2SFCA methodology.

In fact, when we aggregate the population within the overlapping catchment areas of multiple facilities, the original 2SFCA framework leads to double-counting of the population that tends to increase the level of demand in the healthcare system [55]. Various solutions to the demand and level of service increase have been proposed, including selecting weights based on a travel impedance function in the 3SFCA method [55].

The current work intends to elaborate a viable framework to measure spatial accessibility for the resident population in Spain and Portugal regarding hemodynamics rooms. Through the present study, the municipalities have been classified according to their accessibility degree. Therefore, it was allowed to determine which are the ones that show inadequate accessibility levels.

As for the spatial heterogeneity of border areas, by using an adjusted spatial access index, the 3SFCA method indicates strong potential for identifying health professional shortage areas [51]. In this regard, in the borderline region between Spain and Portugal, there is a shortage of hospitals, and as a consequence, there is a shortage in the sanitary services offered. Another point to consider is that the opening hours are 24 h a day. Therefore, for every hemodynamic room, the perception of quality care was taken into account by the doctors who finally decide where the patients will be treated.

In order to carry out such a study, two scenarios will be put forward: (1) the patients could be treated only in hospitals with hemodynamics rooms in their own country; (2) the patients also be treated in hospitals located outside their country. In this regard, the difference between these scenarios will identify the municipalities that improve their accessibility patterns and quantify how people's living standards continue to increase regarding health services.

2. Materials and Methods

Based on official information and the application of the spatial interaction model 3SFCA, the proposed objective could be met. In this regard, the data used comes from publications made by official institutions. Although, they must be differentiated according to the sources used for each of the countries. In the case of Spain, these sources are the Official Road Map of 2021 of the Ministry of Development, the National Cartographic Base at a scale of 1:200,000 (BCN200) of the National Geographic Institute (IGN), the revision of the Municipal Population Register of 2020 of the National Institute of Statistics (INE) and the Minimum Basic Set of Hospital data (CMBD) of 2014, the National Catalog of

Hospitals (CNH) of 2020 prepared by the Ministry of Health, the Ministry of Social Rights and Agenda 2030 and the Ministry of Consumer Affairs.

In the case of Portugal, the data comes from the web portal relating to the Portuguese infrastructure network, the National Geographic Information System (SNIG) and the National Territorial Information System, the PORDATA web portal, and the set of Health Centers in 2012 from the National Institute of Statistics (INE). Likewise, to obtain the hemodynamic room number of each hospital, it was necessary to have Computer-assisted telephone interviewing (CATI) and computer-assisted web interview (CAWI), based on electronic surveys sent to respondents before.

However, there is a common source of information for the two countries, the land use registered by the Corine Land Cover program for the year 2018, to determine the uses of the continuous urban fabric land designated with code 111 serve to determine urban areas.

Likewise, the development of all the tasks and calculations performed was carried out using the R statistical package (created by Ross Ihaka and Robert Gentleman, in Auckland, New Zealand) and the ArcGIS 10.8.1 application (ESRI, Redlands, CA, USA) and its network analysis tool, Network Analyst.

In fact, the tasks carried out are differentiated by five essential phases. Initially, the design of the base cartography, continuing with the determination of the floating catchment areas of the hospitals equipped with some hemodynamic room and continues with the obtaining of the thematic cartography that shows the degree of health coverage for each municipality in two differentiated scenarios and ends with the comparative analysis of the alphanumeric information. In one scenario, the patient can only be treated in hospitals located in the same country where he suffered a myocardial infarction—in the second scenario, taking into account that the patient can also be treated in hospitals in the neighboring country (Figure 1).

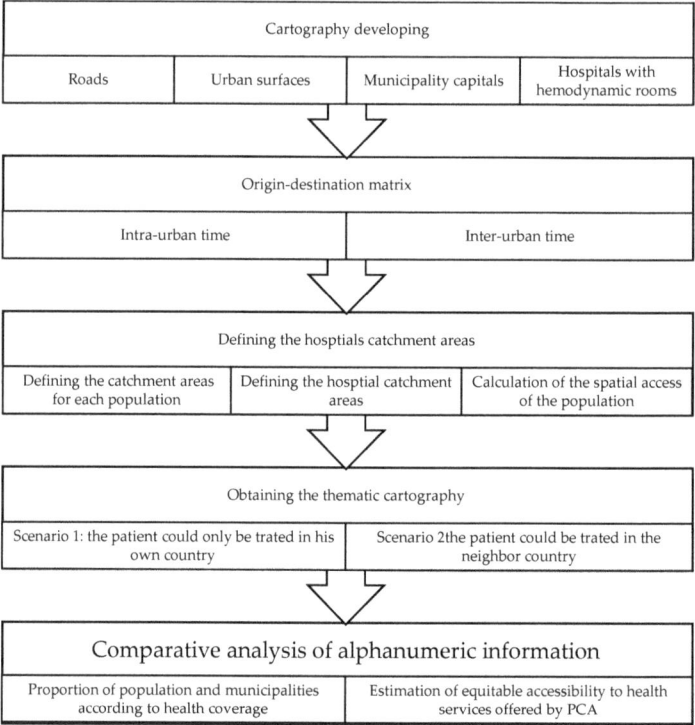

Figure 1. Workflow.

2.1. Developing Cartography

The cartography used is vector and is composed of four layers in Shapefile (shp.) format. Likewise, it has been used in the European Terrestrial Reference System 1989 (ETRS89) in spindle 30.

Firstly, the road network is modeled using graphic entities linear to the entire road network of peninsular highways (Figure 2). The topology generated for this layer is of the arc-node type, on which the impedance is determined in minutes as the time it takes a vehicle to travel each of the network sections. This happens once each section of the road had associated the maximum speed allowed and the distance to travel.

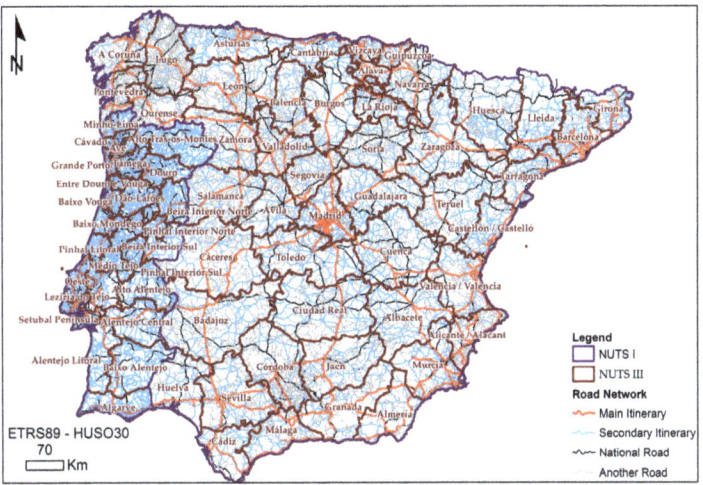

Figure 2. Roads in the Iberian Peninsula.

The second layer of information corresponds to the urban area of cities and towns (Figure 3). Polygonal graphic entities represent these, and the resident population in each one of them composes the associated alphanumeric information.

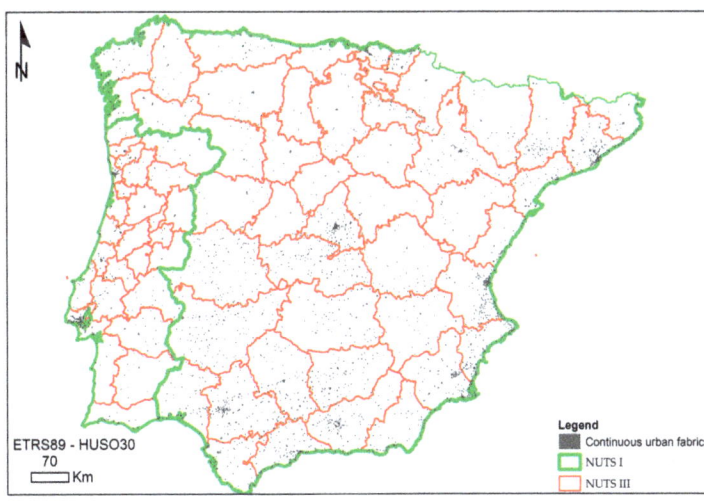

Figure 3. Continuous urban fabric in the Iberian Peninsula.

The third layer of information evokes the municipal capitals represented by dots with the resident population as associated alphanumeric information (Figure 4).

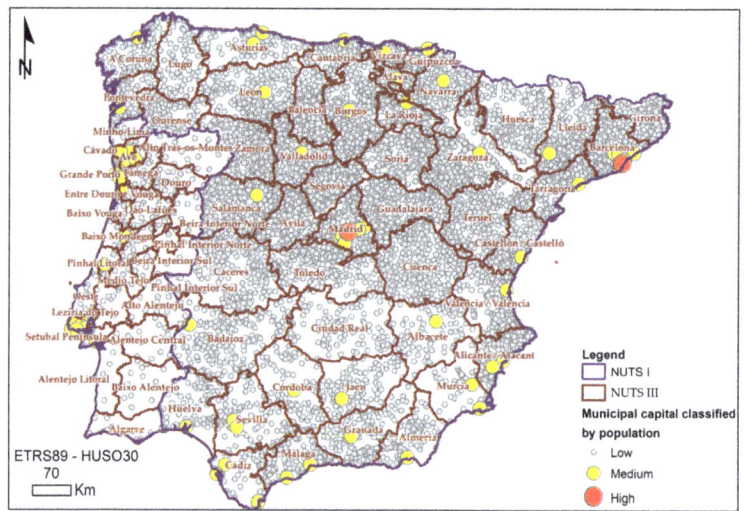

Figure 4. Municipal capitals classified by population.

The last layer represents the cities with hospitals that contain some hemodynamic rooms (Figure 5). Precisely the number of hemodynamic rooms is the alphanumeric information associated with them. The graphic entity that represents them is the centroids of the municipal capitals that contain some hemodynamic room. These were determined by selecting those municipal capitals with a public or subsidized hospital equipped with a hemodynamic room. In this regard, Figure 5 shows a symbol in the cities with hospitals where there are hemodynamics rooms. However, this symbol is also proportional according to the number of hemodynamics rooms in the hospitals.

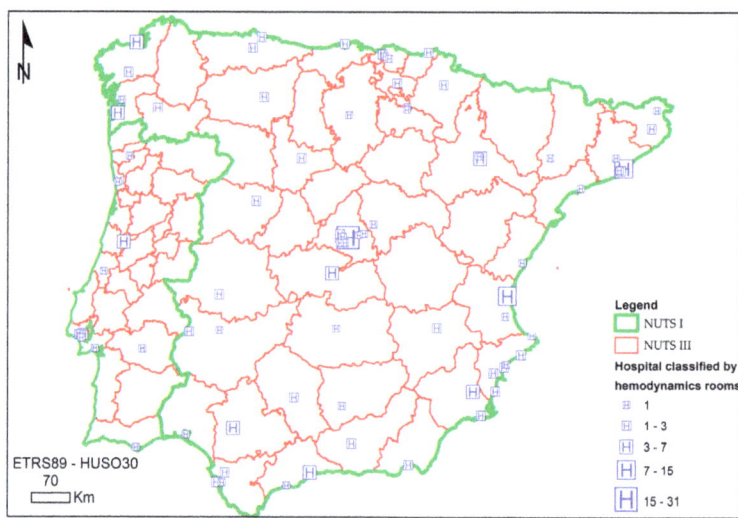

Figure 5. Hospitals classified by number of hemodynamics rooms.

2.2. Origin-Destination Time Matrix

The time from the emergency notification to the balloon implantation in the PCA should not exceed 90 min according to the medical standards [56–60]. Therefore, since the patient suffers acute myocardial infarction, a hemodynamic room is crucial to the treatment in a hospital. In fact, this determines physicians' behavior when selecting the hospital where the patient is to be transferred. As a consequence, a threshold time of 90 min was established in the analysis.

In this regard, the transfer time of the patient to the hospital was determined as the travel time between the municipal capitals that require a PCA and the cities that have a hospital with at least one hemodynamic room. Besides, by calculating the inter-urban travel time between cities or towns, the intra-urban times it takes to traverse the different urban environments are estimated, from the municipality of origin where the patient suffers the myocardial infarction to different hospitals that have a hemodynamic room. Precisely, the population and the urban area are used to estimate these intra-urban times, since in this methodology they are estimated based on the population density of urban areas, through a linear adjustment that gives a maximum of 80 km/h to the areas with the lowest population density and a minimum of 20 km/ha in the most densely populated areas [59]. In this way, the sum of the inter-urban time plus the intra-urban time determines the total time of the journey between the municipal capitals with some patients due to myocardial infarction and the urban centers with a hospital hemodynamic room.

2.3. Defining Hospital Catchment Areas

The relationship between supply and demand for healthcare resources is analyzed by applying the spatial interaction model called 3-step floating catchment area (3SFCA). This model is based on a logical conjecture of the demand for health care [10]. Because it assumes that the population that demands health care from a particular place is influenced by the availability of different nearby sites where medical care is offered, specifically by the time of separation and the services offered. Conceptually, the model assigns a travel-time-based competition weight for each population-medical site pair in addition to the methodology outlined in an enhanced two-step floating catchment area (E2SFCA). This weight is then used to calculate the demand of service sites, thereby minimizing the overestimation [58]. The method is implemented in three steps:

Step 1: Determine the catchment of a population location i based on a 90-min driving zone. A person can suffer a myocardial infarction and where all the services available within the catchment are sought. In this case, all those hospitals have at least one hemodynamic room. Subsequently, a Gaussian weight is assigned to each service site according to the sub-zone in which the site lies (i.e., if a service site is located within the second sub-zone, the Gaussian weight (i.e., W 2) of the sub-zone is assigned to the service site), and calculate a selection weight between each service site and i by:

$$G_{ij} \frac{T_{ij}}{\sum_{k \in \{Dist(i,k) < d_0\}} T_{ij}} \quad (1)$$

where G_{ij} is the weight of the selection between the location i corresponding to the capital of the municipality where a patient could suffer a myocardial infarction, and the place j where there is a hospital with at least one hemodynamic room, $Dist\ (i,j)$ is the cost of the trip (minutes) from i to any service location k within the catchment. Likewise, d_0 is the size of the basin, which in this case is 90 min, taking into account that the maximum time by medical standards [56–60]. The Gaussian weights for j and k were assigned using T_{ij} and T_{ik}, respectively.

Step 2: Determine the 90-min catchment area of each service site *j* and divide the catchment into five sub-zones using the same procedure of step 1. All locations within the catchment are sought and computed the physician-to-population ratio (*R*) of *j* by:

$$R\frac{S_j}{\sum_{k\in D_r} G_{kj}P_k W_r}_j \qquad (2)$$

S_j is the medical capacity of *j*, in this case, it corresponds to the number of hemodynamic rooms available in each hospital. Likewise, W_r is the impedance of the *r*-th sub-zone D_r, was determined through the road network that served to move the patient from each capital of each municipality to a hospital with at least one hemodynamic room. Furthermore, this impedance considers inter-urban time and intra-urban time, and G_{kj} is the selection weight between *j* and population site *k*, and P_k is the population size of *k*.

Step 3: Compute the spatial access of population site *i* by:

$$A_i^F = \sum_{j\in D_r} G_{ij} R_j W_r \qquad (3)$$

where R_j is the physician-to-population ratio of *j* within the catchment, G_{ij} is the selection weight between *i* and *j*, and W_r is the Gaussian weight of the *r*-th sub-zone D_r.

In the case analyzed, the 3SFCA assumes that the demand of a municipality's population is affected by the cost of traveling to the nearest health service that offers the treatment of primary percutaneous coronary angioplasty as by its travel costs to adjacent sites offering the same service. This is a logical assumption because the demand of the people for a medical site will decrease when the adjacent sites are also available since the demand of the population in some cases could exceed the supply of hemodynamic rooms that are offered. In fact, the selection weight, G_{ij}, reflects this change. G_{ij} equals 1 when only one medical site is available for a population site but decreases with an increasing number of available alternatives. The multiplication of G_{ij}, P_i, and W_{ij} represents the adjusted population demand of location *i* on medical site *j*.

2.4. Developing of the Thematic Cartography

All the previous methodological steps were applied, taking into account two scenarios. In the first one, patients suffering from a myocardial infarction can only be transferred to hospitals located in their country to receive a PCA. Second, patients suffering from a myocardial infarction can be transferred to hospitals in their country or to a neighboring country. For this reason, two thematic maps were obtained.

From the results obtained in analyzing the accessibility to the PCA service, five classes were established through equal intervals, considering the maximum value obtained in both scenarios. In this way, they remained constant in both scenarios, allowing the same classification of the values corresponding to the capacity map to be made at the PCA service. Thus, it is possible to compare both thematic maps and, consequently, both scenarios, identifying and locating those municipalities that suffer the greatest and least variation if the patient could have access to health services in the neighboring country.

2.5. Comparative Analysis of Alphanumeric Information

Comparing the alphanumeric information associated with each of the municipalities in the two analyzed scenarios and the results obtained after applying the 3SFCA allows quantitatively determining the municipalities and the population residing in them according to their access coverage they offer hospitals that have a hemodynamic room.

In this regard, the execution of Structured Query Language (SQL) selected the data corresponding to the municipalities classified according to the established levels of health coverage. From this selection, the relative distribution of health coverage concerning the resident population in the analyzed municipalities and the accumulated percentage of the population could be captured, according to the capacity of PCA health services, by the municipality for inhabitants to access to any country or capacity of PCA health services, by the municipality for inhabitants that could only access they own country. Without ambiguity, it is possible to determine which of the scenarios show greater inequality in access to health services.

3. Results

The thematic maps represent the health coverage for each municipality's inhabitants in the two scenarios proposed. For this reason, the first map represents the health coverage of each municipality if the patient can only be transferred to hospitals located in the same country where he suffered a heart attack (Figure 6). The second map shows the health coverage of each municipality if the patient can also be transferred to hospitals in the neighboring country; that is, if the patient suffers a heart attack in Spain, they could also be transferred to Portugal and vice versa (Figure 7).

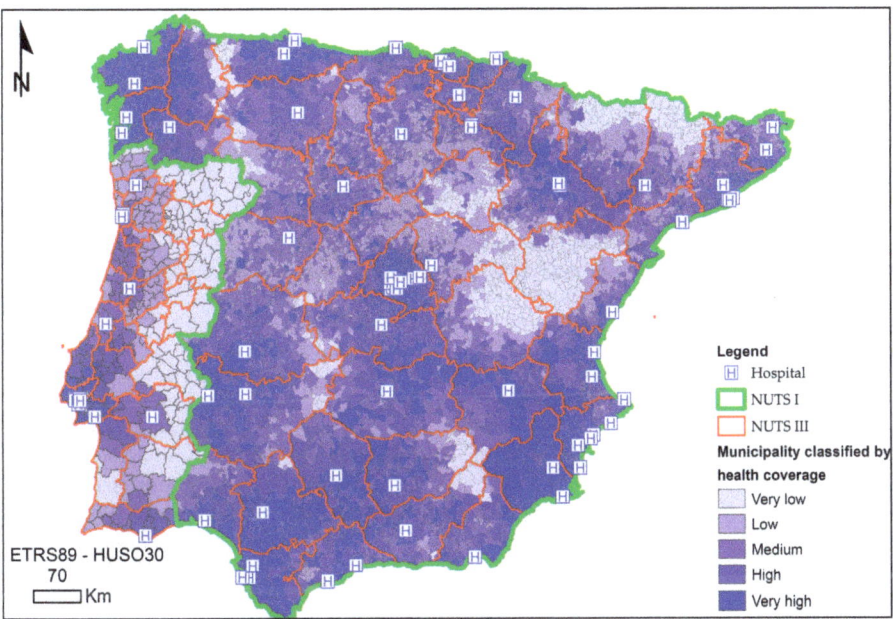

Figure 6. Capacity of health services to make a PCA, by the municipality, if patients that could only access hospitals located in the same country where they suffered a myocardial infarction and are not entitled to be treated in the other country.

The thematic map in Figure 6 shows the situation of each of the hospitals in the Iberian Peninsula that have at least one hemodynamic room to perform a PCA and the health coverage in the municipalities if the patient can only be transferred to hospitals that are in the same country where he suffers the myocardial infarction. Regarding the distribution of hospitals, it can be seen that the distribution in the border area between the two countries is scarce. In fact, there is only one hospital in a cross-border city. This hospital is located in the NUTS III of Badajoz, located in the southwestern part of Spain (Figures 5 and 6). Likewise, also in Spain, in the northwest region, there are three hospitals in areas close to the border located in the NUTS III of Ourense and Pontevedra (Figures 5 and 6).

On the contrary, in Portugal, there is no hospital in a cross-border city. However, there are areas close to the border, in the north in the NUTS III of Cávado, in the southern half in the NUTS III of Alentejo Central, and in the south at NUTS III in Algarve (Figures 2 and 6). This spatial distribution of hospitals reveals that both countries have developed health policies without coordination to achieve greater coverage in the cross-border area.

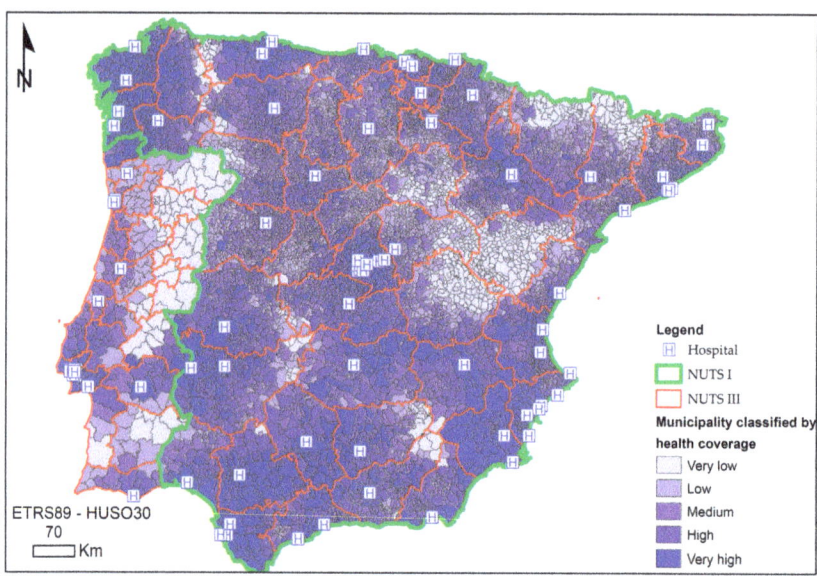

Figure 7. The municipality's capacity of PCA health services for patients that could access hospitals located in the same country where they suffered a myocardial infarction and hospitals in the neighboring country.

Regarding the health coverage observed in each of the countries, in Spain, no pattern is observed (Figure 6). Although, there is a predominance of municipalities with medium, high, or very high health coverage. Even in the cross-border area with Portugal. However, it is true that in Peninsular Spain, there are also some areas with some isolation from access to hospitals. The largest area located between the NUTS III of Soria, Guadalajara, Teruel, and Cuenca stands out. However, the cross-border area with France in the north of the NUTS III of Huesca and Lleida, between the NUTS III of Cáceres, Toledo, Badajoz, and Ciudad Real (Figures 2 and 6) are also noteworthy. In Portugal, a pattern is observed, since in the eastern part and bordering with Spain; there seems to be a low health coverage in the vast majority of municipalities (Figure 6). However, at the western end, coverage is greater, highlighting a center-periphery model around Lisbon. Therefore, Portugal seems to have developed a distribution of health resources in the coastal areas in the northern half and the southern half centered on the NUTS III of Grande Lisboa, south of the NUTS III West and in the NUTS III of Algarve, existing a great contrast between areas with optimal health coverage and those that practically suffer from inadequate coverage (Figures 2 and 6). Precisely, the comparison of this health coverage in the cross-border area indicates that Portugal would benefit more if there were a common policy between both countries, since it has a greater extension of territory with little health coverage, and Spain has adequate health coverage in this cross-border area.

The thematic map in Figure 7 shows, as in Figure 5, the same distribution of hospitals. However, in this case (Figure 7), the patient who suffers a myocardial infarction can also be transferred to hospitals in the neighboring country. As might be expected, the variation in health coverage occurs in the border area and not in the rest of the territory of both countries. However, the comparison of the two scenarios proposed (Figures 6 and 7) in the cross-border area shows that the effects of the variation in health coverage are different in both countries.

In this regard, in Spain, the NUTS III of Ourense (Figures 2 and 7) improves the health coverage of most of the municipalities located in the south of this NUTS III. In Portugal, in the NUTS III of Minho-Lima, some municipalities have low or medium health coverage (Figure 6) to have very high coverage (Figure 7). Possibly, because the accessibility to the hospitals located in the NUTS III of Pontevedra and Ourense is adequate, possibly made possible by an optimal network of roads.

Likewise, in the northern part of the country and in the eastern direction, several municipalities within Tras-os-Montes NUTS III improve their health coverage, going from very low (Figures 2 and 6) to low (Figures 2 and 7). In the case of Spain, some municipalities located to the south within the NUTS III of Ourense improve. Therefore, it is shown that those patients in the Portuguese municipalities located in the northwestern part of the hospital located in the NUTS III of Alto Trás-os-Montes, if they could be transferred to Spanish hospitals, they would have the same health coverage as the Portuguese municipalities closest to the hospital located in Alto Trás-os-Montes. The road network to access Spanish hospitals could be more adequate than the road network to access the hospital located in the NUTS III Alto Trás-os-Montes located in the same country (Figures 2 and 7).

Furthermore, in the NUTS III of Alentejo Central and Alto Alentejo, the health coverage of some municipalities in Portugal improves. Possibly, due to the proximity in access time to the Badajoz hospital, since the road network allows an access time consistently below 90 min in the municipalities indicated above and, also, because this Spanish hospital has a greater number of hemodynamics rooms. On the contrary, in Spain, the variation in health coverage is inexistent. Therefore, there is no improvement in this coverage, even with the possibility of transferring the patient to Portuguese hospitals—possibly, because the access time to the hospital located in Central Alentejo does not compensate for treating the patient when in the hospital located in the NUTS III of Badajoz (Spain) there is a greater number of hemodynamic rooms.

Finally, in the southern border area, the effect produced by the improvement of health coverage in both countries is non-existent. Possibly, each country has adequately endowed that part of the territory and transferring the patient to the neighboring country is not appropriate. Due to the location of the hospitals and the resources available in them, and because of the road network to reach them. In other words, in this case, contrary to what happened in the cross-border northern half, the attractiveness produced by the healthcare resources offered in the neighboring country does not overcome the inconvenience of having to transfer the patient and travel more kilometers to reach them to the hospital.

Also, from the thematic maps, the number of municipalities and the resident population were represented in percentages grouped according to the five levels of health coverage (very low, low, medium, high, and very high) previously used in the thematic maps (Figures 8 and 9).

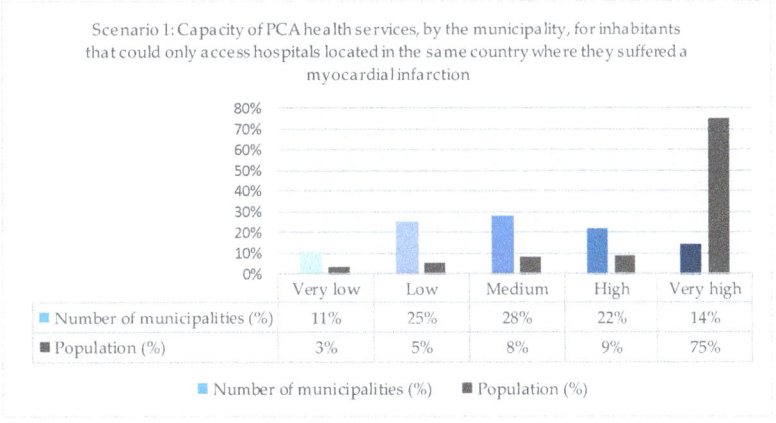

Figure 8. Number of municipalities and population for patients that could only access hospitals located in the same country where they suffered a myocardial infarction.

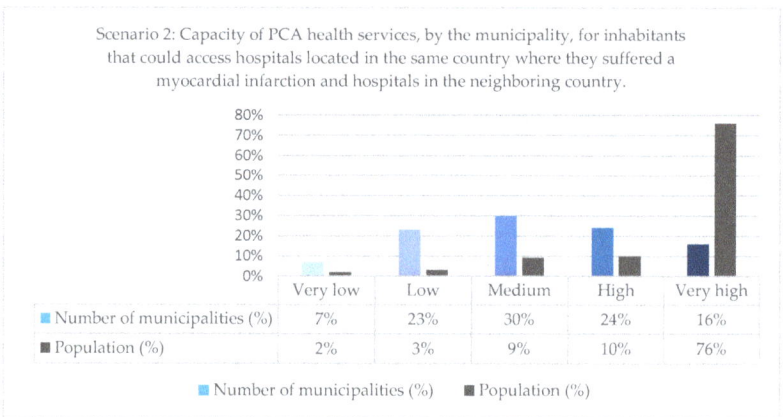

Figure 9. Number of municipalities and population for patients that could access hospitals located in the same country where they suffered a myocardial infarction and hospitals in the neighboring country.

Figure 8 shows these percentages if the patient who suffers a myocardial infarction can only be transferred to a hospital in the same country where he suffered said infarction. Thus, it stands out that, although only 14% of the municipalities have very high health coverage, they host three-quarters of the population. Therefore, it can be stated that a scarce 14% of the municipalities host 75% of the population and have excellent health coverage in the Iberian Peninsula. However, there are also municipalities where there are health coverage problems. On the contrary, 11% of the municipalities with a low population of 3% have health coverage problems.

Consequently, it can be established that the most unpopulated municipalities are those with the greatest health coverage problems. In this sense, it stands out that the population increases progressively from the levels with the worst health coverage to those with the highest health coverage, from 3% to 75%. Therefore, the planning of health services has obeyed, among other criteria, the fundamental criterion of the existing population in each country's regions.

In order to be able to compare health coverage in the two scenarios, Figure 9 was made using the same criteria as in Figure 8. However, in this case, assuming that the patient could be transferred well to hospitals located in the same country where he suffered the heart attack of the myocardium or to a hospital located in the neighboring country. Nevertheless, the comparison of both figures (Figures 8 and 9) allows us to affirm that the pattern is maintained in terms of the health coverage offered. Most of the population, 76%, would continue to have better health coverage and a small population with poor health coverage. Even the same trend is observed in terms of population increase as the level of accessibility increases.

Nonetheless, the comparison of both scenarios (Figures 8 and 9) allows us to observe some patterns. In the first place, at the lowest levels of health coverage (very low and low), the number of municipalities and the population decreased slightly. On the contrary, the number of municipalities and the population with the best levels of health coverage increase (medium, high, and very high). Therefore, it seems that municipalities and their population are being removed from specific sanitary isolation. However, there are still municipalities and populations with little health coverage.

Figure 10 represents the percentage of the accumulated population in percentage values according to the percentage of accumulated health coverage. For this reason, the blue line evokes an equitable ideal distribution of health coverage for the realization of PCA for the entire population of the Iberian Peninsula. Likewise, the red line represents health coverage for the population, considering that the patient can also be transferred to a hospital located in the neighboring country where they have suffered the myocardial infarction. Furthermore, the green line represents the capacity of the health service if the patient can only be treated in a hospital located in the same country where he suffered this myocardial infarction. Thereby, the curve representing the possibility that the patient can be transferred to hospitals located in both countries is closer to the curve that represents the ideal equitable distribution. As a consequence, it can be affirmed that health coverage for PCA would be more equitably distributed if a patient suffering from myocardial infarction can be treated in a hospital independent of the country where they came from, simply taking into account the access time and the number of hemodynamic rooms at the different hospitals.

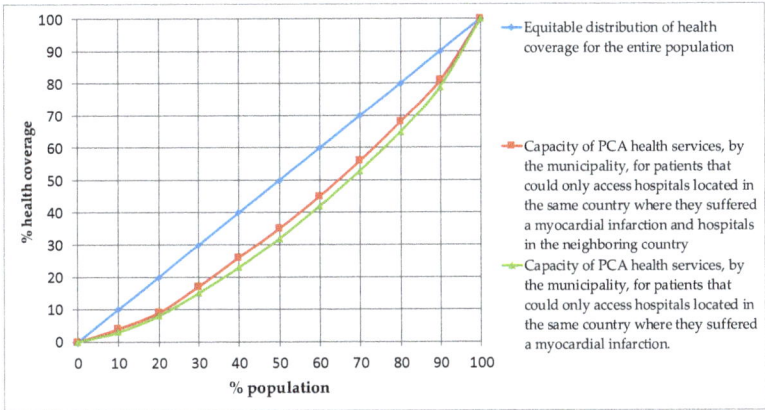

Figure 10. Comparison analysis through a Lorenz curve.

4. Discussion

Policies on health infrastructure between two countries that are part of the European Union should be coordinated. However, this study shows that, to some extent, this is not the case between Spain and Portugal.

The border region is made up of mostly sparsely inhabited municipalities. When it comes to health matters as a primary right of citizens, in both countries, the location of hospitals has been prioritized in those more inhabited places, or at least the establishment of those hospitals better equipped with high-tech sanitary equipment, such as hemodynamic rooms to apply a PCA.

However, greater health cooperation between the two would achieve a more equitable distribution of health coverage for all the inhabitants of the Iberian Peninsula. Although Portugal could benefit more, there would also be inhabitants of Spanish border municipalities that would benefit. Likewise, it must be taken into account that both in the border area and the interior of both countries, considering the two scenarios analyzed, there are areas with little health coverage. One would expect to apply specific mitigating measures to alleviate this possible sanitary isolation of high-tech sanitary resources on these territories.

Additionally, even if current health collaborative environments are now populated mainly of a great diversity of cooperation alternatives, the fact is that we still miss the use of specific tools providing essential and effective strategies regarding the use of medical facilities located along the border. However, as Morales et al. [48] mentioned, communication links enable information collection that can be accessed and/or used by shared infrastructures and services in these territories. Mainly, in medical and clinical environments, resource and service sharing can promote countless potential benefits, supporting very often territories in which medical specialists and infrastructures are very often reduced or limited, enhancing collaboratively gathering vital health opportunities for patients living in these cross-border territories—which are the territories inserted near the borderland, in this case, along the Spanish-Portuguese border.

This fact is increasingly vital in a scenario in which most of the renew equipment and/or construction processes of health infrastructures are supported and financed by European Community funds, that should benefit all the European populations regardless of existing frontiers, bearing in mind the objective to grant better health care for every citizen.

5. Conclusions

Through the present investigation, a series of conclusions were reached, taking into account the access time and the number of hemodynamic rooms to the different hospitals.

Firstly, Spain and Portugal have developed health policies without consideration of the status in the other neighboring country—as shown by the poor distribution of hospitals in the cross-border area—the territories located near the Portuguese-Spanish borderland. However, it is also true that it has been shown that in Portugal, there is a greater concentration of population in the coastal area; this country may require a greater concentration of hospitals here.

Secondly, Portugal would benefit more from developing greater coordination and cooperation in health policy between the two countries—once this country has a more extensive territory where health coverage is low or very low. On the contrary, Spain has a higher level of adequate health coverage in most cross-border areas.

Thirdly, the variation in health coverage that would occur if the patient could also be treated at a hospital in the neighboring country where he suffered the myocardial infarction shows a different effect in both countries. In Portugal, in most of the affected municipalities, they could achieve better health coverage, in some cases equating them to the municipalities closest to hospitals in Portugal. However, in Spain, which already has adequate health coverage, the number of municipalities where better health coverage would be produced is scarce.

Both countries show excellent health coverage for most of the population, as 75% of the population has more than optimal health coverage. Therefore, both have followed a health policy in favor of those most populated municipalities. However, we must not forget that there is still a significant part of the population that has health coverage problems, and for these, it would be necessary to try to apply mitigating measures.

In this regard, the collected data enable us to put forward unique ideas considering that health departments and facilities located along the Portuguese-Spanish border can meet public health needs within their common jurisdictions as long as we enable border regions and their complex environment to be considered as a single European region, regardless of national boundaries. In fact, resource sharing across jurisdictions is a critical opportunity to cross-border regions enabling these territories, sometimes in disadvantaged positions to improve competitiveness, gain effectiveness and increase efficiency.

Additionally, the collected data enabled us to conclude that cross-border health resource sharing constitutes a viable and desirable process to overcome fundamental challenges within scenarios of increasing constraints posed by restricted budgets. Indeed, even if this is not the only reason for cross-border cooperation, limited health resources and budgets associated with low-density territories as the ones characteristic from the majority of the Portuguese-Spanish border, should consider, augmenting resource sharing not only to address emerging challenges but to grant better health services to local populations.

Lastly, although the pattern of health coverage is not broken in the two compared scenarios, it can be established that it is more favorable for the whole of the Iberian Peninsula in the second scenario. In this sense, the municipalities and the population fall for the most precarious levels of health coverage, increasing these in better levels of health coverage. Likewise, health coverage would be distributed more equitably regardless of the country where the patient suffers the myocardial infarction.

The originality and relevance of this study should be emphasized on its findings—once it is possible to find an issue for such a relevant issue as is the case of the emergency health problems of the Portuguese-Spanish borderland populations. Nevertheless, if this study outcome gives us a significant contribution to this thematic field of cross-border cooperation, some improvements and future research lines persist. Among the various research lines that persist, we can use different testing tools—i.e., use a Gini coefficient instead of a Lorenz curve. Therefore, the results from the analysis would be more informative; consequently, more insights could be obtained.

Author Contributions: Conceptualization, José Manuel Naranjo Gómez and Rui Alexandre Castanho; methodology, José Manuel Naranjo Gómez; software, José Manuel Naranjo Gómez; validation, José Cabezas Fer-nández., Rui Alexandre Castanho and Luís Loures; formal analysis, José Manuel Naranjo Gómez; investigation, José Manuel Naranjo Gómez and Rui Alexandre Castanho; resources, José Cabezas Fernández; data curation, José Manuel Naranjo Gómez; writing—original draft preparation, José Manuel Naranjo Gómez; writing—review and editing, Rui Alexandre Castanho; visualization, Luís Loures; supervision, José Cabezas Fernández; project administration, Rui Alexandre Castanho; funding acquisition, José Cabezas Fernández, Rui Alexandre Castanho and Luís Loures. All authors have read and agreed to the published version of the manuscript.

Funding: This publication has been made possible thanks to funding granted by the Consejería de Economía, Ciencia y Agenda Digital from Junta de Extremadura and by the European Regional Development Fund of the European Union through the reference grants GR18052 and GR18054.The project is funded under the program of the Minister of Science and Higher Education titled "Regional Initiative of Excellence" in 2019–2022, project number 018/RID/2018/19, the amount of funding PLN 10 788 423,16. Besides, the authors would like to acknowledge the financial support of the National Funds Fundação para a Ciência e a Tecnologia, I.P. (Portuguese Foundation for Science and Technology) by the project UIDB/05064/2020 (VALORIZA—Research Centre for Endogenous Resource Valorization).

Institutional Review Board Statement: Not applicable.

Informed Consent Statement: Not applicable.

Data Availability Statement: The data presented in this study are openly available. Also, it is possible to contact one of the study authors.

Conflicts of Interest: The authors declare no conflict of interest.

References

1. Gazzeh, K.; Abubakar, I.R. Regional disparity in access to basic public services in Saudi Arabia: A sustainability challenge. *Util. Policy* **2018**, *52*, 70–80. [CrossRef]
2. Borrell, C.; Artazcoz, L. Las políticas para disminuir las desigualdades en salud. *Gac. Sanit.* **2008**, *22*, 465–473. [CrossRef]
3. Castanho, R.; Loures, L.; Fernández, J.; Pozo, L. Identifying critical factors for success in Cross Border Cooperation (CBC) development projects. *Habitat Int.* **2018**, *72*, 92–99. [CrossRef]
4. Faka, A. Assessing Quality of Life Inequalities. A Geographical Approach. *ISPRS Int. J. Geo-Inf.* **2020**, *9*, 600. [CrossRef]
5. Dodson, Z.M.; Agadjanian, V.; Driessen, J. How to allocate limited healthcare resources: Lessons from the introduction of antiretroviral therapy in rural Mozambique. *Appl. Geogr.* **2017**, *78*, 45–54. [CrossRef]
6. Costa, C.; Tenedório, J.A.; Santana, P. Disparities in Geographical Access to Hospitals in Portugal. *ISPRS Int. J. Geo-Inf.* **2020**, *9*, 567. [CrossRef]
7. Xiao, Y.; Chen, X.; Li, Q.; Jia, P.; Li, L.; Chen, Z. Towards healthy China 2030: Modeling health care accessibility with patient referral. *Soc. Sci. Med.* **2021**, *276*, 113834. [CrossRef]
8. Joseph, A.E.; Phillips, D.R. *Accessibility And Utilization: Geographical Perspectives on Health Care Delivery*; Harper & Row: London, UK, 1984.
9. Cromley, E.K.; McLafferty, S.L. *GIS and Public Health*; Guilford Press: New York, NY, USA, 2011.
10. Naranjo, J.M.; Loures, L.; Castanho, R.; Cabezas, J.; Panagopoulos, T. Assessing the feasibility of GIS multimethod approach to ascertain territorial accessibility to hemodynamics rooms in Spain mainland. *Habitat Int.* **2018**, *71*, 22–28.
11. Weiland, M.; Santana, P.; Costa, C.; Doetsch, J.; Pilot, E. Spatial Access Matters: An Analysis of Policy Change and Its Effects on Avoidable Infant Mortality in Portugal. *Int. J. Environ. Res. Public Health* **2021**, *18*, 1242. [CrossRef]
12. Corcoran, M.; Byrne, M. Evaluating a primary care psychology service in I reland: A survey of stakeholders and psychologists. *Health Soc. Care Community* **2017**, *25*, 1080–1089. [CrossRef]
13. Holguín, J.M.; Escobar, D.A.; Tamayo, J.A. Servicio de urgencias versus infraestructura de transporte. Un análisis de accesibilidad enfocado en las desigualdades sociales. Caso de estudio: Manizales, Colombia. *Inf. Tecnol.* **2017**, *28*, 125–134. [CrossRef]

14. Carpentieri, G.; Guida, C.; Masoumi, H.E. Multimodal accessibility to primary health services for the elderly: A case study of Naples, Italy. *Sustainability* **2020**, *12*, 781. [CrossRef]
15. Shah, T.I.; Milosavljevic, S.; Bath, B. Measuring geographical accessibility to rural and remote health care services: Challenges and considerations. *Spat. Spatio-Temporal Epidemiol.* **2017**, *21*, 87–96. [CrossRef]
16. Castanho, R.A. The Relevance of Political Engagement and Transparency in Cross-Border Cooperation (CBC) Environments. Analyzing Border cities in Europe. *Lex Localis-J. Local Self-Gov.* **2020**, *18*, 487–502. [CrossRef]
17. Hui, E.C.M.; Dong, Z.; Jia, S.; Lam, C.H.L. How does sentiment affect returns of urban housing? *Habitat Int.* **2017**, *64*, 71–84. [CrossRef]
18. Pan, J.; Zhao, H.; Wang, X.; Shi, X. Assessing spatial access to public and private hospitals in Sichuan, China: The influence of the private sector on the healthcare geography in China. *Soc. Sci. Med.* **2016**, *170*, 35–45. [CrossRef] [PubMed]
19. Comisión para Reducir las Desigualdades Sociales en Salud en España. Propuesta de políticas e intervenciones para reducir las desigualdades sociales en salud en España. *Gac. Sanit.* **2012**, *26*, 182–189. [CrossRef]
20. Elízaga Corrales, J. La angioplastia primaria es la terapéutica dereperfusión de elección en el tratamiento delinfarto agudo de miocardio. Argumentos a favor. *Rev. Española Cardiol.* **1998**, *51*, 939–947. Available online: https://www.revespcardiol.org/es-la-angioplastia-primaria-es-terapeutica-articulo-X0300893298003855 (accessed on 11 July 2021). [CrossRef]
21. Saugel, B.; Bendjelid, K.; Critchley, L.A.; Rex, S.; Scheeren, T.W. Journal of Clinical Monitoring and Computing 2016 end of year summary: Cardiovascular and hemodynamic monitoring. *J. Clin. Monit. Comput.* **2017**, *31*, 5–17. [CrossRef]
22. Saugel, B.; Bendjelid, K.; Critchley, L.A.H.; Scheeren, T.W.L. Journal of Clinical Monitoring and Computing 2017 end of year summary: Cardiovascular and hemodynamic monitoring. *J. Clin. Monit. Comput.* **2018**, *32*, 189–196. [CrossRef]
23. Fotheringham, S.; Wegener, M. *Spatial Models and GIS: New Potential and New Models*; Taylor & Francis: Oxford, UK, 2000.
24. García, J. La medida de la accesibilidad. *Estud. Construcciín Y Transp.* **2000**, *88*, 95–110.
25. Monzón, A.; Gutiérrez, J.; López, E.; Madrigal, E.; Gómez, G. Infraestructuras de transporte terrestre y su influencia en los niveles de accesibilidad de la España peninsular. *Estud. Construcción Y Transp.* **2005**, *103*, 97–112.
26. Gutiérrez, J.; Monzón, A.; Piñero, J.M. Accesibilidad a los centros de actividad econémica en España. *Rev. Obras Públicas* **1994**, *141*, 34–49.
27. Brocard, M. *Transports Et Territoires: Enjeux Et Débats*; Ellipses Marketing: Paris, France, 2019.
28. Gutierrez-Gallego, J.A.; Gómez, J.M.N.; Jaraíz-Cabanillas, F.; Labrador, E.E.R.; Jeong, J.S. A methodology to assess the connectivity caused by a transportation infrastructure: Application to the high-speed rail in Extremadura. *Case Stud. Transp. Policy* **2015**, *3*, 392–401. [CrossRef]
29. Chen, Z.; Yeh, A.G.-O. Accessibility Inequality and Income Disparity in Urban China: A Case Study of Guangzhou. *Ann. Am. Assoc. Geogr.* **2018**, *109*, 121–141. [CrossRef]
30. Jokar Arsanjani, J.; Vaz, E. Special issue editorial: Earth observation and geoinformation technologies for sustainable development. *Sustainability* **2017**, *9*, 760. [CrossRef]
31. Vicente Galindo, P.; Vaz, E.; De Noronha, T. How corporations deal with reporting sustainability: Assessment using the multicriteria logistic biplot approach. *Systems* **2015**, *3*, 6–26. [CrossRef]
32. Gray, D.; Shaw, J.; Farrington, J. Community transport, social capital and social exclusion in rural areas. *Area* **2006**, *38*, 89–98. [CrossRef]
33. Higgs, G. The role of GIS for health utilization studies: Literature review. *Health Serv. Outcomes Res. Methodol.* **2009**, *9*, 84–99. [CrossRef]
34. Arrivillaga, M.; Borrero, Y.E. A comprehensive and critical view of conceptual models for access to health services, 1970–2013. *Cad. De Saude Publica* **2016**, *32*, e00111415. [CrossRef]
35. Khan, A.A. An integrated approach to measuring potential spatial access to health care services. *Socio-Econ. Plan. Sci.* **1992**, *26*, 275–287. [CrossRef]
36. Kelly, C.; Hulme, C.; Farragher, T.; Clarke, G. Are differences in travel time or distance to healthcare for adults in global north countries associated with an impact on health outcomes? A systematic review. *BMJ Open* **2016**, *6*, e013059. [CrossRef]
37. Lang, W.; Radke, J.D.; Chen, T.; Chan, E.H. Will affordability policy transcend climate change? A new lens to re-examine equitable access to healthcare in the San Francisco Bay Area. *Cities* **2016**, *58*, 124–136. [CrossRef]
38. Chen, T.; Hui, E.C.-M.; Lang, W.; Tao, L. People, Recreational facility and physical activity: New-type urbanization planning for the healthy communities in China. *Habitat Int.* **2016**, *58*, 12–22. [CrossRef]
39. Pathak, E.B.; Reader, S.; Tanner, J.P.; Casper, M.L. Spatial clustering of non-transported cardiac decedents: The results of a point pattern analysis and an inquiry into social environmental correlates. *Int. J. Health Geogr.* **2021**, *10*, 1–11. [CrossRef] [PubMed]
40. Skiles, M.P.; Cunningham, M.; Inglis, A.; Wilkes, B.; Hatch, B.; Bock, A.; Barden-O'Fallon, J. The effect of access to contraceptive services on injectable use and demand for family planning in Malawi. *Int. Perspect. Sex. Reprod. Health* **2015**, *41*, 20–30. [CrossRef] [PubMed]
41. Luo, W.; Wang, F. Measures of spatial accessibility to health care in a GIS environment: Synthesis and a case study in the Chicago region. *Environ. Plan. B Plan. Des.* **2003**, *30*, 865–884. [CrossRef] [PubMed]
42. Frew, R.; Higgs, G.; Harding, J.; Langford, M. Investigating geospatial data usability from a health geography perspective using sensitivity analysis: The example of potential accessibility to primary healthcare. *J. Transport. Health* **2017**, *6*, 128–142. [CrossRef]

43. Yang, N.; Chen, S.; Hu, W.; Wu, Z.; Chao, Y. Spatial distribution balance analysis of hospitals in Wuhan. *Int. J. Environ. Res. Public Health* **2016**, *13*, 971. [CrossRef]
44. Delamater, P.L.; Shortridge, A.M.; Kilcoyne, R.C. Using floating catchment area (FCA) metrics to predict health care utilization patterns. *BMC Health Serv. Res.* **2019**, *19*, 1–14. [CrossRef]
45. Ashik, F.R.; Mim, S.A.; Neema, M.N. Towards vertical spatial equity of urban facilities: An integration of spatial and aspatial accessibility. *J. Urban. Manag.* **2020**, *9*, 77–92. [CrossRef]
46. Luo, W.; Qi, Y. An enhanced two-step floating catchment area (E2SFCA) method for measuring spatial accessibility to primary care physicians. *Health Place* **2009**, *15*, 1100–1107. [CrossRef]
47. Haynes, K.E.; Fotheringham, A.S. *Gravity and Spatial Interaction Models*; Regional Research Institute, West Virginia University: Morgantown, WV, USA, 2020.
48. Chen, X. Take the edge off: A hybrid geographic food access measure. *Appl. Geogr.* **2017**, *87*, 149–159. [CrossRef]
49. Crawford, T.W.; Pitts, S.B.J.; McGuirt, J.T.; Keyserling, T.C.; Ammerman, A.S. Conceptualizing and comparing neighborhood and activity space measures for food environment research. *Health Place* **2014**, *30*, 215–225. [CrossRef]
50. Delamater, P.L. Spatial accessibility in suboptimally configured health care systems: A modified two-step floating catchment area (M2SFCA) metric. *Health Place* **2013**, *24*, 30–43. [CrossRef] [PubMed]
51. Wan, N.; Zou, B.; Sternberg, T. A three-step floating catchment area method for analyzing spatial access to health services. *Int. J. Geogr. Inf. Sci.* **2012**, *26*, 1073–1089. [CrossRef]
52. Wu, J.; Cai, Z.; Li, H. Accessibility of medical facilities in multiple traffic modes: A study in Guangzhou, China. *Complexity* **2020**, *2020*, 8819836. [CrossRef]
53. McGrail, M. Spatial accessibility of primary health care utilising the two step floating catchment area method: An assessment of recent improvements. *Int. J. Health Geographics.* **2012**, *11*, 50. [CrossRef]
54. Wang, F. Measurement, Optimization, and Impact of Health Care Accessibility: A Methodological Review. *Ann. Assoc. Am. Geographers.* **2012**, *102*, 1104–1112. [CrossRef] [PubMed]
55. Paez, A.; Higgins, C.D.; Vivona, S.F. Demand and level of service inflation in Floating Catchment Area (FCA) methods. *PLoS ONE* **2019**, *14*, e0218773. [CrossRef]
56. Palanca Sanchéz, I.; Castro Beiras, A.; Macaya Miguel, C.; Elola Somoza, J.; Bernal Sobrino, J.; Paniagua Caparrós, J. Grupo de Expertos. In *Unidades Asistenciales Del Área Del Corazón: Estándares Y Recomendaciones*; Ministerio de Sanidad, Política Social e Igualdad: Madrid, Spain, 2011; p. 28.
57. Rose, K.M.; Foraker, R.E.; Heiss, G.; Rosamond, W.D.; Suchindran, C.M.; Whitsel, E.A. Neighborhood socioeconomic and racial disparities in angiography and coronary revascularization: The ARIC surveillance study. *Ann. Epidemiology* **2012**, *22*, 623–629. [CrossRef] [PubMed]
58. Márquez Calderón, S.; Jiménez, A.; Perea Milla, E.; Briones, E.; Aguayo, E.; Reina, A. Variaciones en la hospitalización por problemas y procedimientos cardiovasculares en el Sistema Nacional de Salud. *Atlas Var. Pract. Med. Sist. Nac. Salud* **2017**, *2*, 151–174.
59. Condeço-Melhorado, A.; Gutiérrez, J.; López, E.; Monzón, A. El Valor Añadido Europeo De Los Proyectos Transnacionales (Ten-T): Una Propuesta Metodológica Basada En Los Efectos De Desbordamiento, Accesibilidad Y Sig. In *Congreso Nacional de Tecnologías de la Información Geográfica*; Secretariado de Publicaciones de la Universidad de Sevilla: Sevilla, Spain, 2010.
60. Morales, R.; Candolfi, N.; Serna, J.; Mejía, D.A.; Villegas, J.M.; Nieto, J.I.; Medina, M. Resource Sharing in Collaborative Environments: Performance Considerations. In *International Symposium on Distributed Compu-ting and Artificial Intelligence*; Abra-ham, A., Corchado, J.M., González, S.R., De Paz Santana, J.F., Eds.; Springer: Berlin/Heidelberg, Germany, 2011; Volume 91. [CrossRef]

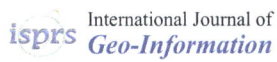

Article

Exploring Equity in Healthcare Services: Spatial Accessibility Changes during Subway Expansion

Maohua Liu, Siqi Luo and Xishihui Du *

School of Transportation Engineering, Shenyang Jianzhu University, Shenyang 110168, China; cemhliu@sjzu.edu.cn (M.L.); yogalinrose@163.com (S.L.)
* Correspondence: daisy_duxi@126.com

Abstract: The unequal allocation of healthcare resources raises many fundamental problems, one of which is how to address inequity in population health. This paper focuses on disparities in public transport healthcare accessibility, with a special focus on an expanding subway system. Based on a vulnerability index, including factors that are likely to limit healthcare opportunities, a two-step floating catchment area method was used to assess the distribution of supply and demand for healthcare. Quantity, quality, and walking distance accessibility were aggregated into hexagonal grids. The Theil index was used to measure inequity and understand the influence of subways on spatial disparities in healthcare accessibility. The ongoing construction of the subway has heterogeneous impacts on healthcare accessibility for different parts of the city and exacerbates spatial inequity in many areas. In an environment where people in peri-urban areas are excluded from healthcare access because of low subway coverage, the results suggest that the potential for subways to address inaccessibility is limited. The findings highlight the requirement of efficient public transport services and are relevant to researchers, planners, and policymakers aiming to improve accessibility to healthcare, especially for populations who dwell in winter cities.

Keywords: geospatial health; spatial disparities; accessibility; GIS; subway expansion; public transport network

1. Introduction

Equity matters for every social group because it raises opportunities and supports the rights that should be available to every individual within a population. If equity among the population is high, the society benefits overall [1]. However, many public transport (PT) systems do not provide adequate services for citizens to easily access public resources or to meet complex travel needs. For example, in many cases, low-income subdistricts are more heavily dependent on PT [2], and a simple PT system may not provide adequate access to groups with high service requirements, such as complex journeys [3]. In high demand regions, inadequate PT may limit access to resources and opportunities, making them more susceptible to social and economic marginalization [4,5]. Equity has attracted considerable attention in relation to public resources and urban infrastructure because a mobility gap often exists between PT availability and population demand. This gap has brought to prominence two key research topics addressing the spatial equity of public resources. First, accessibility based on sociodemographic attributes (e.g., age, gender, race, income), which can highlight inequities in individuals' access to public resources [6–8]; and secondly, in response to this, analysis of locations through spatial optimization of both facilities and transport networks [9,10].

Spatial equity analysis focuses on differences in the services used by different regions or social groups from the perspective of supply and demand; and is, to some extent, an extension of the concept of accessibility [11]. Therefore, quantifying spatial accessibility is an important foundation for measuring spatial equity, hence assessing social equity [12,13]. In the field of health and transportation, measuring accessibility plays an important role in

Citation: Liu, M.; Luo, S.; Du, X. Exploring Equity in Healthcare Services: Spatial Accessibility Changes during Subway Expansion. *ISPRS Int. J. Geo-Inf.* **2021**, *10*, 439. https://doi.org/10.3390/ijgi10070439

Academic Editors: Fazlay S. Faruque and Wolfgang Kainz

Received: 29 April 2021
Accepted: 24 June 2021
Published: 27 June 2021

Publisher's Note: MDPI stays neutral with regard to jurisdictional claims in published maps and institutional affiliations.

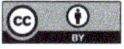

Copyright: © 2021 by the authors. Licensee MDPI, Basel, Switzerland. This article is an open access article distributed under the terms and conditions of the Creative Commons Attribution (CC BY) license (https://creativecommons.org/licenses/by/4.0/).

comprehensively evaluating the equity of service distribution within a region [14,15]. Wee and Geurs [16] proposed that lack of access to opportunities is the most important indicator of transport-related inequity. Measures of access include both the availability of an activity (such as work, education, shopping, healthcare, or recreation) and the ease of access to the location of the activity from a given origin, usually a residential location. Accessibility is mainly influenced by two factors: the balance of supply and demand relative to origin and destination points, and the suitability for purpose of the transportation network. Urban transportation systems are gradually upgraded, and reconfigured, in response to ongoing rapid urbanization and increasingly complex distributions of urban functions, service resources, and diverse people's demands. Estimates of accessibility depend on the factors themselves but are also substantially influenced by the choice of accessibility measure. Four measures are commonly used to evaluate place-based accessibility: gravity-based accessibility, cumulative opportunity accessibility, utility-based accessibility, and emerging measures based on real-time individual data [17]. Gravity-based measures utilize a distance/time decay function to normalize the cost of travel between the origin and destination. This approach follows the gravity model's assumption that the interactions between activities are directly proportional to their size and inversely proportional to the cost of traveling between them [18]; however, the cost decay is uncertain for every group or individual [19]. The cumulative opportunity measure assumes that individuals will utilize the opportunities nearest to them, and more nearby opportunities translate into more choices for individuals. There is no limit to the capacity of these opportunities [20]. However, people often compete for the same opportunities and, in the case of employment, one job can only be taken by a single person. Thus, the assumption that more opportunities will translate to more choices, without considering the potential demand and hence competition for those opportunities, can be misleading [5]. Utility-based measures estimate the value of opportunities based on the assumption that users/consumers of a transport system seek to maximize the utility of their behavioral choices. This is a cross-disciplinary approach utilizing economic, social, land use, and transport data, and is still considered an emerging method that requires substantial research and development [21,22]. The final category is real-time-based accessibility measurements. Influenced by temporal geography, some scholars have researched spatiotemporal accessibility available to individuals, which is expected to accord with social reality [4,23]. They focus on the impact of the scale of public service facilities, transportation mode choices, and real demands on the equity of access to those facilities [10,24,25]. The above four measures have in common either distance/time cost or approach opportunities as indicators. However, accessibility estimation is likely to be influenced by the measurement method, which may limit the assessed access possibilities through limits to distance or accessibility opportunities. In general, commuters are usually concerned about commuting time and distance, which can be measured by gravity-based accessibility. When shopping, consumers are more interested in the variety of goods, their quality, and their prices than by distance [26,27]. In healthcare or education, users are sensitive to the quality of public services in addition to the travel options and costs [28–30]. Therefore, discussing accessibility from a single perspective is only a partial solution, and a customized measurement method should be developed for different behavioral activities. Therefore, in this study, we propose measuring accessibility to healthcare services from diverse perspectives, based on citizens' concerns and interests, and the consequences for social equity.

As important public facilities, a reasonable spatial distribution of healthcare services is influential in people's livelihood and security. Many studies have demonstrated that poor access to healthcare services contributes to lower levels of service utilization, which in turn leads to poorer health outcomes [31–33]. The provision of adequate and equitable healthcare access across the whole population has become a concern for governments and societies [34–36]. Public healthcare plays an important role in meeting the health needs of the population, and seniors especially are considered to be among the most vulnerable groups in the population [37]. Although the elderly are the main demand group for healthcare, their overall health status in China is poor. Nearly 180 million elderly people suffer from chronic diseases, and the proportion of those suffering from one or more chronic diseases is as high as 75%. The number of people aged 60 years and over in the city of Shenyang is estimated to have reached 2.019 million by the end of 2020, accounting for 26.52% of the total population. Consequently, it is vital for Shenyang to make provisions for equal access to healthcare services. Especially in winter, large numbers of people in Shenyang (a designated "winter city") face difficulties walking outdoors, and residents rely on PT for daily travel. Based on data from Shenyang's comprehensive traffic survey conducted in the downtown area in 2017, 32.8% of all journeys were made by PT. The rapid development of China's subway systems has provided a new transportation alternative to citizens in winter cities and has additionally helped mitigate multiple urban health and environmental challenges such as congestion, traffic injuries, air pollution, greenhouse emissions, and noise. Owing to its cost and speed advantages, the subway has become the preferred mode of transportation for most residents, especially when individuals seek healthcare alone. While subways have been undergoing revitalization as one of the country's primary PT modes, inequity in healthcare services has remained a major concern for health planners and policymakers.

We propose an approach for measuring healthcare accessibility from the perspective of subway expansion. We use a vulnerability index and accessibility measures to compare healthcare access equity and so the influence of subway expansion. For this purpose, vulnerability factors that are likely to limit healthcare opportunities have been proposed, including income, recent immigration, population age distribution, and physical conditions. Based on the obtained population vulnerability and healthcare data, the distribution of the supply–demand balance of facilities was visualized using a two-step floating catchment area (2SFCA) method. Furthermore, a comprehensive accessibility measure was used relating quantity, quality, and walking distance in the context of subway upgrading. Finally, the Theil index was used to measure the equity of healthcare resources. The proposed method will provide a more nuanced understanding of spatial disparities in healthcare accessibility, and the results of this empirical study will offer new insights into the ways in which variations in PT influence healthcare accessibility. Officials in the fields of public health and planning can reduce local disparities by designing targeted interventions.

2. Materials and Methods

2.1. Study Area

Shenyang is the capital of Liaoning Province and is an important city in northeastern China. Our study area (Figure 1) includes the central urban area based on the third ring road of Shenyang City (Figure 1c), and incorporates nine districts: Heping, Shenhe, Dadong, Huanggu, Tiexi, Sujiatun, Hunnan, Yuhong, and Shenbei New District, with a total land area of 12,860 km^2. The Hun River runs through central Shenyang from east to west and divides the central area into two parts. According to demographic data from the Shenyang Statistics Bureau (2019), the number of permanent residents in Shenyang was 8.32 million in 2019. However, the populations' requirements for medical care are addressed by a relatively small number of general hospitals, with only 181 in Shenyang's central urban area. According to Shenyang's comprehensive traffic survey, which surveyed the pathways used by residents to access social resources such as healthcare services, the majority chose to use PT [38]. The PT system is known as the Shenyang Rail Transit, and included 478 bus lines and four built subway lines at the end of 2020. Its first subway line commenced operation on 27 September 2010, making it the first in northeastern China. By April 2020, there were four lines in operation (metro lines 1, 2, 9, and 10) with 92 stations and 117.06 km of operating distance, covering the central urban area. Subway lines 3 and 4, as well as extensions to lines 1 and 2, are due to be completed by the end of 2025. By then, Shenyang's main and sub-cities will be connected by the subway network, promoting interaction between subdistricts.

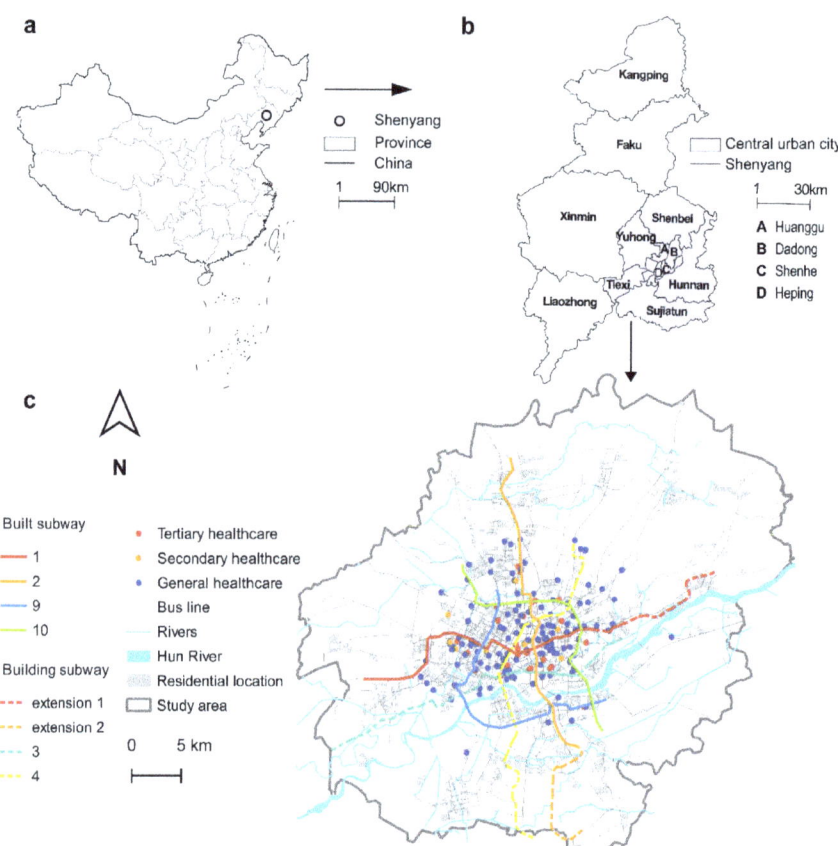

Figure 1. Spatial context of the central urban core of Shenyang: (**a**) location of Shenyang in China; (**b**) administrative boundaries in Shenyang; (**c**) overview of the study area.

2.2. Data Sources and Preprocessing

Generally, healthcare accessibility at any given location depends on three components: the capacity of the healthcare services (e.g., the number of physicians or beds), the potential demand for healthcare services (i.e., population), and transport network performance (i.e., travel impedance from locations with demand for healthcare services). The data used in this study consisted of three categories: population-based demand, healthcare services, and PT data. Population-demand data were extracted from the Shenyang Statistical Yearbook provided by the Shenyang Bureau of Statistics in 2019 and included data related to social identities (e.g., recent immigrants), health inequalities (e.g., elderly population and mortality), and socioeconomic determinants (e.g., tax revenue). Furthermore, healthcare services data (including geographical locations, hospital rank, and the number of beds) were mainly collected from an online medical service website called 99 Hospital Library (https://yyk.99.com.cn/, accessed on 25 December 2019). The hospitals selected in this study were 181 public general hospitals with high-quality medical services, which are economical and more advanced medical equipment; these hospitals are more likely to be included in the social insurance system than private hospitals, specialized hospitals, and other medical institutions [39]. Considering the limitations of adding large-scale public hospitals for decades, public hospitals in 2019 were selected to investigate accessibility. In addition, data on PT connections between various origins and destinations were derived from the AutoNavi Open Platform (https://lbs. amap.com, accessed on 10 January 2020) by implementing Python-based web crawling technology, and were supplemented by material from the Shenyang Metro website (http://www.symtc.com/, accessed on 15 January 2020). The program used basic information on the 478 bus lines and six subway lines in the central urban city of Shenyang.

2.3. Methodology
2.3.1. Supply and Demand of Subdistricts for Healthcare Services

The vulnerability index, for healthcare facilities, of every subdistrict was calculated using weighted factors, which vary by region. As this study focused on accessibility via PT, the vulnerability index draws on characteristics that increase the likelihood of an individual's demand for PT. Following the study by Boisjoly et al. [40] and the characteristics of the study area, we selected the following indicators as the relevant variables for the vulnerability index: (i) tax value (I), (ii) number of elderly (U), (iii) number of immigrants (M), and (iv) mortality (N). The final vulnerability index is given by Equation (1), where Z_x represents the z-score of the variable X.

$$V = -Z_I + Z_U + Z_M + Z_N \tag{1}$$

Subsequently, the 2SFCA method was used to analyze the supply and demand of healthcare services, which is essentially a summation of the service-to-demand rate at residential locations [41]. The demand–supply ratio R_i is given by Equation (2) as follows:

$$R_i = \sum_{j\in\{d_j \leq d_0\}} T_j = \sum_{j\in\{d_j \leq d_0\}} \frac{S_j}{\sum_{k\in\{d_i \leq d_0\}} V_k}, \quad d_0 = 1.5 \text{ km} \tag{2}$$

where V is the vulnerability index at a residential location i that can reach a given service by PT, j denotes a healthcare service, S_j represents the capacity of each healthcare service j (number of beds), and d_i and d_j are the shortest walking distance from residential location i and healthcare service j to a PT station, and d_0 denotes a walking threshold that represents the distance from each residential location or healthcare service to the nearest PT stop. The application of Equation (2) involves two steps: the first step determines T_j as the service capacity of each bed, and the second step calculates the summation of the service-to-demand rate for each subdistrict (R_i). The larger the value, the better the supply relative to the demand.

2.3.2. Accessibility of Population Residential Location to Healthcare Services

As shown in Figure 2, the OD cost matrix and spatial connection in a geographic information system (GIS) were used to evaluate spatial accessibility for citizens in Shenyang to obtain healthcare services that find the best accessibility path from origin to destination in the transport network [42–44]. The service radius of PT stations is 0.5–1 km, and walking speed of residents is 4.5–5 km/h [45–48]. Considering the suburb residents and acceptable distance of 0.5–1.5 km for elderly to PT station in the study area, we used 1.5 km as walking threshold to analyze accessibility using OD cost matrix. Based on the 1.5 km OD's search radius, we evaluated accessibility from the perspectives of the quantity, quality, and walking distance. Quantity accessibility, A_v, refers to the number of healthcare resources that can be accessed by PT from each residential location, which can be divided into none, low, moderate, and high accessibility at equal intervals. However, healthcare equality is a relatively comprehensive concept, which should be evaluated by the number of beds, professional physicians, nurses, and grades; according to China's healthcare services standards, healthcare conditions such as beds or professional physicians partly represent the scale and quality of medical institutions [49,50]. Therefore, the total number of healthcare beds available to individuals represents the quality accessibility (A_w), which can be divided into none (0), low (1–100), moderate (100–500), and high (>500) accessibility based on China's hospital classification standards. Walking to PT stations is the main obstacle for the elderly in using PT services [51]. Hence, walking distance accessibility, A_x, can be represented as the total walking distance when taking PT from the origin or destination. Considering the acceptable distance to PT stations and walking speed, walking distance accessibility can be divided into none (>3 km), low (2.5–3 km), moderate (1.5–2.5 km), and high (0–1.5 km). The A_v, A_w, and A_x are given in Equation (3).

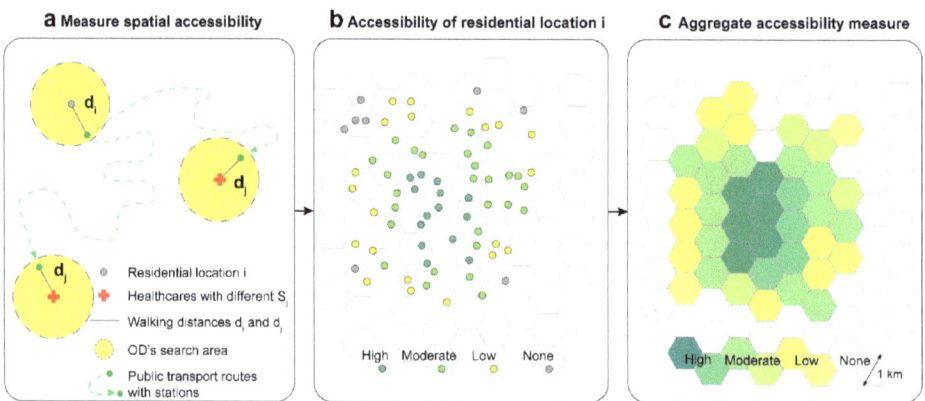

Figure 2. Schematic diagram of measurement of spatial accessibility to healthcare services: (**a**) measure spatial accessibility; (**b**) the accessibility of residential location i; (**c**) aggregate accessibility measure.

Finally, residential location accessibility to hexagonal cells was integrated to minimize orientation bias from edge effects and clearly identify the differences between grids [52,53]. Through experiments, ideal hexagonal diameter was determined to be 1 km, including an average of 2.2 residential locations, thereby providing sufficient accuracy to summarize the results.

$$
\begin{aligned}
A_v &= \sum_i f(d_i, d_j) \\
A_w &= \sum_i S_j f(d_i, d_j) \quad f(d_i, d_j) = \begin{cases} 1 \text{ if } d_i \leq d_o, d_j \leq d_o \\ 0 \text{ else} \end{cases} \\
A_x &= d_i + d_j \quad\quad\quad\quad\quad d_0 = 1.5 \text{ km}
\end{aligned}
\tag{3}
$$

2.3.3. Equity Evaluation

To better understand both inter- and intra-regional variations in accessibility, the Theil index was adopted to identify disparities in equity. This index reflects the relationship between demand among the population living in the study area and accessibility using the PT system [54,55]. In general, the degree of relative advantage or disadvantage among groups in a population can be estimated using the Theil index (T), which ranges from 0 to 1 (Equation (4)). The larger the T, the greater the difference between regions, suggesting more unbalanced development. According to the equity principle, ideally all citizens in the subdistricts have equal access to healthcare services. Therefore, the ideal for planners is to minimize T:

$$T = \sum_j^m \frac{V_j}{V_{tot}} \cdot \frac{A_j}{\overline{A_g}} \cdot ln\left(\frac{A_j}{\overline{A_g}}\right) \tag{4}$$

where m is the number of subdistricts and their districts, V_j is the vulnerability index of group j, V_{tot} is the sum of the m vulnerability indexes, A_j is the accessibility, and $\overline{A_g}$ represents the average of the A_j values in the study area.

3. Results

3.1. Spatial Distribution Characteristics of Healthcare Supply and Demand

This section presents the results of the subdistrict supply and demand analysis for the central urban core of Shenyang. Vulnerability indicators were variable across the nine districts (Table 1). The elderly population ranged from approximately 250 thousand in Tiexi District to approximately 76 thousand in Hunnan District. The mortality rate also varied greatly, from 10.34‰ to 6.42‰. Heping District had the highest tax value, followed by Shenhe District. Interestingly, despite having the lowest tax value and the worst economic development level, Yuhong District was the most popular migration option. The high diversity of regions inevitably led to varying needs for PT. Accordingly, this section reviews the distributions of supply and demand for healthcare services in Shenyang.

Table 1. List of vulnerability factors and vulnerability index in each district.

District	Tax Value (10,000)	Number of the Elderly (10,000)	Number of Arrivals (10,000)	Mortality Rate (‰)	Vulnerability Index
Heping	77,092	17.93	2.03	8.33	146.70
Shenhe	67,900	20.31	1.11	9.37	169.10
Dadong	29,083	18.97	0.74	10.34	129.84
Huanggu	27,022	21.72	1.65	8.97	197.85
Tiexi	44,552	25.15	1.74	9.82	269.21
Sujiatun	12,872	11.10	0.36	9.42	19.57
Hunnan	35,597	7.66	2.37	6.42	116.46
Yuhong	8498	10.21	2.25	7.93	90.50
Shenbei	9093	7.83	0.81	9.04	41.37

As shown in Figure 3, there were several subdistricts on the edge of the central core that have the lowest supply–demand ratio. There are very few healthcare services in these areas, posing challenges to residents. On the one hand, these districts have the lowest populations in the region, but their vulnerability index is high relative to their counterparts. On the other hand, PT stations in these regions are sparsely located; therefore, residents find it harder to access healthcare services. Of the subdistricts with high vulnerability for social services, 60.2% showed lower levels of supply and demand despite having considerable geographical advantages and good PT coverage within the central urban area. Residents in the central region had a moderate level of supply–demand ratio, while their need was moderate or low. Finally, subdistricts with a higher supply–demand ratio, including the group with the highest ratio, were mainly in the northeast of the core area, which has an intensive transport network. Accordingly, the state of supply and demand was in disequilibrium in that area, and most subdistricts likely lacked the healthcare resources to match their needs. Hence, it is important to assess whether upgrading of the subway system in this area can improve access and equity.

3.2. Accessibility across the Central Urban Area after Introducing Subways

Although the supply and demand analysis provided insights into the distribution of healthcare sources and PT, it failed to elaborate on how extending subway services affects accessibility. In this section, quantity, quality, and walking distance are calculated to assess the spatial distribution of accessibility, and to compare differences following expansion of the subway.

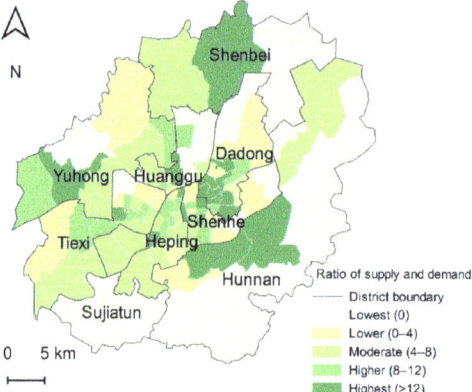

Figure 3. Spatial distribution of supply–demand to healthcare services in the main urban area of Shenyang.

3.2.1. Quantity Accessibility

As shown in Figure 4, quantity accessibility radially decreased with distance from the city center. However, the highest accessibility was not found in the center, but rather near the surrounding metro transfer stations. In areas influenced by metro lines 9 and 10, quantity accessibility exhibited (Figure 4b) a dual-core distribution centered on metro interchanges (metro lines 1 and 9; metro lines 1 and 10). The construction of new subway extensions is projected to clearly expand the dual-core range (Figure 4c). Zones with moderate quantity accessibility are scattered across the heartland. With subway extension the number of metro transfer stations that surround the periphery increases more obviously in the north (Huanggu and Shenhe Districts) than in the south (Hunnan District). Zones with low accessibility are mainly located outside the metro core area and are minimally influenced by the new subway building.

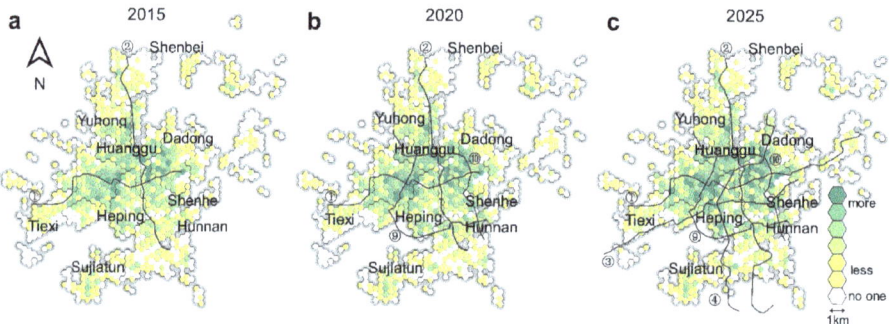

Figure 4. Spatial quantity accessibility to healthcare services at different stages of subway system development: (**a**) accessibility in 2015; (**b**) accessibility in 2020; (**c**) accessibility in 2025.

Quantity accessibility changed over time in every district (Figure 5). Residential locations with high accessibility increased from 13.89% to 32.45% over the study period, and 94.96% of the area showed improved quantity accessibility caused by changes in the subway system. As the subway gradually formed a network, the Tiexi District showed the most notable increase (19.16%) in accessibility. As a result, zones of moderate quantity accessibility were evenly distributed, except in Sujiatun District, which showed a strong change over a decade. The percentage of moderate stage area decreased from 66.64% to 48.08%, and inaccessible zones within each district were reduced by 5.04%.

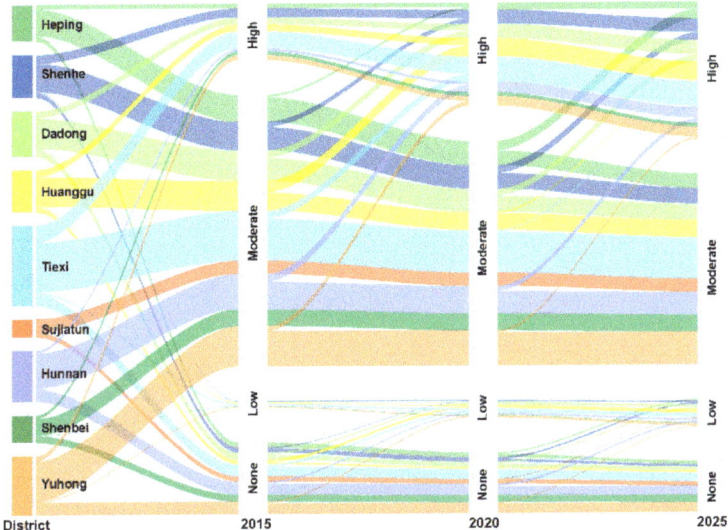

Figure 5. Spatial changes in residential zones with quantity accessibility ranking.

3.2.2. Quality Accessibility

The spatial distribution of quality accessibility (Figure 6) is similar to quantity accessibility, and the healthcare quality available to residents increases as the subway expands. The healthcare quality in residential areas around metro line 1 is the highest, followed by successive decreases outside the core. Upgrading of the subway expands the highest-quality accessibility zones to the north with metro line 3 and west with metro line 10. Notably, the southern region changes little over the study period, which indicates that the healthcare quality available to the southern population is inadequate. This outcome is likely related to the Hun River obstructing subway construction and the concentration of healthcare services in the heartland.

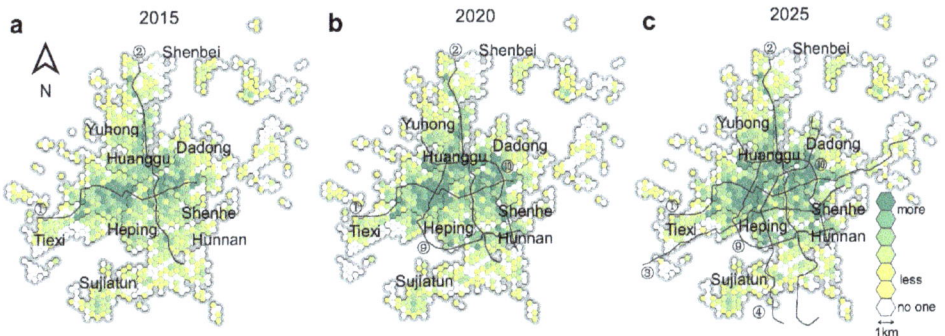

Figure 6. Spatial quality accessibility to healthcare services at different stages of subway system development: (**a**) accessibility in 2015; (**b**) accessibility in 2020; (**c**) accessibility in 2025.

Quality accessibility occurs in every district following subway upgrades (Figure 7). In particular, Heping and Shenhe Districts were influenced by metro lines 3 and 4. Because of the expanded subway, 6.19% of residential locations improved from low healthcare quality accessibility. In addition, 19.62% of residential locations experienced an increase in quality accessibility from moderate to high; most of these locations are in southern Hunnan and Huanggu Districts and are influenced by metro lines 9 and 10. In the dual-core region, the high-quality range expanded; specifically, 18.47% of residential locations newly achieved high-quality access to over the study period.

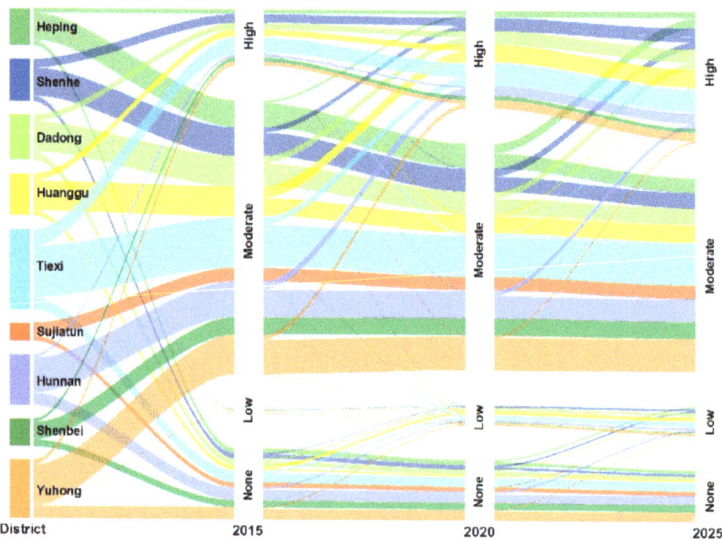

Figure 7. Spatial changes in residential zones with quality accessibility ranking.

3.2.3. Walking Accessibility

As expected, walking accessibility increases dramatically as a result of subway expansion, and residential locations with high walking accessibility generally occurring on both sides of the subway lines (Figure 8). Viewed holistically, the high walking accessibility coverage expanded from the surroundings of metro lines 1 and 2 to the whole enclosed area of old and new metro lines. The addition of lines 9 and 10 clearly reduce walking distances in many districts, apart from Shenbei New District. However, most districts appeared to have been minimally influenced by the construction of lines 3 and 4, although a substantial reduction in walking distance was observed in Heping District (from 2767.37 m to 806.05 m).

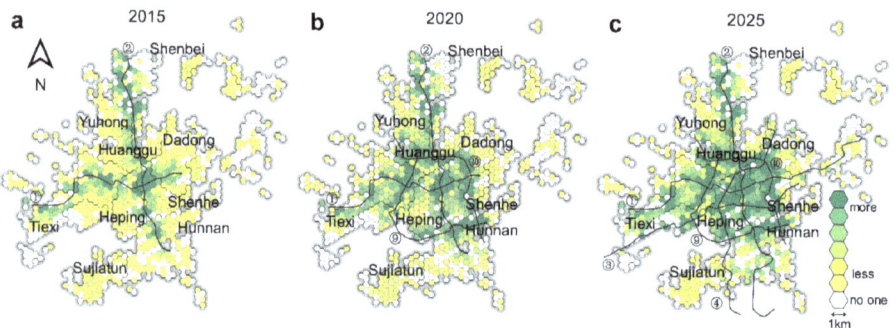

Figure 8. Spatial walking accessibility to healthcare services at different stages of subway system development: (**a**) accessibility in 2015; (**b**) accessibility in 2020; (**c**) accessibility in 2025.

Overall, subway extensions increase walking accessibility (Figure 9). Most districts in the center city become highly walkable, with Dadong and Tiexi Districts showing increases owing to metro lines 9 and 10, and Heping District influenced by metro lines 3 and 4. However, much of Sujiatun District was beyond the acceptable walking range. Approximately 31.48% of residential locations showed a rise in high walkability as subway lines were extended, with 13.89% of residential locations being within the convenient walking threshold (≤1 km). Residential locations with moderate walkability only increased by 2.75%; these locations were distributed within the area enclosed by metro lines 1, 3, 9, and 10. Furthermore, 29.19% of residential locations with previously low walkability, which is far beyond the acceptable walking threshold, had improved walkability.

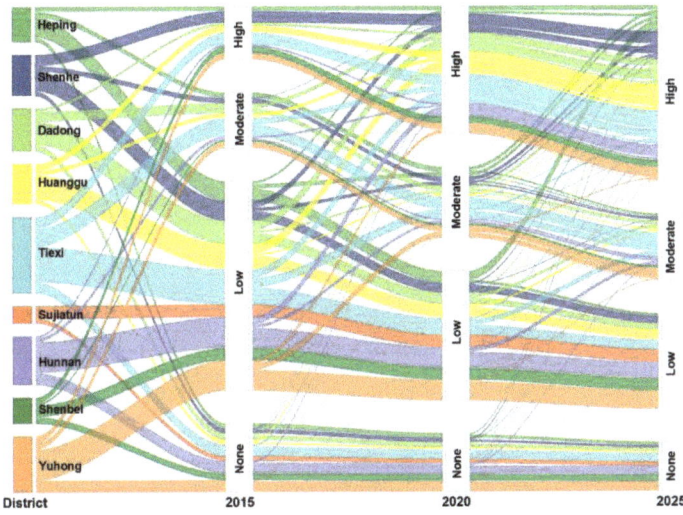

Figure 9. Spatial changes in residential zones with walking accessibility ranking.

3.3. Equity Changes with Subway Line Extensions

While clear regional differences were observed in the temporal and spatial characteristics of accessibility, it is less easy to estimate equity across subdistricts or districts. The Theil index shows the degree of inequity within regions, based on the vulnerability index and accessibility.

3.3.1. Equity between Subdistricts

Although subway services have increased access to healthcare services in Shenyang, there are two ways in which inequity between regions may change. As shown in Figure 10, the impacts of subway lines 9 and 10 on equity were mixed; these lines increased the equity of quantity accessibility in 39 subdistricts, most of which were located in the extreme north or south of study area (Figure 10a). However, inequity increased for 30 subdistricts in the urban core. Further changes in equity occurred when the subway lines were further extended (Figure 10b). Equity between subdistricts clearly improved within the northeast as a result of extension of subway line 1. In contrast, inequity increased in 50 subdistricts mostly north of the Hun River. Only 12 subdistricts were not affected by building subways, mostly on the periphery.

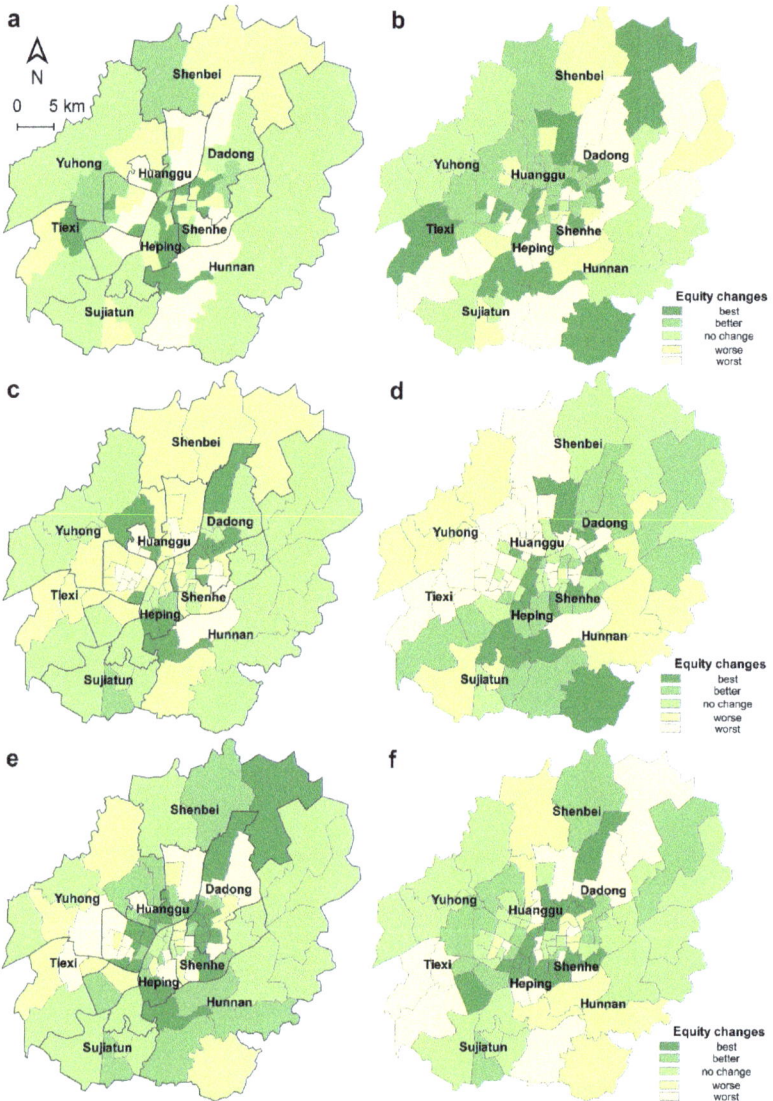

Figure 10. Variations in equity of accessibility to healthcare services during development of subway system: (**a**) changes in equity of access quantity after introduction of metro lines 9 and 10; (**b**) changes in equity of access quantity after introducing metro lines 3, 4, and extension lines; (**c**) changes in equity of access quality after introducing metro lines 9 and 10; (**d**) changes in equity of access quality after introducing metro lines 3, 4, and extension lines; (**e**) changes in equity of walking access after introducing metro lines 9 and 10; (**f**) changes in equity of walking access after introducing metro lines 3, 4, and extension lines.

The influences of subway lines 9 and 10 on equity of access quality were mainly concentrated within the central strip of Shenyang (Figure 10c). Specifically, subway lines 9 and 10 improved equity within 52 subdistricts, with 15 subdistricts located in the heartland having the most obvious improvements. However, 29 subdistricts near the east and west extremes of Shenyang were little influenced by the subway lines in this regard. In addition, there were 17 scattered subdistricts in which the presence of the subway exacerbated the gap in access quality suggesting that building subways is capable exaggerating social inequity (Figure 10d). There were 19 subdistricts far from the subway, where equity in access quality did not change, and only 34 subdistricts showed reduced disparity. Notably, access quality gaps widened within 45 subdistricts largely located in the northwest, which has a high population density and considerable healthcare needs.

Subway lines 9 and 10 reduced equity among subdistricts in terms of walkability. However, they had a positive impact on groups to the north of the Hun River, where the population needs are more diverse than in other areas (Figure 10e). Equity did not change, with subway lines 9 and 10, for 22 subdistricts located mainly in the suburbs and 11 subdistricts in the northwest were unaffected by subway building. There were 31 subdistricts with a large increase in walking distance equity, all of which were near building subways. The remaining 34 subdistricts, however, experienced aggravated walking disparity, with the largest gaps being in urban cores well supplied with PT (Figure 10f).

3.3.2. Equity between Districts

As shown in Figure 11a, the addition of metro lines 9 and 10 increased inequity, as measured by the Theil index, in most districts; the variation was between 0.037 and 0.015 (except for Sujiatun District, which has no subway running through it). Furthermore, the access quantity to healthcare services in 2025 is expected to be more uneven in Yuhong District than in 2015, while the Dadong and Sujiatun Districts are the opposite. The maximum intra-district variation was in Yuhong (0.053), and the district with the least intra-district variation was Shenhe (0.035), which demonstrates that the addition of the subway has a minimal impact on quantity equity. The district with the largest inequity was the Sujiatun District (0.274), followed by Hunnan District (0.219), probably because the periphery of the urban core is sparsely populated.

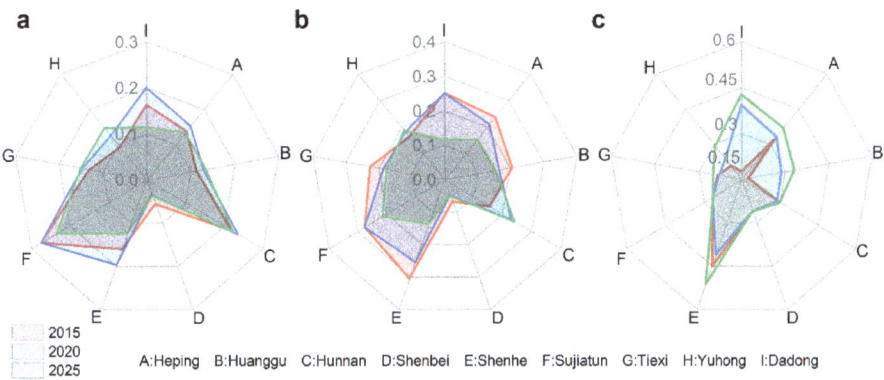

Figure 11. Comparison of equity of healthcare services through development of subway system: (**a**) the Theil index of quantity; (**b**) the Theil index of quality; (**c**) the Theil index of walking distance.

As shown in Figure 11b, metro lines 9 and 10 had a less effect on equity of healthcare quality (the Theil index declined in most districts). However, building subways can also increase regional inequalities. The difference between the Shenhe (0.305) and Sujiatun Districts (0.274) was greatly increased by the addition of the subway. Metro lines 3 and 4 ensured accessibility improvements while also generally narrowing the gap between vulnerability groups (maximum variation was from 0.305 to 0.135 in Shenhe District). Conversely, the addition of subway services exacerbated the inequity of healthcare quality among subdistricts in Hunnan District (the Theil index changed from 0.155 to 0.244).

Finally, the disparity in overall walking access was remarkably greater than that of the other indexes (the maximum variation was 0.252–Figure 11c). Metro lines 9 and 10 decreased walking inequity in Shenhe District (from 0.451 to 0.409) and Yuhong District (from 0.210 to 0.238). However, the Theil index in the Dadong and Huanggu Districts clearly increased after adding metro lines 9 and 10. In addition, the building subway lines are likely to increase the inequity between subdistricts, suggesting that increases in quantity and quality to healthcare is accompanied by a greater walking disparity.

4. Discussion

Improving equity in access to healthcare resources using PT can potentially improve the well-being of individuals and have implications for the equalization of social resources. This study considers subway expansion in Shenyang, China as a case study to explore the ways in which subway extensions can influence accessibility and equity in healthcare facilities. When people relied on bus lines for access to healthcare resources supply and demand values in the main urban area were generally low and had a vast range. As the underground railway was built, differences in supply and demand for healthcare services were disproportionately influenced by the subway system; these findings are similar to previous research in the same context [28,56]. However, Shenyang's centralized urban structure, in relation to the locations of healthcare facilities, creates an imbalance for low-income citizens. These conditions are endemic to many cities in China and lead to marked spatial and social health divides that translate into resource inequity and exclusion for citizens [39,57,58]. Low accessibility in peri-urban areas is a clear example, with people in peri-urban areas being excluded from healthcare options owing to the low coverage of subway lines. Our results suggest that subway expansion, on its own, has limited potential to address problems of accessibility, and its effect is only important in regions with dense PT networks. In previous studies, the influences of PT, including subways, on accessibility were multiple. The expected positive effects of PT on service access have been observed in many metropolitan areas [59]. Although PT plays a role in areas far from healthcare services along metro lines and bus routes, in some areas it may not increase access to healthcare services as much as previously thought [60,61]. Therefore, we analyzed accessibility to healthcare facilities, as a consequence of subway extension, to investigate the system's impact.

Sociodemographic diversity in each region has led to a focus on access to healthcare services. For example, in areas with a low population density and a long distance from healthcare services, people are concerned about both the walking distance to healthcare services as well as quality of the accessible services. With the addition of metro lines 9 and 10, walking distance and quality in Hunnan District clearly improved. In areas with inadequate healthcare services and unmet population needs, quantity accessibility (limited choices) is a key problem (Huanggu District). Tiexi and Shenhe Districts, which have large elderly populations, also have the highest density of healthcare services; however, the elderly have reduced walking capability. Therefore, the subway system must effectively improve walking access for areas with large elderly populations.

We suggest that analysis of the influence of a subway on healthcare accessibility should follow periods of subway extension, as well as focusing on various equities for sociodemographic diversity. Regions with unique locational advantages and highly developed transportation networks generally do not have excessive disparities in access quantity, quality, or walking distance, and typically have higher overall equalization [49,62]. However, costs are higher in areas that are far from urban centers and have larger rural populations, as these areas typically have low economic development levels and are far from hospitals [61,63]. These areas often face extreme inequalities. Therefore, the pursuit of equity in access quality is the primary requirement for such areas under limited conditions. However, the subway system has exacerbated the access quantity and quality inequalities in certain locations, such as Hunnan District, indicating that extension of a subway system does not necessarily improve social resource equity, including healthcare. The analysis confirms that, as with road infrastructure, a disproportionate concentration on high accessibility may lead to spatial inequity in transportation, as suggested by earlier studies. This explains how equity of opportunity can be influenced by the existence of PT [17,40]. Therefore, bridging gaps in healthcare access requires more than just a subway as a mode of transportation, and PT becomes a non-obvious option to obtain the necessary access to medical assistance.

This study focused on improving the delivery of healthcare services by PT and reducing disparities; these are two key goals for planners and policymakers. On the one hand, solutions should address spatial variations in accessibility. Specifically, policies should be introduced to increase the supply capacity of healthcare services by building additional hospitals and encouraging the hiring of more doctors and nurses in suburban areas with high demand. Moreover, planning departments should introduce new PT options in these areas, as they can lead to shorter travel times for citizens when accessing healthcare services. On the other hand, targeted suggestions based on specific needs arising from population diversity should be considered by health authorities. For example, increasing geriatric hospitals in areas with high elderly needs, or new and appropriate hospital departments, may alleviate the imbalance between supply and demand. Further, planners and policymakers should be aware of the impact of subway systems on healthcare equity. Awareness of temporal variations in healthcare accessibility, using diverse measures, during PT system development gives planners and policymakers greater insight into accessibility issues. Each location can have a profile of healthcare demand and supply, hence, specific problems that require specific solutions.

It is important to acknowledge the limitations of this study, which we hope to address in the future. First, the mode of transportation used in this study was PT. Despite Shenyang's cold climate, citizens can also drive and walk for movement. Thus, the results may not completely reflect the real healthcare accessibility conditions. All available modes of travel should be considered. Second, healthcare services and population demand have changed in a decade, which should be taken into consideration. Finally, the situations in which healthcare services may be sought was incomplete; we only considered cases in which people seek healthcare services on their own. Although this is a high proportion of cases, emergency medical services should also be considered. Enrichment of the analysis to include other modes of transport and modes of hospitalization is the next step in future studies.

5. Conclusions

This study comprehensively examined spatial accessibility and equality in healthcare services in the central region of Shenyang, following an extension of its subway network. A vulnerability index was calculated to indicate the required conditions for sufficient access to healthcare services. Citizen accessibility and equity was further assessed in terms of quantity, quality, and walking distance. These factors were compared over a period of subway extensions. The results showed that upgrading the subway had spatially heterogeneous impacts on healthcare accessibility, especially walking accessibility. Construction of the subway also exacerbated spatial inequity in healthcare accessibility. There are multiple influences on the equity of proximity to healthcare services. The issues identified can be largely explained by a lack of healthcare services in the urban peripheries and by high disequilibrium in the PT network in the inner city. This reflects the suburbanization of poverty that many cities around the world have been experiencing.

Author Contributions: Conceptualization, Maohua Liu and Xishihui Du; methodology, Xishihui Du; software, Maohua Liu; resources, Maohua Liu; writing—original draft preparation, Siqi Luo; writing—review and editing, Xishihui Du and Siqi Luo; visualization, Siqi Luo; supervision, Maohua Liu. All authors have read and agreed to the published version of the manuscript.

Funding: This work was supported by the Social Science Planning Fund of Liaoning Province under Grant number L19CSH001.

Institutional Review Board Statement: Not applicable.

Informed Consent Statement: Not applicable.

Data Availability Statement: The data presented in this study are available on request from the corresponding author.

Acknowledgments: The authors acknowledge the contribution of all the anonymous reviewers that improved the quality of the paper.

Conflicts of Interest: The authors declare no conflict of interest.

References

1. Rekha, R.S.; Wajid, S.; Radhakrishnan, N.; Mathew, S. Accessibility Analysis of Health care facility using Geospatial Techniques. *Transp. Res. Procedia* **2017**, *27*, 1163–1170. [CrossRef]
2. Sanchez, T.W. Equity Analysis of Personal Transportation System Benefits. *J. Urban Aff.* **1998**, *20*, 69–86. [CrossRef]
3. Borrell, L.N.; Talih, M. A symmetrized Theil index measure of health disparities: An example using dental caries in U.S. children and adolescents. *Stat. Med.* **2011**, *30*, 277–290. [CrossRef]
4. Kain, J.F.; Meyer, J.R. *Transportation and Poverty. The 100*; ERIC: Online, 1970.
5. Sun, Z.; Zacharias, J. Transport equity as relative accessibility in a megacity: Beijing. *Transp. Policy* **2020**, *92*, 8–19. [CrossRef]
6. Mouter, N.; van Cranenburgh, S.; van Wee, B. An empirical assessment of Dutch citizens' preferences for spatial equality in the context of a national transport investment plan. *J. Transp. Geogr.* **2017**, *60*, 217–230. [CrossRef]
7. Pereira, R.H. Future accessibility impacts of transport policy scenarios: Equity and sensitivity to travel time thresholds for Bus Rapid Transit expansion in Rio de Janeiro. *J. Transp. Geogr.* **2019**, *74*, 321–332. [CrossRef]
8. Rong, P.; Zheng, Z.; Kwan, M.-P.; Qin, Y. Evaluation of the spatial equity of medical facilities based on improved potential model and map service API: A case study in Zhengzhou, China. *Appl. Geogr.* **2020**, *119*, 102192. [CrossRef]
9. Wang, C.-H.; Chen, N. A geographically weighted regression approach to investigating the spatially varied built-environment effects on community opportunity. *J. Transp. Geogr.* **2017**, *62*, 136–147. [CrossRef]
10. Shin, K.; Lee, T. Improving the measurement of the Korean emergency medical System's spatial accessibility. *Appl. Geogr.* **2018**, *100*, 30–38. [CrossRef]
11. Siegel, M.; Koller, D.; Vogt, V.; Sundmacher, L. Developing a composite index of spatial accessibility across different health care sectors: A German example. *Health Policy* **2016**, *120*, 205–212. [CrossRef]
12. Foster, A.; Dunham, I.M. Volunteered geographic information, urban forests, & environmental justice. *Comput. Environ. Urban Syst.* **2015**, *53*, 65–75. [CrossRef]
13. Schultz, C.L.; Stanis, S.A.W.; Sayers, S.P.; Thombs, L.A.; Thomas, I.M. A longitudinal examination of improved access on park use and physical activity in a low-income and majority African American neighborhood park. *Prev. Med.* **2017**, *95*, S95–S100. [CrossRef]
14. El-Geneidy, A.; Levinson, D.; Diab, E.; Boisjoly, G.; Verbich, D.; Loong, C. The cost of equity: Assessing transit accessibility and social disparity using total travel cost. *Transp. Res. Part A Policy Pract.* **2016**, *91*, 302–316. [CrossRef]
15. Foth, N.; Manaugh, K.; El-Geneidy, A.M. Towards equitable transit: Examining transit accessibility and social need in Toronto, Canada, 1996–2006. *J. Transp. Geogr.* **2013**, *29*, 1–10. [CrossRef]
16. Wee, G.; Geurs, K. Discussing Equity and Social Exclusion in Accessibility Evaluations. *Eur. J. Transp. Infrastruct. Res.* **2011**, *11*. [CrossRef]
17. Deboosere, R.; El-Geneidy, A. Evaluating equity and accessibility to jobs by public transport across Canada. *J. Transp. Geogr.* **2018**, *73*, 54–63. [CrossRef]
18. Hansen, W.G. How Accessibility Shapes Land Use. *J. Am. Inst. Planners* **1959**, *25*, 73–76. [CrossRef]
19. Luo, W.; Wang, F. Measures of Spatial Accessibility to Health Care in a GIS Environment: Synthesis and a Case Study in the Chicago Region. *Environ. Plan. B Plan. Des.* **2003**, *30*, 865–884. [CrossRef]
20. Shen, Q. Location characteristics of inner-city neighborhoods and employment accessibility of low-wage workers. *Environ. Plan. B Plan. Des.* **1998**, *25*, 345–365. [CrossRef]
21. Curtis, C.; Scheurer, J. Planning for sustainable accessibility: Developing tools to aid discussion and decision-making. *Prog. Plan.* **2010**, *74*, 53–106. [CrossRef]
22. Geurs, K.T.; van Eck, J.R. Accessibility measures: Review and applications. In *Evaluation of Accessibility Impacts of Land-Use Transportation Scenarios, and Related Social and Economic Impact*; RIVM: Bilthoven, The Netherlands, 2011.
23. Kwan, M.-P.; Murray, A.T.; O'Kelly, M.E.; Tiefelsdorf, M. Recent advances in accessibility research: Representation, methodology and applications. *J. Geogr. Syst.* **2003**, *5*, 129–138. [CrossRef]
24. Neutens, T. Accessibility, equity and health care: Review and research directions for transport geographers. *J. Transp. Geogr.* **2015**, *43*, 14–27. [CrossRef]
25. Xia, N.; Cheng, L.; Chen, S.; Wei, X.; Zong, W.; Li, M. Accessibility based on Gravity-Radiation model and Google Maps API: A case study in Australia. *J. Transp. Geogr.* **2018**, *72*, 178–190. [CrossRef]
26. Niedzielski, M.A.; Kucharski, R. Impact of commuting, time budgets, and activity durations on modal disparity in accessibility to supermarkets. *Transp. Res. Part D Transp. Environ.* **2019**, *75*, 106–120. [CrossRef]
27. Widener, M.J.; Farber, S.; Neutens, T.; Horner, M. Spatiotemporal accessibility to supermarkets using public transit: An interaction potential approach in Cincinnati, Ohio. *J. Transp. Geogr.* **2015**, *42*, 72–83. [CrossRef]

28. Herskovic, L. The Effect of Subway Access on School Choice. *Econ. Educ. Rev.* **2020**, *78*, 102021. [CrossRef]
29. Islam, M.S.; Asktar, S. Measuring physical accessiblity to health facilities: A case study on Khunla City. *World Health Popul.* **2011**, *12*, 123–127. [CrossRef]
30. Perry, B.; Gesler, W. Physical access to primary health care in Andean Bolivia. *Soc. Sci. Med.* **2000**, *50*, 1177–1188. [CrossRef]
31. Dai, D. Black residential segregation, disparities in spatial access to health care facilities, and late-stage breast cancer diagnosis in metropolitan Detroit. *Health Place* **2010**, *16*, 1038–1052. [CrossRef] [PubMed]
32. Hiscock, R.; Pearce, J.; Blakely, T.; Witten, K. Is Neighborhood Access to Health Care Provision Associated with Individual-Level Utilization and Satisfaction? *Health Serv. Res.* **2008**, *43*, 2183–2200. [CrossRef]
33. Wan, N.; Zhan, F.B.; Zou, B.; Wilson, J.G. Spatial Access to Health Care Services and Disparities in Colorectal Cancer Stage at Diagnosis in Texas. *Prof. Geogr.* **2013**, *65*, 527–541. [CrossRef]
34. McGrail, M.R.; Humphreys, J.S. Measuring spatial accessibility to primary health care services: Utilising dynamic catchment sizes. *Appl. Geogr.* **2014**, *54*, 182–188. [CrossRef]
35. Wang, F. Measurement, Optimization, and Impact of Health Care Accessibility: A Methodological Review. *Ann. Assoc. Am. Geogr.* **2012**, *102*, 1104–1112. [CrossRef] [PubMed]
36. Mansour, S. Spatial analysis of public health facilities in Riyadh Governorate, Saudi Arabia: A GIS-based study to assess geographic variations of service provision and accessibility. *Geo-Spat. Inf. Sci.* **2016**, *19*, 26–38. [CrossRef]
37. Chang, H.-T.; Lai, H.-Y.; Hwang, I.-H.; Ho, M.-M.; Hwang, S.-J. Home healthcare services in Taiwan: A nationwide study among the older population. *BMC Health Serv. Res.* **2010**, *10*, 274. [CrossRef]
38. Wang, Y.; Cao, M.; Liu, Y.; Ye, R.; Gao, X.; Ma, L. Public transport equity in Shenyang: Using structural equation modelling. *Res. Transp. Bus. Manag.* **2020**, 100555. [CrossRef]
39. Chen, G.; Wang, C.C.; Jin, P.; Xia, B.; Xiao, L.; Chen, S.; Luo, J. Evaluation of healthcare inequity for older adults: A spatio-temporal perspective. *J. Transp. Health* **2020**, *19*, 100911. [CrossRef]
40. Boisjoly, G.; Deboosere, R.; Wasfi, R.; Orpana, H.; Manaugh, K.; Buliung, R.; El-Geneidy, A. Measuring accessibility to hospitals by public transport: An assessment of eight Canadian metropolitan regions. *J. Transp. Health* **2020**, *18*, 100916. [CrossRef]
41. Rao, Y.; Lin, G. Rationality of the Geographical Distributio of Urban Education Resources from the Perspective of Balancing Supply and Demand: A Case Study of Wuhan City. *J. South-Central Univ. Natl. Soc. Sci.* **2021**, *41*, 147–152. (In Chinese)
42. Giuliano, G.; Kang, S. Spatial dynamics of the logistics industry: Evidence from California. *J. Transp. Geogr.* **2018**, *66*, 248–258. [CrossRef]
43. Hickman, R. Cultural perspectives on transport, urban planning and design. *J. Transp. Geogr.* **2017**, *63*, 50–52. [CrossRef]
44. Sukaryavichute, E.; Prytherch, D.L. Transit planning, access, and justice: Evolving visions of bus rapid transit and the Chicago street. *J. Transp. Geogr.* **2018**, *69*, 58–72. [CrossRef]
45. Duan, M.; Hang, Z.; Long, L.; Ou, R. The evaluation of allocation fairness to urban transit system service to elderly in mountainous city. *J. Geo-inf. Sci.* **2021**, *23*, 617–631. (in Chinese) [CrossRef]
46. Jiang, H.; Zhang, W.; Wei, S. Public service facility accessibility as influenced by public transportation in Beijing. *Prog. Geogr.* **2017**, *36*, 1239–1249. (In Chinese) [CrossRef]
47. Luo, X.; Yue, B.; Lin, A. The research of accessibility and fairness of pension service facilities based on multiple modes of transportation-a case study of Wuhan. *J. Cent. China Norm. Univ. Sci.* **2018**, *52*, 883–893. (In Chinese)
48. Li, M.; Long, Y. The Coverage Ratio of Bus Stations and an Evaluation of Spatial Patterns of Major Chinese Cities. *Urban Plan. Forum* **2015**, *6*, 30–37. (In Chinese)
49. Chen, B.Y.; Cheng, X.-P.; Kwan, M.-P.; Schwanen, T. Evaluating spatial accessibility to healthcare services under travel time uncertainty: A reliability-based floating catchment area approach. *J. Transp. Geogr.* **2020**, *87*, 102794. [CrossRef]
50. Luo, J.; Chen, G.; Li, C.; Xia, B.; Sun, X.; Chen, S. Use of an E2SFCA Method to Measure and Analyse Spatial Accessibility to Medical Services for Elderly People in Wuhan, China. *Int. J. Environ. Res. Public Health* **2018**, *15*, 1503. [CrossRef]
51. Hess, D.B. Walking to the bus: Perceived versus actual walking distance to bus stops for older adults. *Transportation* **2011**, *39*, 247–266. [CrossRef]
52. Kang, J.-Y.; Michels, A.; Lyu, F.; Wang, S.; Agbodo, N.; Freeman, V.L.; Wang, S. Rapidly measuring spatial accessibility of COVID-19 healthcare resources: A case study of Illinois, USA. *Int. J. Health Geogr.* **2020**, *19*, 1–17. [CrossRef] [PubMed]
53. Jue, W.; Mei-Po, K. Hexagon-Based Adaptive Crystal Growth Voronoi Diagrams Based on Weighted Planes for Service Area Delimitation. *Isprs Int. J. Geo. Inf.* **2018**, *7*, 257.
54. Caggiani, L.; Colovic, A.; Ottomanelli, M. An equality-based model for bike-sharing stations location in bicycle-public transport multimodal mobility. *Transp. Res. Part A Policy Pract.* **2020**, *140*, 251–265. [CrossRef]
55. Theil, H. *Economics and Information Theory*; North-Holland: Amsterdam, The Netherlands, 1967.
56. Liu, X.; Macedo, J.; Zhou, T.; Shen, L.; Liao, Y.; Zhou, Y. Evaluation of the utility efficiency of subway stations based on spatial information from public social media. *Habitat Int.* **2018**, *79*, 10–17. [CrossRef]
57. Wang, Y.; Li, Y.; Qin, S.; Kong, Y.; Yu, X.; Guo, K.; Meng, J. The disequilibrium in the distribution of the primary health workforce among eight economic regions and between rural and urban areas in China. *Int. J. Equity Health* **2020**, *19*, 1–10. [CrossRef] [PubMed]
58. Yin, C.; He, Q.; Liu, Y.; Chen, W.; Gao, Y. Inequality of public health and its role in spatial accessibility to medical facilities in China. *Appl. Geogr.* **2018**, *92*, 50–62. [CrossRef]

59. Ahn, K.; Jang, H.; Song, Y. Economic impacts of being close to subway networks: A case study of Korean metropolitan areas. *Res. Transp. Econ.* **2020**, *83*, 100900. [CrossRef]
60. Zhou, Q.; Dai, D.; Wang, Y.; Fan, J. Decade-Long Changes in Disparity and Distribution of Transit Opportunity in Shenzhen China: A Transportation Equity Perspective. *J. Adv. Transp.* **2018**, 1–16. [CrossRef]
61. Qian, T.; Chen, J.; Li, A.; Ang, L.; Shen, D. Evaluating Spatial Accessibility to General Hospitals with Navigation and Social Media Location Data: A Case Study in Nanjing. *Int. J. Environ. Res. Public Health* **2020**, *17*, 2752. [CrossRef]
62. Yohan, F.; Delphine, P.; Béatrice, F.; Isabelle, R.-C.; Jean-Yves, B.; Françoise, D.; Guy, F.; Elodie, F. Beyond the map: Evidencing the spatial dimension of health inequalities. *Int. J. Health Geogr* **2020**, *19*, 46.
63. Subal, J.; Paal, P.; Krisp, J.M. Quantifying spatial accessibility of general practitioners by applying a modified huff three-step floating catchment area (MH3SFCA) method. *Int. J. Health Geogr.* **2021**, *20*, 1–14. [CrossRef]

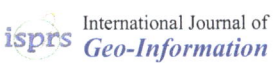

Article

LionVu 2.0 Usability Assessment for Pennsylvania, United States

Nathaniel R. Geyer [1,*], Fritz C. Kessler [2] and Eugene J. Lengerich [1,3]

1. Department of Public Health Sciences, Penn State College of Medicine, Penn State University, Hershey, PA 17033, USA; elengerich@psu.edu
2. Department of Geography, College of Earth and Mineral Sciences, Penn State University, PA 16801, USA; fck2@psu.edu
3. Penn State Cancer Institute, Hershey, PA 17033, USA
* Correspondence: nrg139@psu.edu; Tel.: +1-717-531-7178

Received: 28 August 2020; Accepted: 22 October 2020; Published: 23 October 2020

Abstract: The Penn State Cancer Initiative implemented LionVu 1.0 (Penn State University, United States) in 2017 as a web-based mapping tool to educate and inform public health professionals about the cancer burden in Pennsylvania and 28 counties in central Pennsylvania, locally known as the catchment area. The purpose of its improvement, LionVu 2.0, was to assist investigators answer person–place–time questions related to cancer and its risk factors by examining several data variables simultaneously. The primary objective of this study was to conduct a usability assessment of a prototype of LionVu 2.0 which included area- and point-based data. The assessment was conducted through an online survey; 10 individuals, most of whom had a masters or doctorate degree, completed the survey. Although most participants had a favorable view of LionVu 2.0, many had little to no experience with web mapping. Therefore, it was not surprising to learn that participants wanted short 10–15-minute training videos to be available with future releases, and a simplified user-interface that removes advanced functionality. One unexpected finding was the suggestion of using LionVu 2.0 for teaching and grant proposals. The usability study of the prototype of LionVu 2.0 provided important feedback for its future development.

Keywords: usability assessment; web GIS; cancer; service area; geospatial health

1. Introduction

In 2015, the Penn State Cancer Initiative (PSCI) implemented LionVu 1.0, a web-based mapping tool (Figure 1). LionVu 1.0 was designed to educate and inform the public health professionals about the risk of cancer within 28 counties located in central Pennsylvania, locally known as the catchment area. More specifically, LionVu 1.0 was designed to help answer research questions regarding the person–place–time nature of epidemiology related to cancer. The original targeted audience for LionVu 1.0 was PSCI health practitioners such as program managers, epidemiologists, and clinicians, but not the general public. The data sources used in LionVu 1.0 came from the United States Census Bureau, Pennsylvania Department of Health, and the County Health Rankings.

LionVu 1.0 has received criticism from users within PSCI, including not addressing the needs, i.e., of the PSCI catchment area and the lack of help documentation. These issues rendered LionVu 1.0 as unsatisfactory, with the need for revisions. Other criticisms focused on the user interface design, which permitted only one map to be displayed at a time. This map design was criticized for not using ColorBrewer 2.0 (Penn State University, United States) color scheme standards, which were developed to aid in visualization. Another criticism was the lack of comprehensive help documentation and tutorials for how to navigate through LionVu 1.0.

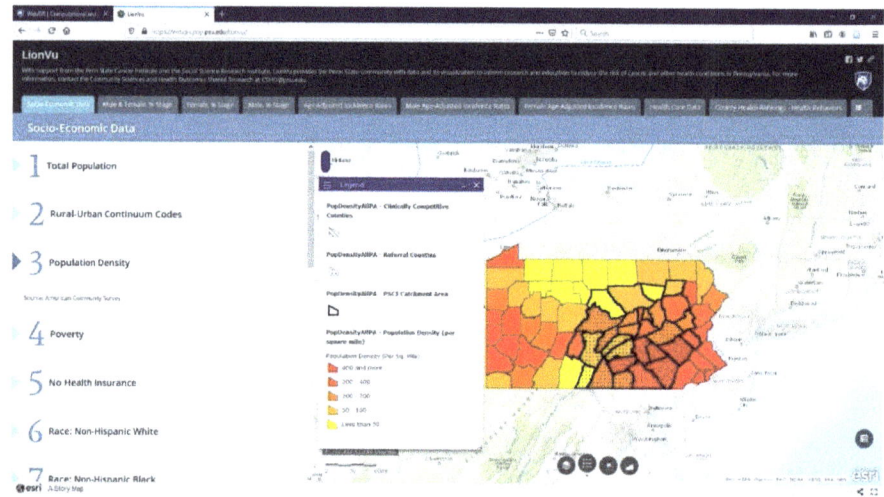

Figure 1. Original Design of LionVu 1.0 for population density (per square miles) within Pennsylvania. The 28 county Catchment Area is outlines in a thick black line.

In response to criticisms of LionVu's 1.0 user interface, the development of LionVu 2.0 began in 2020. The criticisms of LionVu 1.0 were used as a framework guiding the redesign of LionVu 2.0, which included the following issues: mapping Pennsylvania and the catchment area side-by-side, updating the datasets, and including additional functionality, such as the ability to print. Figure 2 shows a redesigned LionVu 2.0 interface where Pennsylvania and the catchment area are mapped side-by-side. After exploring various data sources for Pennsylvania, revised data from the United States Census Bureau, Pennsylvania Department of Health, County Health Rankings, and Medicare were used. Advanced functionality, such as the ability to print and help documentation (i.e., read me first section) and color schemes based on ColorBrewer 2.0 were added. Based on the recommendations of Brewer and Pickle, the quantile classification was used as the default classification, since it had the most accurate epidemiological mapping applications [1]. Once initial criticisms were addressed in a prototype, a usability survey was conducted to guide the further development of LionVu 2.0, which is the focus of this paper.

1.1. Literature Review

The focus of this literature review was to examine research on usability assessment methodologies, focusing on the health and geospatial disciplines, to help develop the LionVu 2.0 usability assessment. We searched three databases: PubMed, Web of Science, and Cochrane for usability assessment methodology articles, using keywords: usability study, user feedback, (GIS) systems design, prototyping, web mapping, spatial analysis software, cancer, health, ecology, participants as investigators, usability metrics, and policy makers. Google Scholar's cited-by function was also employed to find additional sources published between 2015 and 2020. Seminal work that was published prior to 2014 was also reviewed.

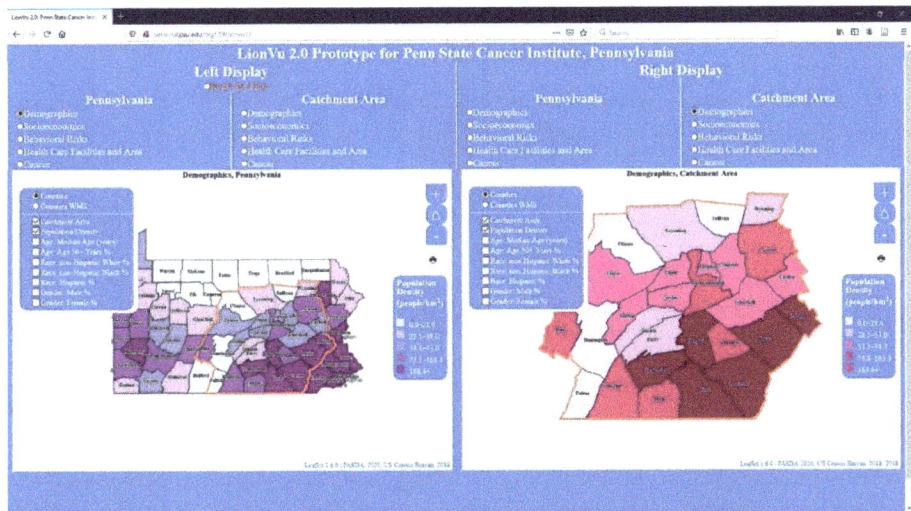

Figure 2. LionVu 2.0 used in usability assessment. Left Display: population density (people/km^2) within Pennsylvania. Right display: population density (people/km^2) within catchment area. Layer list was not collapsed in order to clarify what fields were available for selection.

Usability studies in the health field included methodologies such as concordance or consensus building [2,3], discordance or tension [4], qualitative weight and sum method [5], mixed methods [6], focus groups [7], or surveys [8]. One of the more relevant investigations was a two-part study that analyzed existing Missouri printed maps (InstantAtlas) in a web mapping tool, which were developed by the Missouri Department of Health [9,10]. This usability assessment was conducted during two time periods with part one being completed by a subset of college students first, followed by a second usability assessment including a subset of health professionals. The two-part usability studies of InstantAtlas were designed to evaluate user friendliness and user satisfaction, and test whether the usability improved by modifying InstantAtlas web maps on an ongoing process comparable to our development of LionVu 2.0. Based on the results of part one, the InstantAtlas web map was revised and the new version went through a second usability assessment in part two. A select group of policymakers and clinicians examined InstantAtlas in part two to determine if the modified maps improved the usability according to the suggestions of part one. Part two found that the InstantAtlas web maps were effectively utilized by participants with limited mapping experience. Some additional suggestions were to simplify the printed maps and improve the help documentation on how to interpret the information in the web maps.

Geospatial usability assessments are critical for determining the quality of a user's interaction with internet-based mapping applications and measuring how accessible web maps are to participants. One study used eye-tracking to measure how well a mapping prototype, mimics real-life applications, stressing the importance of a properly designed user interface when completing tasks online [11]. Web maps that went through a usability assessment also need to have responsive web design that works in all platforms: desktop, mobile, and laptops, while balancing customization of functionalities [12]. In addition to a well-defined user interface, it is also critical for using a survey instrument (i.e., system usability scale (SUS) and participatory GIS usability scale (PGUS)) to insure that the scale can differentiate between usable and unusable systems [13,14]. The SUS uses 10 Likert scale-based questions that are easy to administer with small sample sizes and can effectively differentiate between usable and unusable systems [13]. The PGUS uses 25 Likert scale-based questions in five domains (i.e., user interface, spatial interface, learnability, effectiveness, and communication) and seven demographic and participants questions [14]. The PGUS was first used in a marine spatial planning group and was more applicable to geospatial usability assessments than SUS and can better facilitate rapid evaluation for web mapping projects.

Key components of the usability assessment were an evaluation of completion time, efficiency, and effectiveness. Measures to evaluate the effectiveness include baseline performance usability metrics such as satisfaction, efficiency, and effectiveness [15]. Effectiveness is the ratio of task completion to number of errors. Efficiency is the ratio of task completion to task time in minutes [16]. Although these studies focused on efficiency and effectiveness there was little to no assessment on learnability, which was measured as part of the PGUS survey questions.

Based on the results of this literature review, several themes emerged that focused on: (a) having a well-designed user interface; (b) displaying visually appealing maps; (c) using a usability assessment scale (i.e., SUS and PGUS); and (d) using a survey with both open-ended and close-ended questions. When developing the usability assessment, we started with the PGUS survey tool. The PGUS contains seven sections and roughly 30 questions on demographic characteristics, participant's characteristics, and five Likert-scale sections (i.e., user interface, interaction, learnability, effectiveness, and communication). For our assessment, we adapted a total of 20 PGUS Likert-scale questions from Ballatore et al. [14]. Specifically, we adapted five PGUS questions on demographic characteristics (i.e., gender, race, ethnicity, age, and educational attainment) and four on employment characteristics. One question from each of the five Likert-scale sections was selected to evaluate the user interface, accessibility of information, how to perform tasks, reliability, and whether the maps are easy to understand was included as individual tasks. The LionVu 2.0 usability assessment built on these themes assessed how well the user interface displays visually appealing maps, to an audience with limited mapping experience.

1.2. Objectives

The primary objective of this study was to conduct a usability assessment of a prototype of LionVu 2.0 using domain expertise related to cancer data. To complete the usability assessment, we developed 50 survey assessment questions, based on the literature review section, including both open- and close-ended questions. The usability assessment was distributed via REDCap (Research Electronic Data Capture) survey system. The qualitative survey data was analyzed in two ways: content analysis and item analysis for evaluating patterns in survey data (i.e., task completion, effectiveness, efficiency, and time). A discussion of key findings from the usability assessment will be addressed, including limitations, recommendations, and conclusions.

2. Materials and Methods

After reviewing the various methodological approaches, we decided that a survey was the preferred method to reach participants from various organizations and geographic areas. We targeted professionals located in the 28-county catchment area. Since the professionals were spread out in organizations throughout the 28 counties, the survey had to be conducted asynchronously with participants being given the opportunity to do the assessment in multiple settings.

2.1. Survey Question Development

The online survey of LionVu 2.0 contained 10 sections: (1.) Demographics Characteristics; (2.) Employment Characteristics; (3.) United States Cancer Statistics (USCS) Web Map; (4.) Task 1: Demographics; (5.) Task 2: Cancer; (6.) Task 3: Health Care Facility and Area; (7.) Task 4: Behavioral Risk and Socioeconomic; (8.) Likert Scale; (9.) Purpose, Data, Help Documentation, and Functionality Feedback Questions; and (10.) General Feedback. Each had five questions, for a total of 50 questions. In addition to tallying responses to the 50 questions, time for completion was recorded for each participant on 10 of the questions. The survey was expected to be completed in 30–45 min. We discuss the survey question development and REDCap and ethical considerations in separate sections.

This survey contains 10 sections with 5 questions each totaling 50 questions (Table A1 in Appendix A). In the demographics section we asked the participants about gender, race, ethnicity, and highest educational attainment. In the employment characteristics section, we asked the participants about employment and a self-reported web-mapping proficiency question based on the National Institutes of Health's Competencies Proficiency Scale [17]. In the USCS web map section, we asked the participants five task-specific questions about a Centers for Disease Control and Prevention web map [18]. The first task-related question prompted the participant about the 5-year time period for new cancer diagnoses in Pennsylvania based on the USCS web mapping environment. The four other questions asked the participants about the strengths, limitations, expectations, and capabilities of the USCS map. The purpose of this section was to orient the user about other web maps that were outside of our control. The four other task-related sections involve assessing the participant on specific tasks using the LionVu 2.0. For example, in task 1, we asked the participants to determine population density and Hispanic population in Luzerne County. In this task, the population density required the user to select demographic layers from LionVu 2.0's user interface and to respond to multiple-choice questions. There were three additional open-ended questions on determining how the user was able to find the answers and applying the results to the entire state of Pennsylvania and the catchment area. Other task-related sections asked users to interpret cancer data, to identify health care providers using point data, and to evaluate the side-by-side functionality. The intent of these task-related questions was to ensure that LionVu 2.0 was comprehensively reviewed. The Likert Scale section asked the participant questions based on the five target areas of the PGUS (i.e., user interface, interaction, learnability, reliability, and communication). The last two sections asked the participant open-ended questions about the general purpose, help documentation, functionality, and general feedback questions about areas of improvement about the LionVu 2.0.

2.2. REDCap and Ethical Considerations

We collected survey data for the usability assessment and managed using REDCap, a secure web application designed to support data capture for research studies. The advantage of REDCap over other survey systems is that it allows for surveys to be ethically compliant and for participants to finish where they started. Doing so provides a user-friendly web-based platform to capture and validate data for quality assurance purposes. The data used for this survey are hosted at the Penn State Health and College of Medicine data center. The data are protected under the Health Insurance Portability and Accountability Act of 1996 (HIPAA), which is protected from disclosure without consent. REDCap gives the investigator the opportunity to download a statistical software and do more complex analyses [19]. REDCap also allow us to preload a list of emails for invitations to send to participants asking to complete a survey. Using the REDCap system for this usability assessment required a review by the Penn State College of Medicine's institutional review board (IRB) and was determined to be non-human subjects research (IRB # STUDY00015009).

2.3. Sample Population and Procedures

We initially sought a response rate of 33% from a sample frame of 25 PSCI members and 20 people from the Pennsylvania Department of Health. The initial invitation was sent on 13 May 2020. On 18 May, we sent an invitation to the entire membership of the PSCI cancer control program, as requested by the director of the PSCI. On 15 June, we closed the survey with 23 responses, 10 of which completed the entire survey.

2.4. Analyses Performed

We performed a content analysis of participant responses to all open-ended questions that were reported on the usability assessment. We also performed an item analysis of participant responses to the closed-ended questions identifying skewness of the demographic characteristics, employee characteristics, and accuracy measurements for the task related questions. The time intervals of completion time were estimated using a web calculator [20]. In addition, we analyzed and reported the measures of effectiveness and efficiency using the definitions adapted by Gómez Solórzano et al. [16]. Given the small sample size for this survey, there was not enough statistical power to perform complex analyses, but it did help inform the future directions for developing LionVu 2.0.

3. Results

We sent invitations to the LionVu 2.0 usability survey to 123 individuals; 23 started and 10 completed the survey. The response rate was 19% and completion rate was 43%. The completion time (geometric mean: 51.41 min; median: 50.5 min; 95% Confidence Interval: 37, 71.5) was over the 30–45 min time estimate, which was adjusted for people who stopped and came back to the survey at a later time period. The results discussion is organized based on the 10 sections of the survey, with an additional summary that reported the effectiveness and efficiency of LionVu 2.0.

3.1. Demographic Characteristics

We asked five demographic questions about age, race, ethnicity, gender, and highest educational attainment. The median age of the subset was 56 years. The self-reported race, which was defined using the United States Census Bureau's categories, was 71% White, 19% Asian, and 10% Black. The self-reported ethnicity, as defined by the United States Census Bureau was 15% Hispanic. The self-reported gender was 55% female. The highest educational attainment earned was 65% Doctorate (e.g., PhD, EdD, DrPH), 15% Professional (e.g., MD, DDS, DVM), 15% Masters (e.g., MA, MS, MEd, MPH), and 5% Bachelors (e.g., BA, BS) degrees.

3.2. Employment Characteristics

We asked the users to identify their work location, type, organization, title, and proficiency of web mapping. The employment location was 65% Hershey, 20% state college, and 15% Harrisburg; work type was 70% faculty, 15% manager, 10% clinician, 5% staff; while the organization type was 45% Penn State College of Medicine, 20% Penn State Health, 20% Penn State University Park, 10% Pennsylvania Department of Health, and 5% Penn State Harrisburg. Common work titles included: 42% assistant professor, 31% professor, 7% administer, 5% program director, 5% research project 5% manager, and 5% physician. The web map proficiency was found to be 45% fundamental awareness (e.g., beginner), 25% limited experience, 20% intermediate, 10% advanced, and 0% expert. In addition, we had 20 people who completed the questions in this section, who were grouped based on job title to either academics or professionals, which were evenly split at 10 for this section. In the following sections there was non-completion in roughly half of the participants leading to a sample of six academic and four non-academic professionals by the time the Likert scale questions were asked.

3.3. United States Cancer Statistics (USCS) Web Map

These questions asked participants to visit the USCS web map to determine the 5-year age-adjusted rate of new cancers in Pennsylvania [18]. The response accuracy to the 5-year rate of new cancers, was low (13%). This low accuracy was largely due to the poorly designed web map interface which displayed the 1 year rate by default, while the survey instructions required the participant to click an obscure radio button to change the map to the 5 year timeframe. Other limitations reported by the participants were poor data availability (i.e., data were out of date), hard to navigate, and the interface was not intuitive. On the other hand, reported strengths of the web map from the participants included: the ability to manipulate data and easy interpretation the web map. To most of the participants the USCS's web map met their expectations, but some individuals noted the limited capability to map data at the state level.

3.4. Task 1: Population Densities and Hispanic Populations within Luzerne County

In task 1, we asked the participants to use choropleth maps to determine the population density and color value for Hispanics in Luzerne County (Figure 3). The response showed that 92% answered the population density question correctly, but only 58% provided the correct color value. This low accuracy on identifying the color value was due to a contrasting blue background on the legend, white on the map, and yellow on the survey. In the REDCap survey, participants were given a multiple-choice answer with various color values and asked to click the answer that best fit the situation. The wording of the task asking about the color value could have been confusing to the participants. The intent was to have the participant match the color value on the map to the data class on the legend. One positive comment was that the visualization of the choropleth maps appeared to show an increased population density in Philadelphia and Pittsburgh. One negative comment was the inability to find help documentation (i.e., read me first section).

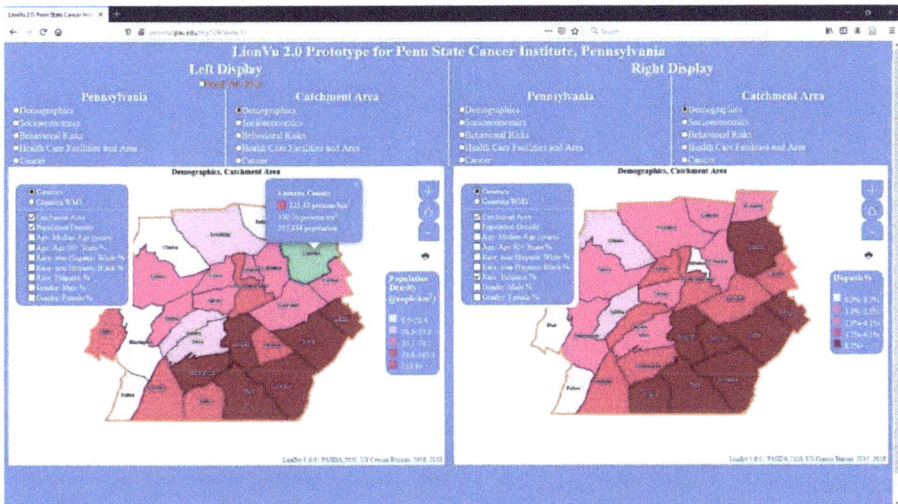

Figure 3. Screenshot of task 1. Left display: Population density (people/km^2) within catchment area. Right Display: Percent Hispanics residing within catchment area. Layer list was not collapsed in order to clarify what fields were available for selection.

3.5. Task 2: Assessing Cancer Patterns

In task 2, we asked participants to use choropleth maps to determine the mortality and percentage of colorectal cancer in the Centre County that were diagnosed at a late stage (Figure 4). The participants answered the two cancer-related questions (92% mortality; 100% late stage percentage) correctly. This high rate of accuracy was likely because most participants were from the cancer field, which made them more critical towards the quality of LionVu 2.0. This task was praised for the maps and including a variety of cancer mortality and stage information for colorectal, breast, and all cancers. However, the web map was criticized for the lack of data on cancer survivorship and other types of cancer.

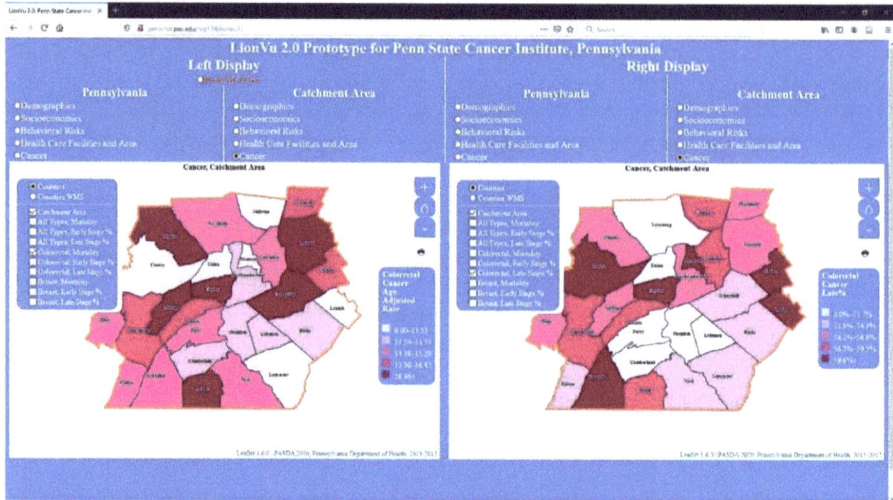

Figure 4. Screenshot of task 2. Left display: Colorectal cancer mortality age—adjusted rate within catchment area. Right display: Late stage incidence percentage of colorectal cancer within catchment area. Layer list was not collapsed in order to clarify what fields were available for selection.

One map design issue had to do with the county labeling. The Leaflet JavaScript programming language prevented the labels from being added directly to the web map. In the LionVu 2.1, labels were fixed by using the QGIS 3.14 centroid function and then created a tooltip at the centroid to show the county name. Another issue was the lack of user control over classification methods (i.e., quantile, natural breaks, etc.) between the Pennsylvania and catchment area maps. One participant asked for the option to change the color scheme and include the option to export images.

3.6. Task 3: Health Care Facility and Area

In task 3, we asked participants to review choropleth maps to determine the density of endoscopy providers in Lancaster County. Participants were also asked to examine a dot map and indicate the number of providers that were not found in Lancaster County. Of the responses, 90% answered the density of endoscopy question correctly, but only 30% correctly identified Hillside Endoscopy Center which is found in York County (Figure 5). The reason for the 90% accuracy was that endoscopy density is not a widely used measure of density, but since it was a choropleth map it was easy to figure out the density by hovering the mouse over Lancaster County. Whereas the low accuracy of identifying Hillside Endoscopy Center was because the participant had to hover the mouse over each point and view the pop-up, which was confusing and hard to identify. In order to rectify this problem, it was requested to include tabular data, instead of hovering over each point. Part of the technological hurdle here is that the Leaflet JavaScript does not include tabular outputs, so additional plug-ins are needed, which will increase the time needed to process and load the map by the browser. We included tabular data and the option to print the map into the tool. However, the download data were found in the read me first section (e.g., the location was not evident to the participants), and the print button on the map was difficult to locate.

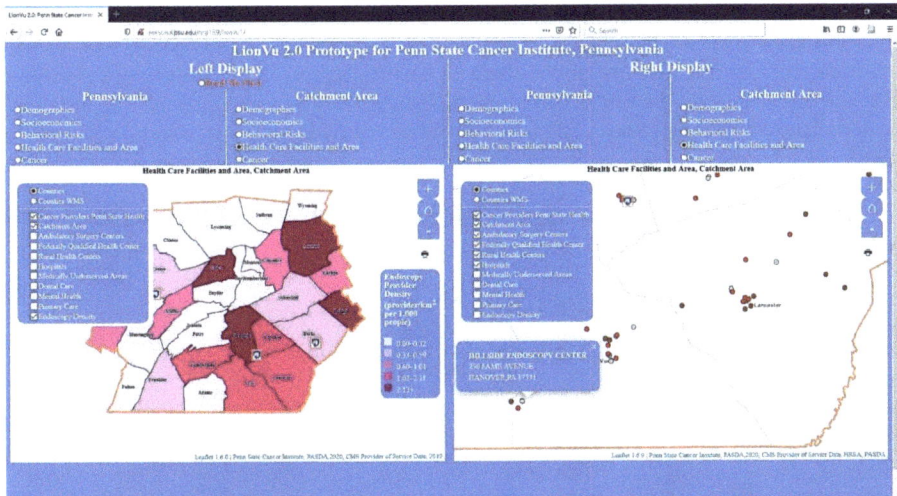

Figure 5. Screen shot of task 3. Left display: Endoscopy density (providers/km^2 per 1000 population) within catchment area. Right display: Health care providers (dots: Gray-Ambulatory Service Centers; Brown-Federally Qualified Health Centers; Red-Hospitals) within catchment area. Layer list was not collapsed in order to clarify what fields were available for selection.

3.7. Task 4: Behavioral Risk and Socioeconomics

In task 4, we asked the participants to use the side-by-side displays of choropleth maps to measure the functionality by comparing two maps of selected characteristics, within Centre and Luzerne Counties. A hint was provided to the participants to use both displays with the left window displaying the behavior risk characteristics for the catchment area, while the right window displaying the socioeconomic characteristics. The first question asked participants about adult obesity % and poverty percentage in Luzerne County, resulting in 90% accuracy (Figure 6). The second question asked about mammogram screening and rurality percentages in Centre County, resulting in 80% accuracy (Figure 7). One reason for the 80–90% accuracy had to do with a participant using the legend instead of the popup to answer the mammogram and rurality questions. Another concern was the widespread distribution (0–23%) with the quantile data classification that resulted in Philadelphia having 0% rurality but being grouped in with the 0–23% group. There is an additional concern about the description of what selection was being measured, such as what do percentage of screening and rurality mean as displayed in the web map.

3.8. Likert Scale Questions

We used Likert scale questions to measure the participants on five target areas: user interface, interaction, learnability, reliability, and communication, with one being strongly disagree and four being strongly agree, as adapted from the PGUS scale [14]. The median score of the 10 participants was highest for both learnability (four) and reliability and lowest (three) for the user interface (Table 1). In addition, the professionals who have job titles other than professor or lecturers tended to rate LionVu 2.0 with a lower score than professors or lecturers did. One major concern with the user interface was the inclusion of the layer list, which was a checkbox, which allowed multiple choropleth layers to be selected, making the map difficult to interpret. Another concern was the over-sensitive ability to zoom in just by clicking the mouse (i.e., zoom by click). There were two general concerns with the interaction question. Here, participants asked for more help documentation to resolve the situation when there was a desire to return to the data source. Additionally, the quantile data classification method was used for each variable. This led to confusion with the participants who felt that switching to a Natural Breaks or another classification method would present the data in a different perspective. Two common concerns with learnability included not having any training videos recorded to aid in using LionVu 2.0 as part of the help documentation. Two focused concerns with reliability included a time delay between selecting a layer and labels as well as screen display glitches especially with the county labels.

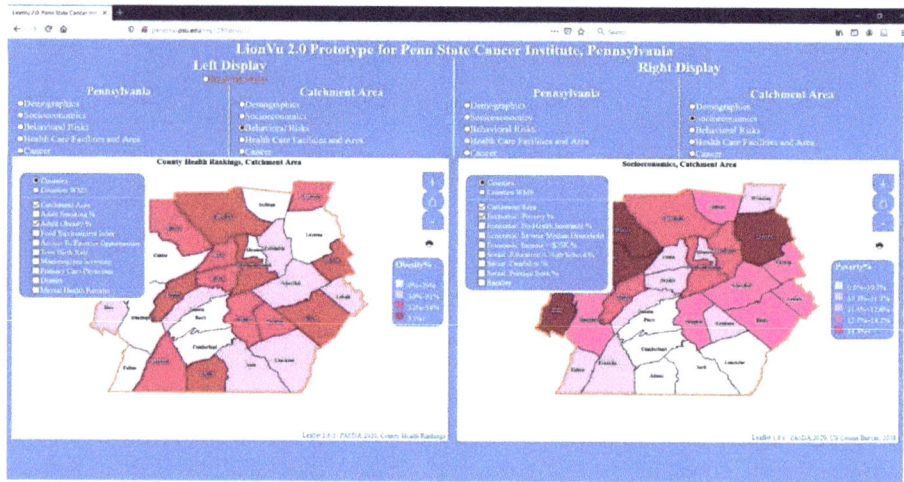

Figure 6. Screen shot of task 4. Left display: Obesity percentage within catchment area. Right display: Poverty percentage within catchment area. Layer list was not collapsed in order to clarify what fields were available for selection.

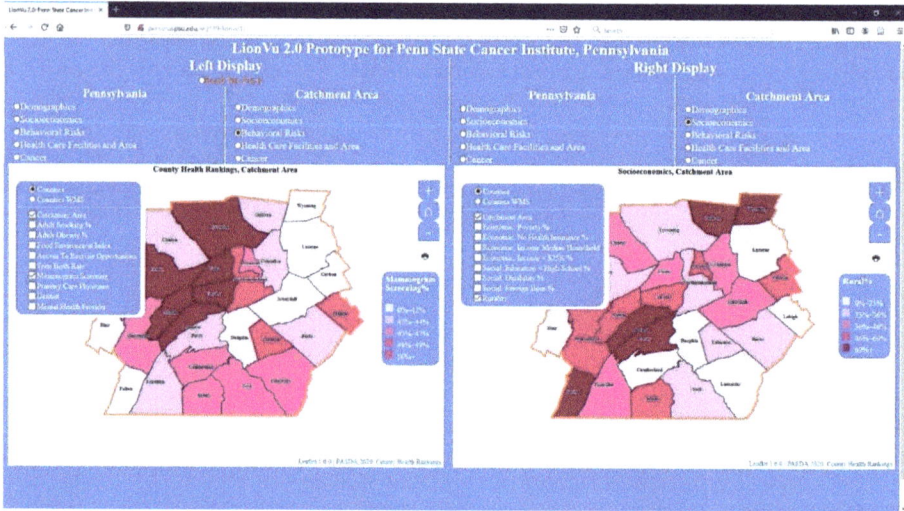

Figure 7. Screen shot of task 4. Left display: Mammogram percentage within catchment area. Right display: Rural percentage within catchment area. Layer list was not collapsed in order to clarify what fields were available for selection.

Table 1. Median score of participatory GIS usability scale responses between academics and professionals (10 Responses).

	User Interface	Interaction with the Web Maps	Learnability	Reliability	Communication
Total (10)	3	3	4	4	3
Professionals (4)	2.5	3	3.5	3.5	3
Academics (6)	3	3.5	4	4	3.5

3.9. Purpose, Data, Help Documentation, and Functionality Feedback Questions

In the next section, we asked participants to provide specific feedback on the purpose of LionVu 2.0, the timeliness and relevancy of the data, the help documentation usefulness, and the overall functionality. The participants considered the primary purpose of LionVu 2.0 to be: providing a quick view of local data, mapping preliminary data for grants, performing basic geographic analyses, visualizing existing data, and using the information for classroom discussion or other teaching purposes. The participants responded to two questions about the addition of more recent data on cancer survivorship and cancer types but did not ask to remove any data from LionVu 2.0. Participants provided comments stating that the help documentation read me first section was mostly ignored prior to reading this question. Possible ways to improve the presence of the help documentation would be to make it more persistent on the home page and the need to be comprehensive, and understandable to the participants. Suggested additional features in LionVu 2.0 include: exporting to an image file, including tables, putting the layer selection in a dropdown menu, and removing the ability to zoom-in the map by clicking the mouse.

3.10. General Feedback

In the final section, we asked participants about strengths, limitations, job applicability, and general comments about both the LionVu 2.0 and the survey instrument. One of the overall strengths was that participants felt that it was easy to visualize and learn about patterns in the data from the choropleth maps. Limitations were the user interface (i.e., radio buttons reduced the space of the displays making it difficult to see on smaller screens), lack of historical data to complete a multiple year assessment, difficulty in exporting an image from LionVu 2.0, and the collapsible layer list made it difficult to select and unselect layers. The lack of adequate training for LionVu 2.0 users meant there is a potential for future growth in this area. Responding to the question about whether LionVu 2.0 provides the tools to complete your job, most of the participants indicated that it did, but added the potential for teaching and classroom discussion. Other participants responded that it may not be applicable to their careers, but it was visually appealing and can be a good introduction to how to view other web maps. There also was a request for the addition of layers of information on county names, catchment area counties, and the Pennsylvania and catchment area counties found in Appalachia [21], which were added to the LionVu 2.1 version.

3.11. Usability Comparison

For the usability comparison, we defined an academic as people who have a job title of any type of professorship or lecturer, and non-professional being people who have any other job title outside of academia. The median time spent by participants to complete the usability assessment differed among academics and non-academic professionals. Of the 23 people who started the survey, 10 were from academia, 10 from professional organizations, and three with missing professional information. Table 2 shows the performance based on the median time in seconds, success rate, and sample size, for total, professional, and academic subsets. Based on the effectiveness non-academic professionals had a higher total effectiveness and efficiency than those who work in any academic positions (Tables 3 and 4). Based on the small sample size of the survey, the times were measured at the beginning of each section, so it is possible to analyze participants who did not complete the survey. The data were not normally distributed, so we report the median times instead of the average times.

Table 2. Performance in median time and success between professionals and academics.

Overall Performance	USCS	Task 1	Task 2	Task 3	Task 4
Time (s)	340	343	293	618.5	410.5
Success	13%	92%	92%	90%	90%
Sample	15	12	12	10	10
Professionals					
Time (s)	402.5	369	266	532	410.5
Success	30%	90%	90%	50%	100%
Sample	7	5	5	4	4
Academics					
Time (s)	325	325	320	1,098	428.5
Success	0%	80%	100%	50%	75%
Sample	9	7	7	6	6

USCS-United State Cancer Statistics Web Map Task.

Table 3. Effectiveness between professionals and academics.

	Professionals			Academics		
Task	Success (%)	Errors	Effectiveness (%)	Success (%)	Errors	Effectiveness (%)
USCS	30%	6	5	0%	9	0
1	90%	1	90	80%	2	40
2	90%	1	90	100%	1	100
3	50%	4	12.5	50%	7	7.14
4	100%	1	100	75%	4	18.75
Total			59.5			33.18

USCS-United State Cancer Statistics Web Map Task.

Table 4. Efficiency between professionals and academics.

	Professionals			Academics		
Task	Success (%)	Time (min)	Efficiency (%)	Success (%)	Time (min)	Efficiency (%)
USCS	30%	6.70	4.48	0%	5.42	0
1	90%	6.15	14.63	80%	5.42	14.76
2	90%	4.43	20.31	100%	5.33	18.76
3	50%	8.89	5.62	50%	18.3	2.73
4	100%	6.84	14.61	75%	7.14	10.48
Total			11.93			6.42

USCS-United State Cancer Statistics Web Map Task.

4. Discussion

The original purpose of this usability assessment was to evaluate how successful the LionVu 2.0 was in serving the needs of PSCI health practitioners. In order to develop an effective web mapping tool for public health purposes, it is important to identify the critical content for facilitating participants' decision making and to develop the optimal interface for ensuring ease of information access and usability [22]. Findings of the usability assessment indicated that most people had a favorable view of LionVu 2.0. While most participants had little to no experience with web mapping, it was not surprising to learn that participants wanted short 10–15 min training videos to be available with LionVu 2.1. One unexpected finding was the idea that LionVu 2.0 would be useful for teaching purposes and writing grant proposals. There was also a suggestion to simplify the interface by removing advanced functionality, which can be done by reducing the number of JavaScript functions thereby decreasing the time needed for the browser to process loading the maps [23]. Another suggestion was to allow the end user to change the data classification method (i.e., equal interval, natural breaks, etc.), color values, based on ColorBrewer 2.0, for the choropleth maps. An ongoing revision plan is to increase the participatory design through a mechanism that provides feedback such as a short survey that is linked to LionVu 2.1's homepage.

4.1. Limitations

The limitations of this usability assessment impacted generalizability, validity, and reliability of the findings. First, the response rate of 19% was lower than the goal of 33%, most likely due to the start of the COVID-19 pandemic, which most likely reduced the response rate. Second, the low completion rate of 43% was due to the design of the survey with 50 questions that may have overwhelmed the participants who have busy schedules. This issue was partially mitigated by allowing the participant to come back later to complete the survey. In hindsight we realized that the survey took longer to complete than we anticipated, which diminished the response rate. A shorter survey could have provided a richer set of feedback. Third, while the survey was being administered, the USCS web maps were updated to newer data and removed the 2012–2016 maps from the website and replaced them with 2013–2017 maps, which had different data values. This issue was mitigated because most participants completed this portion of the survey prior to the USCS updates. A fourth issue was the large number of Department of Health employees with inactive email addresses, due to an outdated contact list which meant that many invited participants never received the formal invitation to participate. This issue was mitigated by the last-minute addition of 83 community members. Some of the challenges for effective evaluation of mapping tools include: (a) the lack of methods for testing usability, (b) analyzing complex workflows, and (c) assessing long-term usage [24]. Therefore, the results are only reflective of this assessment and cannot be validated or generalized to other evaluations. Despite these limitations, we believe that by implementing the recommendations in the next section will produce an improved LionVu 2.1.

4.2. Recommendations

There are seven recommendations to improve the LionVu 2.0 before and after the launch by December 2020. First, there is a need for developing action items for future programming efforts. Second, LionVu 2.1 will include functionality to allow the user to select data, method chose a color schema, modify the legend position, and set the number of data classes, using seven dropdown menus instead of checkboxes, and the addition of button to download the map as an image file (Figure 8). Third, the suggestion of using LionVu 2.1 in a classroom setting could be piloted into existing educational classes, which may expand the user base and offer additional recommendations for functionality not presently integrated into LionVu 2.0. Fourth, there is a need for moving to a server host that is HIPAA compliant rather than the Penn State access account storage space server where it presently sits. Fifth, development of short training videos needs to be completed prior to the anticipated December 2020 launch. Sixth, in LionVu 2.1, we created a separate data class that contained duplicates or rates that are equal to zero, as shown in the left display in Figure 8. Seventh, there is a need for users to see tabular outputs of the mapped data, using a jQuery plug-in DataTables, with buttons to export to comma separate values (.csv) file, adjust page lengths, and change column visibility.

As shown in Figure 8, in the case of years life lost rate, there was a request for five data classes and natural breaks classification, but the first class had a value of zero, which was assigned a white color and a duplicate class value, which was removed from the map. Whereas in the right display the population density value were neither non zeros nor duplicates so the default values of the five classes were mapped. This ensured that the end-user will not be seeing wide ranges or duplicate class values, which was a problem with LionVu 2.0. In addition, in LionVu 2.1, we implemented geostat.js and chroma.js for choropleth maps, which allows the end-user to switch layers of information, classification method, sequential ColorBrewer 2.0 color palettes, or add/remove/adjust the position of a legend. The default was set at five classes or bins, orange color palette, quantile method, and bottom-right legend. However, we did give the user the option to change layers of information; seven classification methods; 1–20 bins/classes; 18 ColorBrewer 2.0 sequential color palettes; option to reverse color palette (i.e., cancer survival uses inverted color palettes) and add, remove, or adjust the position of a legend. Additionally, in LionVu 2.1 we replaced the checkboxes with toggleable displays, using a leaflet JavaScript plugin [25], for Appalachian and catchment county overlays, and county names. Lastly, we also included tabular outputs (i.e., DataTables) below the maps that allow the user to view the data.

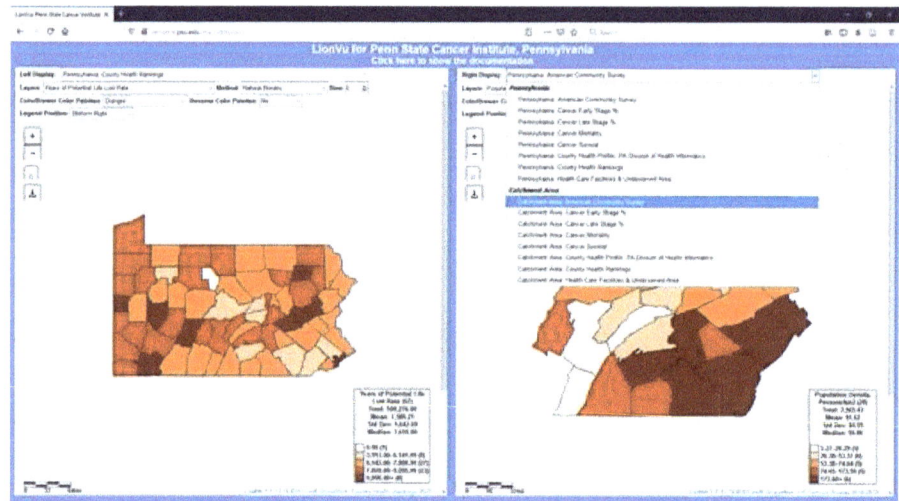

Figure 8. LionVu 2.1 tool using seven dropdown menus and a button to download maps, while preserving side-by-side displays. Left display: Years of potential life lost rate within Pennsylvania. Right display: Population density within catchment area.

5. Conclusions

As noted by Dr. Gerry Rushton in 2003, the future of GIS in public health in the United States will be the development of specialized disease surveillance systems, clinical practice location will broaden to geographic areas, and public health personnel will need to be trained in the GIS environment [26]. In 2020 we are now using specialized surveillance systems, clinical sites are using web GIS, and people are being trained to use the data in web-based platforms. The challenge is that often the products are internally developed and are limited in substance or only perform specific analyses for a limited set of variables. As noted previously, the purpose of this usability assessment began with a very primitive web mapping tool. Unlike previous usability assessments, LionVu 2.0 is being constantly developed to allow for mapping comparisons for a variety of different variables and locations in each dataset for Pennsylvania. For example, the County Health Rankings, are published annually where only a selected number of fields are mapped, even though the datasets have more than 100 variables. In LionVu 2.1, all 100 variables are loaded to a file and presented on a map for both Pennsylvania and catchment area, side-by-side. In addition, other datasets used may be specific to a given geographic area, but the programming can be replicated to a larger area and datasets, potentially increasing the effectiveness and efficiency of the product. Given the massive amount of data being collected, the hope of this assessment was to initiate a communication process to demonstrate the potential value of web GIS and spatial analysis to a wider audience. The question remains; is it relatively unique to display data side-by-side among cancer centers that provides the ability to view data for various datasets and geographical characteristics?

LionVu 2.0 fills a niche in the health community by giving a practitioner the ability to visualize and utilize health data. In the era of big data, there is a need for sharing health data with the public while preserving privacy. LionVu 2.0 presents health-related data spatially in a way that allows people the ability to visualize health data for a given area, while utilizing available health data, at various levels of aggregations and geographical scales (i.e., state, county, zip code, etc.). LionVu 2.0 aims to bridge the gap between data availability and utilization by providing a tool for health practitioners to visualize and utilize health data at the county level, which is small enough to see a difference in a given state, but large enough to minimize data privacy concerns. With the widespread usage of electronic data with various geographical scales there is a need for sharing data that can be used to benefit public health to improve the quality of life. As a result, cancer population researchers are increasingly using geospatial analysis techniques (i.e., exposure assessment, identify spatial associations, proximity analysis, cluster detection and descriptive mapping) to visualize these datasets [27]. LionVu 2.0 includes the most recently available cancer data and includes a wide variety of datasets that can be utilized by anybody who has online access. Although the focus is just on Pennsylvania and the catchment area, it is possible to reuse the code for a wider geographical area. The side-by-side functionality also allows the health practitioner the ability to visualize and compare maps from different layers or datasets. The results of the assessment show that LionVu 2.0 meets the needs by giving the users the ability to provide feedback for further improvements to LionVu 2.1. Based on participants' feedback, the radio buttons were converted to seven dropdown menus, allowing users to adjust the choropleth map displays. In addition, we uncovered feedback to address how to best respond to the issues uncovered by this assessment and ensure that LionVu 2.1 will meet the needs of its health-care professionals and identified new audiences, such as students.

Author Contributions: Conceptualization, Eugene J. Lengerich and Nathaniel R. Geyer; methodology, Nathaniel R. Geyer; software, Nathaniel R. Geyer; formal analysis, Nathaniel R. Geyer; resources, Eugene J. Lengerich; data curation, Nathaniel R. Geyer; writing—original draft preparation, Nathaniel R. Geyer; writing—review and editing, Fritz C. Kessler; visualization, Nathaniel R. Geyer; supervision, Fritz C. Kessler; project administration, Eugene J. Lengerich; funding acquisition, Eugene J. Lengerich. All authors have read and agreed to the published version of the manuscript.

Funding: This study was partially supported by Highmark Incorporation Grant at Penn State Cancer Institute (no key-personnel role). The REDCap survey instrument used was supported by the National Center for Advancing Translational Sciences, National Institutes of Health, through Grant UL1 TR002014. The content is solely the responsibility of the authors and does not necessarily represent the official views of the NIH.

Acknowledgments: The authors acknowledge the contribution of all the anonymous reviewers that improved the quality of the paper.

Conflicts of Interest: The authors declare no conflict of interest. The funders had no role in the design of the study; in the collection, analyses, or interpretation of data; in the writing of the manuscript, or in the decision to publish the results.

Appendix A

Table A1. LionVu 2.0 Usability Survey Questions.

Section	Question
A. Demographic Questions:	1. Please provide your current age in years. 2. Please provide your racial identify. 3. Please provide your ethnic identity. 4. Please provide your current gender. 5. What is your highest level of education?
B. Employment Characteristics, Prior to the COVID-19 Outbreak:	6. Please specify the locations where you were employed, prior to the COVID-19 outbreak. 7. Please specify employee classifications, prior to the COVID-19 outbreak. 8. Please specify official job title, prior to the COVID-19 outbreak (i.e., Research support technologist). 9. What was your primary organization of employment, prior to the COVID-19 outbreak (i.e., Penn State, Pennsylvania Department of Health, etc.)? 10. Please rate your proficiency (e.g., NIH competencies proficiency scale) with using any web mapping tools.

Table A1. *Cont.*

Section	Question
C. Web Mapping Comparison to United States Cancer Statistics:	11. From the rate of new cancers in the United States web map, what was the age-adjusted rate of new cancers within Pennsylvania, 2012–2016? 12. What are some limitations of the United States web map? 13. What are some strengths of the United States web map? 14. What information do expect to see with the web mapping tools, like the United States web map? 15. What capabilities of the United States web map are important to you?
D. Task 1: Using LionVu 2.0 prototype, determine Population Densities and Hispanic Populations within Luzerne County (hint: use catchment area: Demographics thematic layers, legend, and county popups, except where noted).	16. What is the population density (catchment area: Demographics) of Luzerne County (person/km^2)? 17. What bin or color value is Luzerne County Hispanics (catchment area: Demographics)? 18. How did you determine the population density and color value? 19. What are your interpretations of population density across Pennsylvania (Pennsylvania: Demographics)? 20. How could the map interface in LionVu 2.0 be improved to help illustrate the demographic characteristics across Pennsylvania (Pennsylvania: Demographics)?
E. Task 2: Using LionVu 2.0 prototype, determine colorectal cancer mortality and late stage percentage within Centre County (hint: use catchment area: Cancer thematic layers, legend, and county popups, except where noted).	21. What is the age-adjusted mortality rate (per 100,000 people) of colorectal cancer (catchment area: Cancer) in Centre County? 22. What is the percentage of late stage colorectal cancer (catchment area: Cancer) in Centre County? 23. How did you determine the colorectal cancer mortality rate and late stage percentage? 24. What are your interpretations of colorectal cancer mortality across Pennsylvania (Pennsylvania: Cancer)? 25. How could the map interface in LionVu 2.0 be improved to help illustrate the cancer characteristics across Pennsylvania (Pennsylvania: Cancer)?
F. Task 3: Using LionVu 2.0 prototype, determine provider characteristics, within Lancaster County (hint: use catchment area: Cancer thematic layers, legend, and county popups, except where noted).	26. What is the density of endoscopy providers (catchment area: Health care facility and area) within Lancaster County (providers/km^2 per 1000 people)? 27. From the catchment area: Health care facility and area layers, what provider is not found within Lancaster County? 28. How did you determine the selected provider characteristics? 29. How could the map interface in LionVu 2.0 be improved to help illustrate the health care facilities and area characteristics across Pennsylvania (Pennsylvania: Health care facilities and area)? 30. What are your interpretations of the density of endoscopy providers (Pennsylvania: Health care facilities and area—left display) relative to colorectal cancer mortality rates (Pennsylvania: Cancer—right display) across Pennsylvania?
G. Task 4: Using LionVu 2.0 prototype, determine selected characteristics using the side-by-side functionality, within Centre and Luzerne Counties (hint: use both catchment area: Behavioral risks—left display and catchment area: Socioeconomics—right display thematic layers and county popups, except where noted).	31. Using the side-by-side functionality, what is the adult obesity (catchment area: Behavioral risks—left display) and poverty percentages (catchment area: Socioeconomics—right display) in Luzerne County? 32. Using the side-by-side functionality, what is the mammogram screening (catchment area: Behavioral risks—left display) and rurality percentages (Catchment area: Socioeconomics—right display) in Centre County? 33. How did you determine the selected behavioral risks and socioeconomic characteristics? 34. How could the map interface in LionVu 2.0 be improved to help illustrate the behavioral risk characteristics across Pennsylvania (Pennsylvania: Behavioral risks)? 35. How could the map interface in LionVu 2.0 be improved to help illustrate the socioeconomic characteristics across Pennsylvania (Pennsylvania: Socioeconomics)?
H. Rate on your experience using the LionVu 2.0 Prototype (scale: Strongly disagree—strongly agree), based on the participatory GIS usability scale.	36. It is easy to move through different parts of the user interface (Domain: User interface). 37. I can easily access information displayed in the map (Domain: Interaction with the web maps). 38. It is easy to remember how to perform tasks (Domain: Learnability). 39. The system is reliable (Domain: Reliability). 40. The maps are easy to understand (Domain: Communication).

Table A1. *Cont.*

Section	Question
I. Purpose, Data, Documentation, and Functionality Feedback Questions.	41. What do you see as the primary purpose of the LionVu 2.0 prototype? 42. Please specify, what data would you want to remove from the LionVu 2.0 prototype? 43. Please specify, what data would you want to add to the LionVu 2.0 prototype? 44. How can the documentation (read me first), in the LionVu 2.0 prototype, be revised and improved for better comprehension? 45. Please elaborate on your thoughts about what kind of functionality do you consider to be essential for LionVu 2.0.
J. Strengths, Limitations, and General Comments.	46. Other than data, documentation, and functionality, please provide some limitations about the LionVu 2.0 prototype. 47. Other than data, documentation, and functionality, please provide some strengths about the LionVu 2.0 prototype. 48. Please elaborate, whether the LionVu 2.0 Prototype provides you the tools you need to do your job well. 49. Do you have any other feedback, about the LionVu 2.0 Prototype, which was not covered in this usability assessment? 50. Do you have any other comments about this questionnaire or REDCap?

References

1. Brewer, C.A.; Pickle, L. Evaluation of Methods for Classifying Epidemiological Data on Choropleth Maps in Series. *Ann. Assoc. Am. Geogr.* **2002**, *92*, 662–681. [CrossRef]
2. Zelmer, J.; van Hoof, K.; Notarianni, M.; van Mierlo, T.; Schellenberg, M.; Tannenbaum, C. An assessment framework for e-mental health apps in Canada: Results of a modified Delphi process. *JMIR Mhealth Uhealth* **2018**, *6*. [CrossRef] [PubMed]
3. Birken, S.A.; Rohweder, C.L.; Powell, B.J.; Shea, C.M.; Scott, J.; Leeman, J.; Grewe, M.E.; Kirk, M.A.; Damschroder, L.; Aldridge, W.A.; et al. T-CaST: An implementation theory comparison and selection tool. *Implement. Sci.* **2018**, *13*. [CrossRef] [PubMed]
4. Smith, F.; Wallengren, C.; Ohlen, J. Participatory design in education materials in a health care context. *Action Res.* **2017**, *15*, 310–336. [CrossRef]
5. Avila, J.; Sostmann, K.; Breckwoldt, J.; Peters, H. Evaluation of the free, open source software WordPress as electronic portfolio system in undergraduate medical education. *BMC Med. Educ.* **2016**, *16*. [CrossRef] [PubMed]
6. Bourla, A.; Ferreri, F.; Ogorzelec, L.; Peretti, C.S.; Guinchard, C.; Mouchabac, S. Psychiatrists' attitudes toward disruptive new technologies: Mixed-methods study. *JMIR Ment. Health* **2018**, *5*. [CrossRef] [PubMed]
7. Milward, J.; Deluca, P.; Drummond, C.; Watson, R.; Dunne, J.; Kimergård, A. Usability Testing of the BRANCH Smartphone App Designed to Reduce Harmful Drinking in Young Adults. *JMIR MHealth UHealth* **2017**, *5*, e109. [CrossRef]
8. He, X.; Zhang, R.; Rizvi, R.; Vasilakes, J.; Yang, X.; Guo, Y.; He, Z.; Prosperi, M.; Huo, J.H.; Alpert, J.; et al. ALOHA: Developing an interactive graph-based visualization for dietary supplement knowledge graph through user-centered design. *BMC Med. Inform. Decis. Mak.* **2019**, *19*. [CrossRef]
9. Ben Ramadan, A.A.; Jackson-Thompson, J.; Schmaltz, C.L. Usability Assessment of the Missouri Cancer Registry's Published Interactive Mapping Reports: Round One. *JMIR Hum. Factors* **2017**, *4*, e19. [CrossRef]
10. Ben Ramadan, A.A.; Jackson-Thompson, J.; Schmaltz, C.L. Usability Assessment of the Missouri Cancer Registry's Published Interactive Mapping Reports: Round Two. *Online J. Public Health Inform.* **2019**, *11*, e3. [CrossRef]
11. Rzeszewski, M.; Kotus, J. Usability and usefulness of internet mapping platforms in participatory spatial planning. *Appl. Geogr.* **2019**, *103*, 56–69. [CrossRef]
12. Horbinski, T.; Cybulski, P. Similarities of global web mapping services functionality in the context of responsive web design. *Geod. Cartogr.* **2018**, *67*, 159–177. [CrossRef]

13. System Usability Scale (SUS). Available online: https://www.usability.gov/how-to-and-tools/methods/system-usability-scale.html (accessed on 28 April 2020).
14. Ballatore, A.; McClintock, W.; Goldberg, G.; Kuhn, W. Towards a usability scale for participatory GIS. *Cartogr. Maps Connect. World* **2020**, 327–348. [CrossRef]
15. Çöltekin, A.; Heil, B.; Garlandini, S.; Fabrikant, S.I. Evaluating the Effectiveness of Interactive Map Interface Designs: A Case Study Integrating Usability Metrics with Eye-Movement Analysis. *Cartogr. Geogr. Inf. Sci.* **2009**, *36*, 5–17. [CrossRef]
16. Gómez Solórzano, L.S.; Sancho Comíns, J.; Bosque Sendra, J. Atlas Design: A Usability Approach for the Development and Evaluation of Cartographic Products. *Cartogr. J.* **2017**, *54*, 343–357. [CrossRef]
17. Competencies Proficiency Scale. Available online: https://hr.nih.gov/working-nih/competencies/competencies-proficiency-scale (accessed on 15 July 2020).
18. USCS Data Visualizations. Available online: https://gis.cdc.gov/grasp/USCS/DataViz.html (accessed on 15 July 2020).
19. Harris, P.A.; Taylor, R.; Thielke, R.; Payne, J.; Gonzalez, N.; Conde, J.G. Research Electronic Data Capture (REDCap)—A metadata-driven methodology and workflow process for providing translational research informatics support. *J. Biomed. Inform.* **2009**, *42*, 377–381. [CrossRef]
20. MeasuringU: Graph and Calculator for Confidence Intervals for Task Times. Available online: https://measuringu.com/time_intervals/ (accessed on 18 September 2020).
21. Appalachian Counties Served by ARC. Available online: https://www.arc.gov/appalachian-counties-served-by-arc/ (accessed on 18 September 2020).
22. Cao, Y.H.; Boruff, B.J.; McNeill, I.M. The smoke is rising but where is the fire? Exploring effective online map design for wildfire warnings. *Nat. Hazards* **2017**, *88*, 1473–1501. [CrossRef]
23. Hennig, S.; Vogler, R. User-Centred Map Applications Through Participatory Design: Experiences Gained During the "YouthMap 5020" Project. *Cartogr. J.* **2016**, *53*, 213–229. [CrossRef]
24. Unrau, R.; Kray, C. Usability evaluation for geographic information systems: A systematic literature review. *Int. J. Geogr. Inf. Sci.* **2019**, *33*, 645–665. [CrossRef]
25. Leaflet.Legend. Available online: https://github.com/ptma/Leaflet.Legend (accessed on 23 October 2020).
26. Rushton, G. Public Health, GIS, and Spatial Analytic Tools. *Annu. Rev. Public Health* **2003**, *24*, 43–56. [CrossRef]
27. Simkin, J.; Erickson, A.C.; Otterstatter, M.C.; Dummer, T.J.B.; Ogilvie, G. Current State of Geospatial Methodologic Approaches in Canadian Population Oncology Research. *Cancer Epidemiol. Biomark. Prev.* **2020**, *29*, 1294–1303. [CrossRef] [PubMed]

Publisher's Note: MDPI stays neutral with regard to jurisdictional claims in published maps and institutional affiliations.

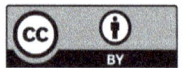

© 2020 by the authors. Licensee MDPI, Basel, Switzerland. This article is an open access article distributed under the terms and conditions of the Creative Commons Attribution (CC BY) license (http://creativecommons.org/licenses/by/4.0/).

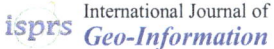

Article

Disparities in Geographical Access to Hospitals in Portugal

Claudia Costa [1,*], José António Tenedório [2] and Paula Santana [1,3]

1   CEGOT, Centre of Studies in Geography and Spatial Planning, University of Coimbra, 3000-043 Coimbra, Portugal; paulasantana@uc.pt
2   Interdisciplinary Centre of Social Sciences (CICS.NOVA), NOVA School of Social Sciences and Humanities (NOVA FCSH), Universidade NOVA de Lisboa, 1069-061 Lisbon, Portugal; ja.tenedorio@fcsh.unl.pt
3   Department of Geography and Tourism–Humanities Faculty–University of Coimbra, 3000-043 Coimbra, Portugal
*   Correspondence: claudiampcosta@uc.pt

Received: 28 August 2020; Accepted: 28 September 2020; Published: 29 September 2020

Abstract: Geographical accessibility to health care services is widely accepted as relevant to improve population health. However, measuring it is very complex, mainly when applied at administrative levels that go beyond the small-area level. This is the case in Portugal, where the municipality is the administrative level that is most appropriate for implementing policies to improve the access to those services. The aim of this paper is to assess whether inequalities in terms of access to a hospital in Portugal have improved over the last 20 years. A population-weighted driving time was applied using the census tract population, the roads network, the reference hospitals' catchment area and the municipality boundaries. The results show that municipalities are 25 min away from the hospital—3 min less than in 1991—and that there is an association with premature mortality, elderly population and population density. However, disparities between municipalities are still huge. Municipalities with higher rates of older populations, isolated communities or those located closer to the border with Spain face harder challenges and require greater attention from local administration. Since municipalities now have responsibilities for health, it is important they implement interventions at the local level to tackle disparities impacting access to healthcare.

Keywords: geographical accessibility; local scale; municipality; healthcare services; spatial planning; decentralization

1. Introduction

Internationally, access to healthcare is one of the primary goals of every country's government [1–5]. Providing access to quality and essential healthcare services and reducing inequalities within countries are, in fact, two of the United Nations' Sustainable Development Goals, set out by world leaders to promote the eradication of poverty and advance economic, social and environmental development on a global scale by 2030 [6]. Moreover, the improvement in accessibility is considered a main driver for smart, sustainable and inclusive growth proposed by the Europe 2020 Strategy and the Territorial Agenda 2020 [7]. Achieving those goals is fundamental to achieving equity in access to healthcare because large inequalities can exacerbate disparities in health outcomes and quality of life [3].

Despite this, there is no consensus on how to define access, mainly due to its multidimensional nature and the vast array of accessibility measures that can be applied [8–10]. The following concepts were adopted for this paper. Penchansky and Thomas [11] define access as a concept representing a degree of fit between patients and the health system; Gulzar [12] considers access as the ability of a population to use health services, whether that ability be affected by access barriers or facilitators.

According to Joseph and Philips [13], access can be realized or potential. The first approach focuses on utilization patterns. The latter considers potential barriers to utilization and measures access as potential utilization.

There is also no agreement regarding the dimensions to define access. Penchansky and Thomas' [11] dimensions are accessibility, availability, accommodation, affordability and acceptability. Availability and accessibility are the two spatial dimensions that together measure the patient's geographical accessibility [3,9,14]. Geurs and Wee [15] stated the four major components of accessibility: (1) land-use, which reflects the location of supply and demand as well as the interactions between them; (2) transportation, which considers the way an individual covers the distance between the origin and the destination; (3) temporal, which focus on the availability of opportunities to move through the day and the time available; (4) individual, regarding the individual characteristics that influence a person's access. This paper will focus on the two spatial dimensions from Penchansky and Thomas' approach and the two first components referred by Geurs and Wee. In this way, the study will consider the relationship between three factors, their spatial distribution and their characteristics: (a) how far people live from healthcare services and are willing to travel, (b) how well transport provides links to the healthcare services, and (c) how long it takes to travel to such services [16–22].

Finally, accessibility measurements are under growing scrutiny. Geurs and Wee [15] categorized accessibility measures based on three perspectives: (1) infrastructure-based accessibility measures, used to analyze the performance of the transport infrastructure; (2) activity-based accessibility measures, used to analyze the range of opportunities with respect to their distribution in space and the travel barriers between users and services; (3) utility-based accessibility measures, used to analyze the benefits individuals derive from using the transport system [22]. Guagliardo [14] classifies them into four categories: (1) provider-to-population ratios that are computed within bordered areas; (2) distance to nearest provider, measured from a patient's residence or from a population centre; (3) average distance to a set of providers that corresponds to a combined measure of accessibility and availability since travel impedance to all providers are summed and averaged; (4) gravitational models of provider influence that represent the potential interaction between any population point and all service points within a reasonable distance.

Geographical accessibility is generally accepted as an important component in evaluating a population's overall access to healthcare and is a basic aim to meet the population's health needs [23–25]. Identifying where the truly underserved populations are located is an essential first step toward meaningful and effective government intervention programs that can narrow gaps in accessing healthcare and promote overall population health [3]. Thus, it is widely recognized as an important spatial barrier to healthcare services [11,26] and, therefore, a significant source of spatial inequality [27] and a major health determinant to be tackled [28]. Its study is essential for evaluating population exposure to local environments [29,30]. According to the literature, geographical constraints on access to services contribute to lower health care utilization, decreased uptake of preventive services and lower survival rates, which may contribute to poorer health outcomes, particularly for those with lower incomes [31–37]. It is also associated with poor utilization of specialization units, such as maternity hospitals, pediatric centers and cancer management institutes, often located in larger cities and not accessible or visible for people living in socio-economically deprived areas, rural communities and remote places [38–41]. This is also of significant concern to ageing societies where geographical access is critical [21,42] and seniors are experiencing more challenges accessing care [43,44]. Thus, a community that needs to travel large distances from their residence to healthcare facilities experiences greater difficulty in gaining access [45]. Users become prone to missing the opportunity to detect illnesses at an early stage, starting treatment at different stages of chronic disease, receiving adequate pharmacological prescriptions and dosages or participating in screening programs [46]. As a consequence, several studies found an association between geographical accessibility to healthcare and the type of treatment and medical intervention [47], the utilization of surgical services [48], cardiac rehabilitation treatment [49] or maternity hospitals [50], hepatitis C detection [51], survival from a cardiac disease [52–54], stage of several cancers at diagnosis [55,56], and access to cancer treatment [57]. Ecological mortality studies have also revealed that a longer distance to travel to healthcare is significantly associated with higher mortality from heart attack [43], asthma [58], perinatal death [59,60], prostate and lung cancers [61] and trauma accidents [62,63]. Therefore, those communities that have poor transportation infrastructures and a lack of public transportation options, also often suffer from increased disadvantage and poorer health status, meaning that they require even greater levels of access than those living in well served areas [64].

Identifying health disparities—in the form of vulnerable territories with poorer geographical access to health services that can be shaped by policies [65]—can be a key input for local authorities during the design and implementation of policies [66,67]. Research highlighted that measuring geographical accessibility enables: (1) to quantify differences in access [35,68]; (2) to identify gaps in service provision [69–71]; (3) to model optimal facility location [72,73]; (4) to identify inequalities in service provision [74,75]; (5) to promote evidence-based health policies [76–79]. Hence, measuring geographical accessibility can be an essential element to support rationing decisions that affect both the process of urban area development and spatial planning of health resources, and reinforce the need for interventions that promote and improve the population health of a community [2,8,9,42,75,80–87]. However, geographical accessibility is often misunderstood and inadequately measured on many studies and local plans [15].

According to the European Commission, Portugal is among the EU countries facing substantial inequalities in the supply of healthcare services between regions and across urban and rural areas [88]. The OECD also points out the uneven geographical distribution of facilities as one of the biggest barriers to accessing healthcare [89]. According to the scientific literature, poor geographical access is affecting the utilization of health services in Portugal and some health outcomes. Santana [90] was the first author to identify an association between distance and use of Emergency Rooms. Recently, Vaz et al. [91] identified that a 10% increase in distance to Emergency facilities results in a 10 to 20% decrease in utilization, especially for low-severity demand. Costa et al. [92] identified a 2% higher risk of dying from an amenable cause of death due to health care services for those living in municipalities where it takes more than 30 min to reach the closest hospital. Therefore, researchers state that it is essential to undertake a comprehensive assessment of geographical inequalities in access, and to ensure that interventions to improve healthcare access are put in practice [93].

Until recently, health policies were only produced by Portugal's central government, so most plans focused on the national level and provided evidence at this level. Nonetheless, legislation from 2018 gave the municipalities the power to plan primary care units, and manage some human resources, services and infrastructure. Moreover, they are now responsible for producing a local health plan and implementing a health strategy to promote community and healthy living and active ageing [94]. Therefore, it is important to have access to clear evidence on inequalities regarding access to healthcare. According to Mizen and colleagues [19], geographical accessibility to healthcare services needs to be accurately assessed and effectively communicated to decision makers so that successful policy and infrastructure planning can be implemented.

Operationalizing and computing a measurement able to quantify geographical accessibility is challenging since it depends on a set of four parameters: definition of residential areas, a method of aggregation, a measure of accessibility and a type of distance [5]. The choice and combination of these parameters is likely to generate different results or lead to significant errors in measurement [5,17,95–99].

The first parameter relies on the definition of residential area. Selecting the appropriate spatial unit of analysis is critical for quantifying geographical accessibility [100]. Aggregation errors arise when, for the purpose of distance calculations, a single point is used to represent a larger spatial unit, which, in turn, represents an aggregation of spatially distributed individuals, leading to a lack of precision and estimation errors [83,101]. This may create the problem of ecological fallacy, since the larger the spatial unit, the higher the error will be [19,98,99]. The census tract unit is often selected due to the low number of people, and the availability of detailed socioeconomic, demographic and housing data, as well as their relative homogeneity [95].

The second focuses on the aggregation method applied. It is important to apply an aggregation method so as to limit errors in the measurement of potential spatial access of larger areas, such as parishes and municipalities [100]. Due to the differences between residential areas, it is inappropriate to ignore who is living there since it introduces ecological fallacy [19]. Therefore, it is important to weigh spatial access based on their number and distribution in the territory [66]. Studies generally choose to consider the number of inhabitants in each residential area [29,66].

The third parameter considers the way geographic accessibility between the residential area and the public service is measured. According to the literature, the five most commonly used measures are: (1) the distance/time to the service [102]; (2) the number of services within n meters or minutes [101]; (3) the mean distance/time to the n closest services [30]; (4) the gravity model [103,104]; (5) the two-step floating catchment area methods and those derived from them [18,20,21,24,85,103,105–108]. Among these, the last two are relatively popular methods for measuring spatial equity [18,82,109]. Still, the most often used method is clearly the distance/time to the closest service, which allows for evaluating geographical access to the healthcare services [27,100].

Finally, the fourth parameter deals with the type of distance, defined as the degree to which two places on the same surface are connected [15]. There are several types of distance that can be implemented [19]. Crow-fly with straight line distance is used in many studies for determining healthcare services catchment areas or for estimating rates of population served [8,18,101]. Public authorities generally use it as a decision tool [74] despite some doubts as to its reliability [101,110,111]. Additionally, very popular among researchers, network-based distance is measured under a network made of lines and nodes computing the length of the shortest path along the transport network, representing the real network system taken by the population to move between locations [8]. Therefore, it is more accurate and realistic [19,82] than the previous option, mainly in regions where roads exhibit high degrees of sinuosity and topographical barriers [5,100,101].

Besides those four parameters mentioned in the literature, a fifth one must be considered in accessibility studies aiming to support decision-making: the outcome of the measurement. The unit can be different according to those parameters, influencing the way results are interpreted. According to previous studies, displaying results in units of analysis that are meaningful to decision-making will increase the likelihood that such results will be embedded in policy [15,77,112,113]. Most studies on geographical accessibility present measurements of distances in kilometers [29,66], time in minutes [114] or scores represented in quintiles [105,106]. Distance metrics offer awareness of geographical access regardless of the transportation mode being used. Still, it does not consider the speed or physical barriers, such as intersections that influence the time to reach healthcare. Time measurement considers both, does not require previous assumptions and it is easily communicated to decision-makers. However, it considers that all the healthcare services are equal. Scores allow for overcoming the aforementioned negative aspects, although they cannot be easily interpreted and require comparison to be understood.

Following the best approaches for each parameter, the population-weighted driving time indicator is considered an adequate choice for measuring geographical accessibility because it allows for overcoming the unrealistic equal access assumption and potential edge effects of the container-based approach, and also uses an intuitive form of a distance-base measure [29], avoiding the modifiable unit area problem [115]. This indicator accounts for the average time between population in a residential area (e.g., census tract) and the healthcare service by considering the shortest distance between them and the share of population within a larger area (e.g., municipality) [66]. This flexibility makes it applicable to individual persons or households, as well as for a geographic area [29]. Previous studies have applied this method to assess access to hospitals [66,111], alcohol sales [29], parks [116] and supermarkets [30]. It was applied to studies at local [30] and national levels [29,66,111,116].

The aim of this paper is to draw on population-weighted driving time to better assess whether there are disparities in geographical access to the reference hospital in Portugal, how it has changed in the past 20 years (1991–2011) and what influenced that change.

Due to the recent decentralization of power from the health sector to the local administration, this is an important policy issue. For this reason, the geographical accessibility of Portuguese municipalities was investigated with the aim of developing policy recommendations regarding which interventions can be implemented to reduce the impact on health disparities.

2. Materials and Methods

2.1. Geographical Scales

Studying geographical accessibility to healthcare in Portugal requires two geographical levels to be considered: the lowest level with population data and the adequate administrative level able to implement changes.

The census tract is the minimal unit of census geographic hierarchy in Portugal. By using the population at its smallest level, the geographic aggregation error is minimized [117]. In addition, census tract-based spatial access metrics provide the flexibility to aggregate the metrics to any higher geographic level that can be linked to geocoded individual or aggregated health outcomes [29].

Although the small-area level is adequate to capture the right level of areal differentiation [77,118], the municipality administrative level is the most appropriate to present a geographical accessibility measurement for Portugal. Four important points justify this choice: (1) it is considered the geographical level that better fits ecological studies in Portugal, based on national registries, such as mortality [99,119–121]; (2) hospitals had a catchment population area based on municipalities (except for main urban areas where delimitation is based on parishes) until 2015 [122]; (3) it is the lowest meaningful administrative level with an elected government with capacity to implement policies and interventions that may impact population health [23,123]; (4) recently, municipalities became responsible for a set of tasks and decisions that were previously taken centrally by the Health Ministry, as well as for the production of a local health plan.

2.2. Method: The Population-Weighted Driving Time Indicator

Population-weighted driving time was the indicator selected to measure the potential geographical accessibility from municipalities to the hospital's catchment area in Portugal in three periods (1991, 2001 and 2011).

This metric is a matter of calculating the accessibility measures on the level of the census tracts and then computing the average time weighted by the population within the municipality.

The process to compute this indicator is straightforward, comprising three steps: (1) computing the travelling time using a private car from the centroid of each small-area level (census tract) to the reference hospital; (2) weighting the time needed for the population living in each small area; (3) aggregating the travel time in order to identify the weighted average travel time of a municipality. These steps can be translated into a formula. By taking a small-area *i* from municipality j:

$$\text{time}_j = \sum_{i=1}^{n} \left(\frac{T_i \times P_i}{\sum_{j=1}^{n}(T_i \times P_i)} \times T_i \right) \quad (1)$$

where P_i is the population living in the small area and T_i is the time (in minutes) needed to reach the hospital. The outcome is measured in minutes, revealing the time that the population from a municipality would need to reach the hospital through private car utilization. Figure 1 presents the workflow implemented, namely the data and the functions, with ArcGIS 10.5 being used.

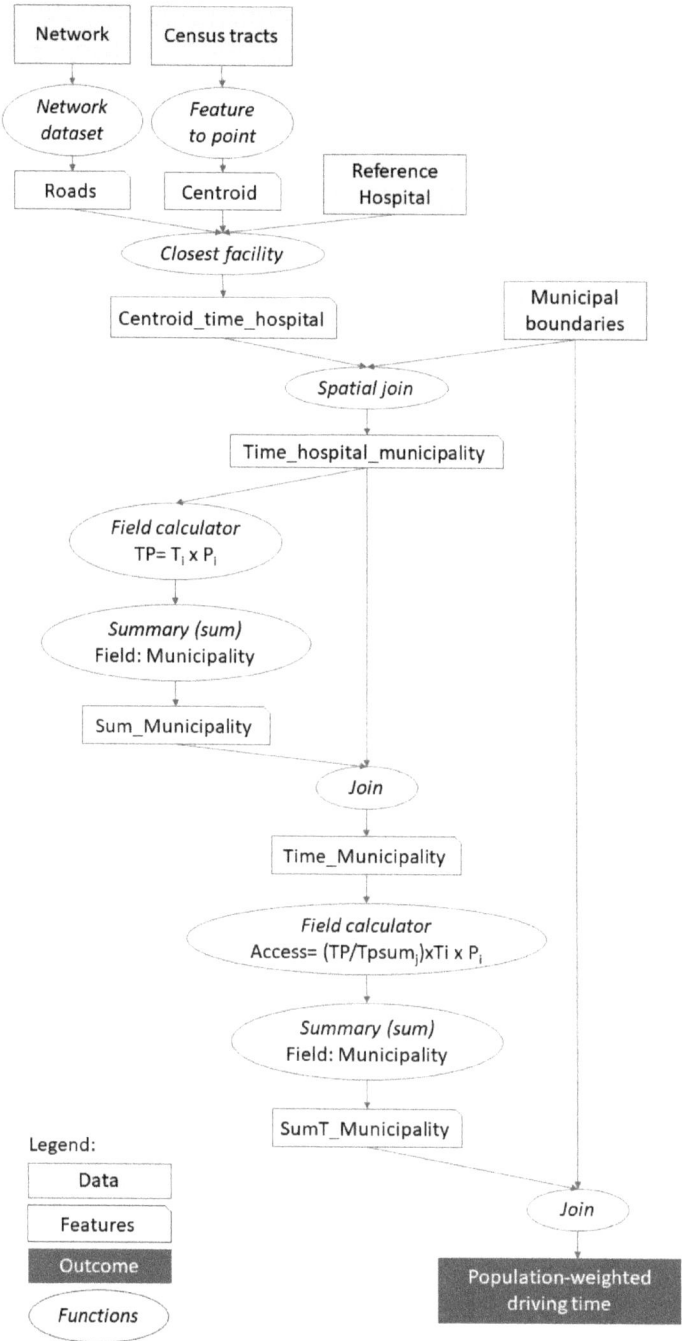

Figure 1. Workflow implemented to build the population-weighted driving time indicator.

2.3. Geographical Data

To build the population-weighted driving time metric, cartographic information was required for (1) the distribution of the population at the small-area level (census tract); (2) the road network, with information about speed limits and general driving conventions (e.g., intersections, traffic lights); (3) the location of the hospital and its catchment area; (4) the boundaries of the municipalities.

The population data by census tract was provided by Statistics Portugal who collect this information through the Census Survey every ten years. The indicator used for this study was the number of permanent residents in the housing unit by census tract in 1991, 2001 and 2011. The quality of the data from the census (population and housing censuses) for 1991, 2001 and 2011 was guaranteed by the international standard that is applied by Statistics Portugal. The 1991 Census initiated the automatic coding of alphabetic expressions; the 2001 census has already made use of the optical questionnaire reading process and the 2011 census introduced the modernization of data collection processes, via the internet response (it was called e-Censuses). The 2011 census followed the regulation of the European Union (regulation EC 763/2008 of the European Parliament and of the European Council, of 9 July 2008; complementary regulations rEG (EC) No. 1201/2009, rEG (EC) No. 1151/2010 and rEG (CE) No. 519/2010). These regulations introduced standards for all Member States, namely the smallest data unit and the census moment. In this investigation, the census tract was used as the smallest data unit. According to Statistics Portugal, the Census data collection corresponds to 97.5% of the Portuguese population in 2011. In 2001, the coverage rates were higher (98.6%) as well as in 1991 (99.6%).

The roads and urban streets data was provided by ESRI Portugal, in the form of vector digital data (Geospatial Data Presentation Form). The data are the TeleAtlas Multinet shapefiles produced by TeleAtlas (now TomTom) as it is widely used in the market, particularly in the navigation sector. This road database not only includes extensive, current and accurate geographical data, but it also includes additional information, such as the legal speed limit, turn-by-turn instructions, street signs, intersections and other transit directions. These data guarantee quality at all levels: attribute accuracy (address attributes pre-standardized based on ESRI Portugal), logical consistency (shapefile), completeness (compared to official Portuguese sources) and positional accuracy (map accuracy standards for 1:100,000-scale maps). According to the company, the positional accuracy of the data is up to one meter. These data were for the year 2011. The 2011 data served as reference to retrospectively build the 2001 and 1991 road network. Due to a lack of data for the previous years, the National Road Plan from 1985, old road maps and historical data from technical reports regarding the opening of highway sections were used to backdate these data from 2011 to 2001 and 1991.

The location of the hospitals and their catchment areas were provided by the Central Administration of the Health System, which manages the public hospitals and defines the catchment population area of each hospital. Since the National Health Service (NHS) was created in 1979, the country has been served by a network of public hospitals with access based on the pre-defined catchment area of each hospital and, until 2015, a strong gate-keeping system [44,122,124]. Hospitals are classified into a three-level administrative hierarchy that reflects differences in scale and scope [125]. Group I comprise local hospitals with a catchment area of 75,000 to 500,000 inhabitants, providing some medical and surgical specialties. Within group I there are some hospitals that are managed by charity trusts. These so-called "social hospitals", have agreements with the NHS and they provide healthcare to users of the system in the same way as public hospitals. Group II comprises district hospitals that provide the group I specialties in their own catchment area and also provide other specialties to some group I hospitals located nearby. Group III comprises central hospitals that provide all medical and surgical specialties in both the direct and indirect catchment areas from groups I and II hospitals located nearby [126]. Therefore, district and central hospitals "accumulate" specialties according to their level, and human resources and beds are allocated to the hospital and not to the different levels. The group I hospitals were considered for this study because they only provide healthcare to those living in their catchment area.

The boundaries of the municipalities were produced by the Directorate General for the Territory, which is responsible for producing accurate information regarding the administrative boundaries of the administrative levels and providing their official delimitation.

3. Results

Through the census years, there was an increase in the number of census tracts and, simultaneously, a decrease in the average population (Table 1). In 2011 there were more than 200,000 census tracts with an average area of 300 square meters and 43 inhabitants.

Table 1. Descriptive statistics of the census tracts and municipalities.

			1991	2001	2011
Smallest level: Census tracts	Number of census tracts		91,615	149,603	232,625
	Area (km^2) *	average	0.9	0.5	0.3
		min–max	0.1–227	0.1–227	0.1–164
	Population (n°)	average	102	65	43
		min–max	1–2585	1–1699	1–1742
Lower Administrative level: Municipalities	Number of census tracts	average	370	612	837
		min–max	50–3700	74–5346	82–4099
	Area (km^2)	average	324	320	230
		min–max	8–1721	8–1720	7–1685
	Population (n°)	average	34,094	35,501	36,143
		min–max	2052–663,394	1924–564,657	1834–547,733

* Only considering census tracts with population.

The time to reach the reference hospital, measured for each census tract, was aggregated to the municipalities from Continental Portugal in order to identify the population-weighted driving time to the reference hospital.

Since the area of the municipalities is large (average: 230 km^2), the first step was to analyze the internal range of values between the closest and the furthest census tract within the municipality to the reference hospital. According to Figure 2, there is still a huge range in travel time. On average, the travel time range is 22 min; 9.1% of the population lives in municipalities with an internal travel time range to the reference hospital longer than 30 min. In 1991, it was slightly higher (23 min) and the share of the population living in municipalities with a travel time longer than 30 min was higher (10.6%).

According to Figure 3, inequalities between the Eastern and Western areas are evident. The population-weighted access pattern follows the population distribution, with the municipalities closer to Atlantic Ocean from North, Centre and the Greater Lisbon Region presenting very good geographic accessibility. Outside this area there are also some pockets with very good accessibility in the regions' capitals. However, due to the greater distance between hospitals, there are 79 municipalities whose population-weighted driving time is more than 30 min. The municipalities closer to the border with Spain are those with the worst accessibility. This was already visible in 1991 and 2001. In 2011, municipalities were, on average, within a 25-min journey to the hospital, accounting for 92.8% of the population living in municipalities with population-weighted driving time lower than 30 min (9,320,793 inhabitants). In 1991 the average population-weighted driving time to the hospital was 28 min.

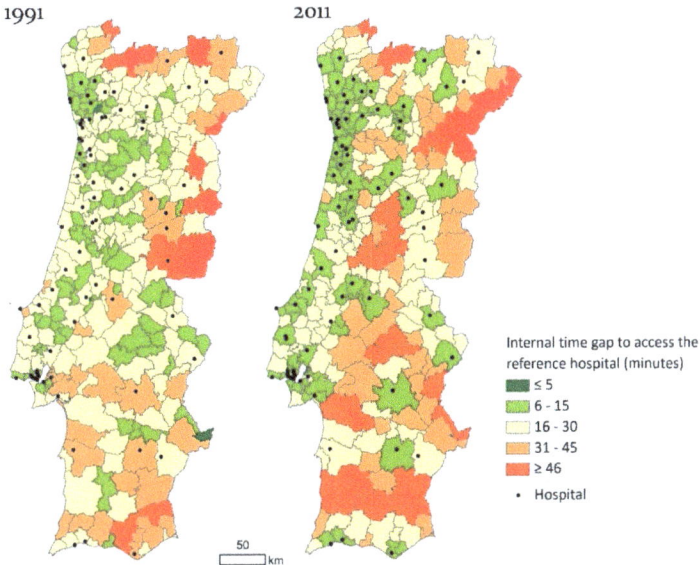

Figure 2. Difference between the maximum and minimum time required by the census tracts within each municipality to reach the hospital in 1991 and 2011.

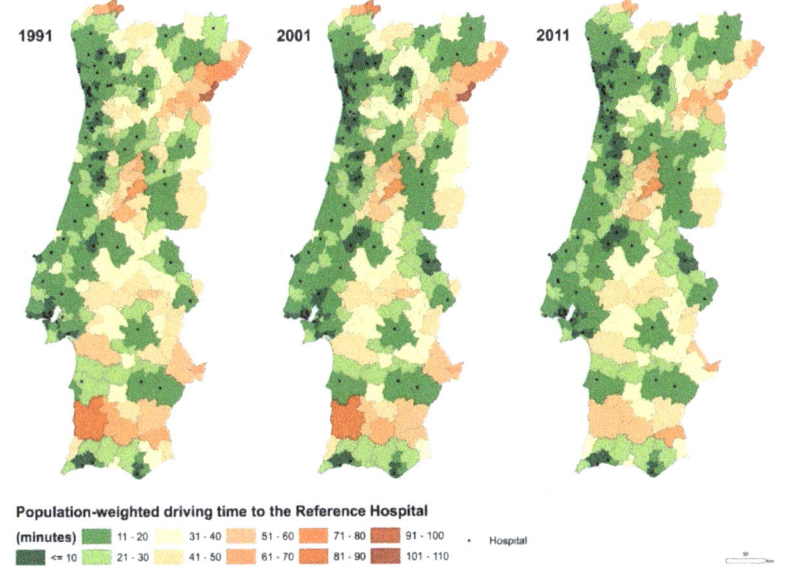

Figure 3. Population-weighted driving time to the reference hospital in Portugal by municipality in 1991, 2001 and 2011. Note: The population-weighted driving time to the reference hospital, by year and municipality, is available here: saudemunicipio.uc.pt.

Comparing 1991 and 2011, almost all municipalities improved accessibility to the hospital within the period of analysis (Figure 4). On average, population-weighted driving time for 2011 is 3 min lower when compared to 1991, corresponding to an average gain of 10% in population-weighted driving time to the hospital. At present, residents of some municipalities need half the time they needed in 1991 to reach the hospital and, for others, the time decreased by more than 20 min. However, the Gini Coefficient reveals that spatial inequalities are still persistent: in 1991, the Gini Coefficient was 0.335 and in 2011, 0.326.

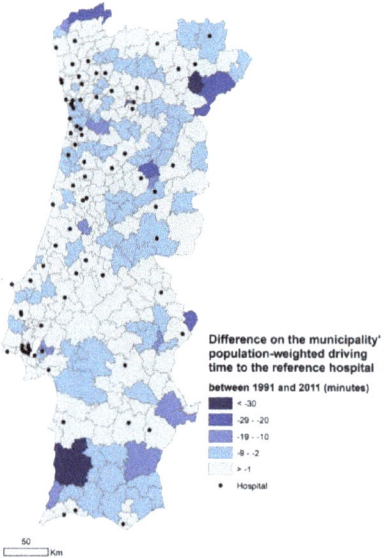

Figure 4. Differences in minutes between 1991 and 2011 of the Population-weighted driving time to the reference hospital by municipality.

Due to the chance that the reference hospital might not be the closest one, it was important to apply the same methodology without considering the catchment areas. Figure 5 reveals that, for most municipalities, there is no significative difference between the population-weighted time to the reference hospital when compared to the closest hospital. However, in 1991 there were four municipalities where the population-weighed driving time to the closest hospital was 30 min or more lower than the population weighted driving time to the reference hospital. In 2011 only one municipality remains in this category, located in the center of the Centro Region.

Figure 6 reveals the relevance of three different factors on the verified evolution of geographical accessibility: changes to the hospital reference catchment area, improvement of the road network and demographic changes to population concentration. Most municipalities were influenced by all three factors: 31.8% of the population live in municipalities where the reference hospital changed, the road network improved, and the external and internal changes of the population were considerable. Only 5% of the 2011 population does not live in a municipality affected by at least one factor. These are mostly located in inland Alentejo and the Centro Region. When looking at each factor individually, it is evident that most people live in municipalities where significant changes to demographic distribution occurred (72.2%), followed by populations living in municipalities where a highway was built (62.4%), and 61.7% of the population live in municipalities where the reference hospital was not the same throughout the study period.

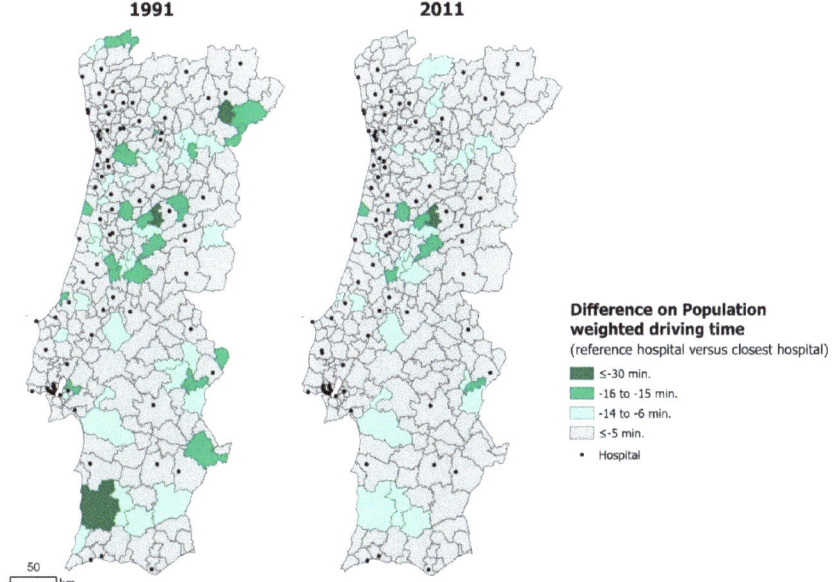

Figure 5. Difference in the population weighted driving time by municipality in 1991 and 2011 when considering the reference hospital and the closest hospital.

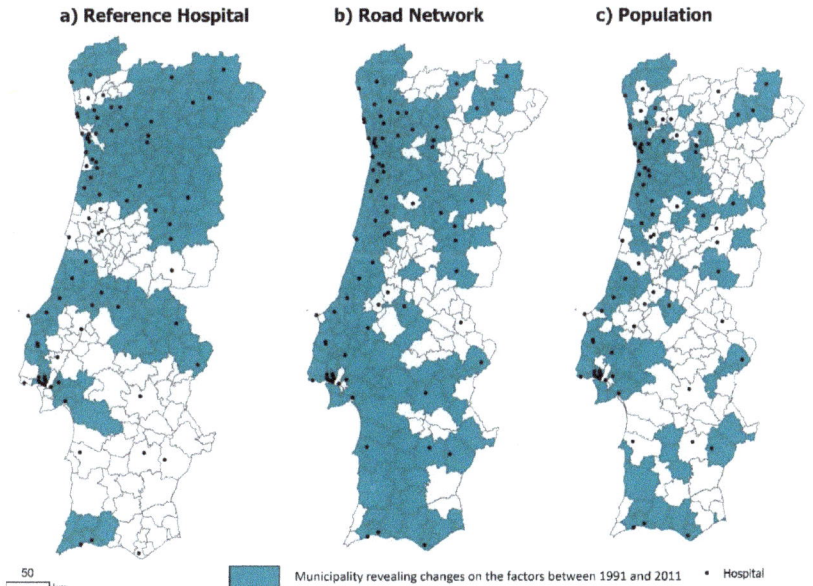

Figure 6. Impact of each factor on the change in population-weighted driving time to the reference hospital by municipality between 1991 and 2011: (**a**) reference hospital (municipality where the reference hospital changed); (**b**) road network (municipality where a road with a legal speed limit equal or higher to 100 km/h was built); (**c**) population (municipality where there was a 10% increase/decrease in the share of population living on predominantly urban parishes).

According to Table 2, in 1991, 16% of the population was living in municipalities where the population-weighted driving time to the hospital was more than 30 min. In 2011 that rate was 7%; a decrease of more than half. The biggest improvement was for those living in municipalities with a population-weighted driving time between 40 and 50 min. Notice that, in 1991, there were municipalities whose population-weighted driving time to reach the hospital was more than 90 min, a situation that does not presently occur.

Table 2. Change in population between 1991 and 2011 interval of population-weighted driving time to the hospital and population by interval in each year.

		2011								Pop. (1991)	
		≤10	11–20	21–30	31–40	41–50	51–60	61–70	≥71	N	%
1991	≤10	90%	10%	-	-	-	-	-	-	3,950,420	39.1%
	11–20	12%	88%	-	-	-	-	-	-	3,522,533	34.9%
	21–30	2%	26%	72%	-	-	-	-	-	1,008,268	10.0%
	31–40	-	3%	47%	50%	-	-	-	-	470,573	4.7%
	41–50	-	5%	6%	56%	33%	-	-	-	854,226	8.5%
	51–60	-	-	-	14%	35%	50%	-	-	129,093	1.3%
	61–70	-	-	6%	-	21%	26%	48%	-	105,546	1.0%
	71–80	-	-	-	-	68%	-	-	32%	17,985	0.2%
	81–90	-	-	-	-	-	100%	-	-	37,963	0.4%
	≥91	-	-	-	-	-	-	-	100%	4914	0.1%
Pop. (2011)	N	4,047,471	4,260,054	1,013,268	398,171	165,120	111,924	43,352	8261		
	%	40.3%	42.4%	10.1%	4.0%	1.6%	1.1%	0.4%	0.1%		

Note: The percentage within the 1991–2011 matrix takes into account the number of people within one time-interval in 1991.

Table 3 reveals that there is a statistical association between the population-weighted driving time and some demographic characteristics: municipalities with bad geographical accessibility to the reference hospital have higher share of elderly population, high rates of premature mortality and lower population density.

Table 3. Association between municipality population-weighted driving time to the reference hospital and characteristics of the municipality.

Variable	Year	R^2	Coefficient (95%CI)	p-Value
Population aged 65 or more (%)	2011	0.41	0.29 [0.25–0.33]	<0.01
	1991	0.33	1.02 [0.84–1.18]	<0.01
Population density (n°/km^2)	2011	0.12	−0.005 [−0.007−−0.004]	<0.01
	1991	0.09	−0.005 [−0.007−−0.004]	<0.01
Premature mortality per 100,000 inhabitants	2011	0.21	0.14 [0.10–0.17]	<0.01
	1991	0.12	0.13 [0.17–0.09]	<0.01

Note: p-value below 0.01 provides evidence that the association is statistically significant.

Figure 7 exhibits that longer travel time is associated with higher share of elderly people. Table 3 reveals that even a one-minute increase in the population-weighted driving time is associated with an increase of 0.3% in the share of the elderly population. This was already visible in 1991 but the association was not so high. Almost all the municipalities with higher rates of elderly population are located outside of the littoral border, between Porto, Lisbon and Algarve, and are mostly those closer to the border with Spain.

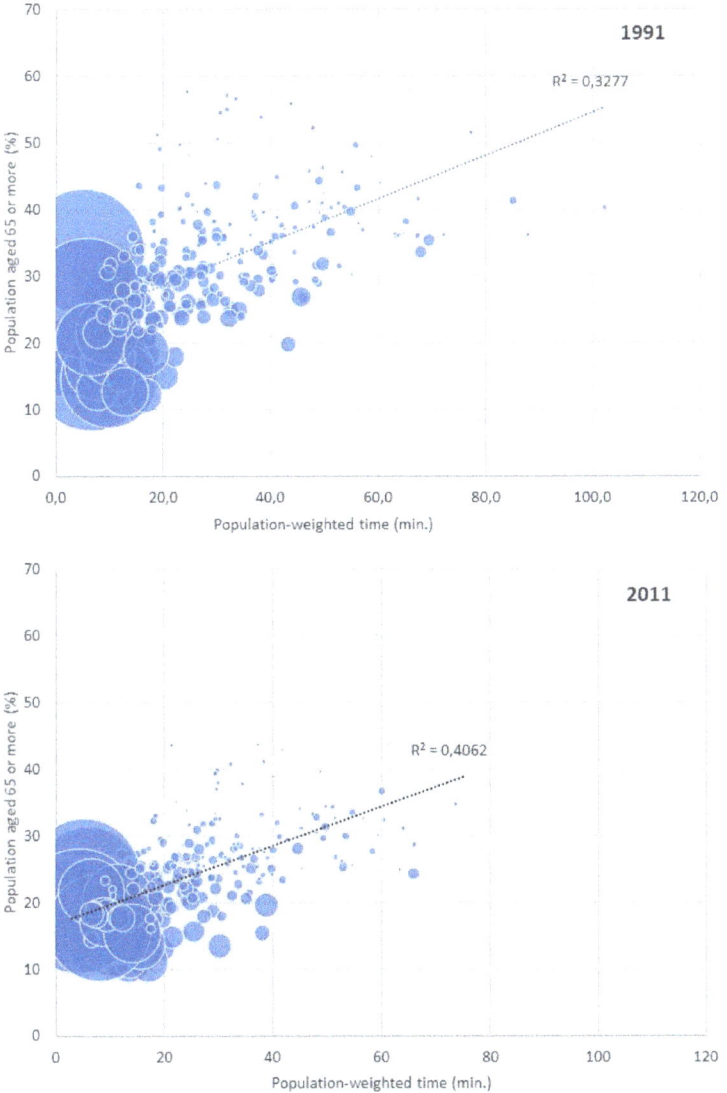

Figure 7. Share of elderly population (*y*-axis), population-weighted driving time to the reference hospital (*x*-axis) and population density (area) by municipality in 1991 and 2011.

Additionally, in Figure 7, it is visible that there is a negative association between population density and time to the reference hospital: the higher the time to reach the reference hospital, the smaller the population density is. As expected, hospitals are mainly located in the most densely populated municipalities and where the share of the elderly population is lower.

The population-weighted driving time to the reference hospital also reveals an association with premature mortality, providing the evidence that areas with a high share of deaths, before the age of 75, might have low levels of geographical accessibility. Results show that a one-minute increase in population-weighted driving time is associated with an increase of 0.14% in premature mortality. In 1991 the association was a fraction lower. The municipalities with higher rates of premature mortality are mostly located closer to the border with Spain and on the central axis that crosses Portugal from North to South.

Most of the municipalities reveal more than one of these demographic characteristics. According to Figure 8, all the municipalities where the population-weighted driving time is higher than 30 min, also have an elderly population which is above the Portuguese average, and/or above average premature mortality. In addition, some municipalities are negatively impacted by their proximity to the border with Spain. Major issues are found in the municipalities closer to the border between the Alentejo and Algarve regions; the central axis that crosses the country North to South in the middle; the Foz Côa Valley; and the municipalities closer to the Spanish border.

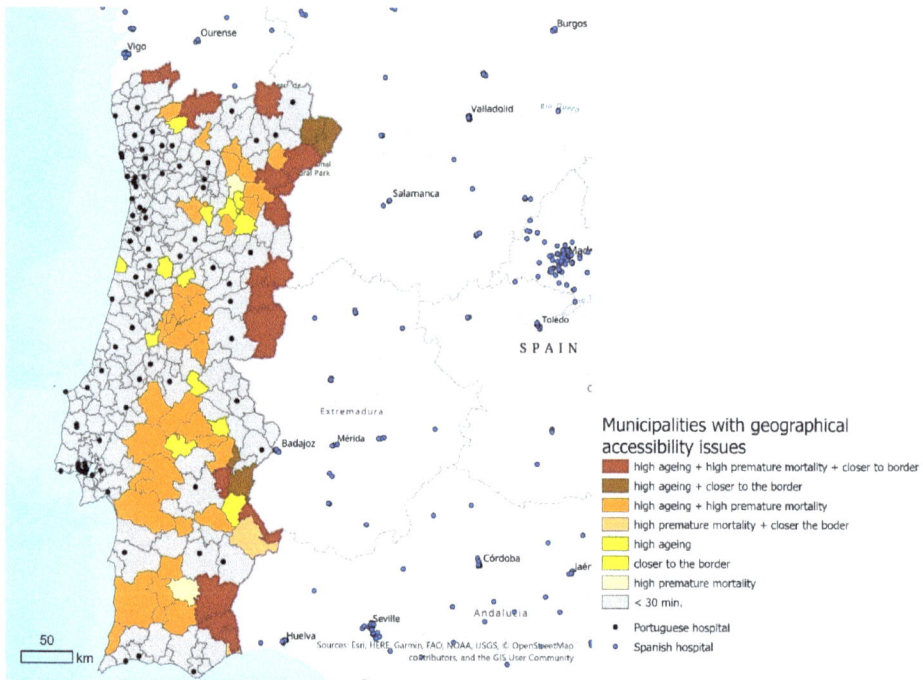

Figure 8. Municipalities with geographical accessibility issues regarding the demographic characteristics analyzed, 2011.

4. Discussion

4.1. Geographical Accessibility to the Reference Hospital in Portugal

The aim of this paper was to assess whether there are disparities in access to a hospital in Portugal and how this has changed in the last 20 years (1991–2011). The results show that geographical accessibility to the reference hospital improved over the years. However, disparities are still visible between municipalities, with ageing and border communities remaining vulnerable and requiring more attention.

Geographical access to the reference hospital mostly improved over time in Portugal with an average gain of 10% in population-weighted driving time. The biggest improvement has been for those living in municipalities with population-weighted driving time between 40 and 50 min and higher than 70 min. In 2011, almost half of the population lives in municipalities with a population-weighted driving time to the hospital lower than 10 min (40%) and 93% lives in municipalities with a travel time lower than 30 min, revealing very good geographical access. On average, municipalities present a population-weighted driving time of 25 min in 2011—3 min less than 20 years ago. Still, there are clearly two distinct realities in Portugal: Western Portugal between the two metropolitan areas, with a high level of accessibility, and the remaining country, with low level of accessibility, with the exception for the district capital regions.

Other authors identified the good levels of access to hospital care and also this dichotomy of the Portuguese territory [27,106,127–129]. However, the levels of accessibility differ among them due to different methods applied. By considering the year 2011 and the measurement of geographical accessibility to the closest hospital, Perista [93] stated that over 90% of the population is deemed to live within a radius of 15 min travel by road; Polzin and colleagues [106] found that 92% of the Portuguese population has good geographical accessibility; Lopes and colleagues [130] concluded that they are 98% of the population; Sá Marques and colleagues quantified 99% of the population requiring until half an hour to reach the hospital.

Several factors influence the decrease in the population-weighted driving time to the reference hospital and the improvement of geographical accessibility between 1991 and 2011, namely (1) the extension of the road network; (2) changes to the hospital distribution and catchment area; (3) demographic changes in population distribution.

First, the significant expansion of the Portuguese road network contributed to a major decrease in distances between main cities located in the littoral and inland areas [131,132]. Between 1991 and 2011 the dimension of the road network with a speed-limit higher than 100 km/h increased from 1358 km to 5045 km. This threefold increase in the road network was one of the main goals of public policies supported by the European Commission and the Portuguese Government [27]. More than half of the population benefited directly from this improvement with the construction of highways. Nonetheless, there is a concentration of these roads along the littoral, linking the metropolitan areas, and West–East highways, built to facilitate the connection between the littoral and Spain.

Second, the distribution of hospitals in Portugal did not have major changes: two new hospitals were built between 1991 and 2011 in both metropolitan areas and in places where existing hospitals did not have enough capacity to address the population health' needs. Over time, preference was given to the reconstruction and construction of hospitals on the outskirts of the cities to replace the previous ones [133]. Still, almost 62% of the population lives in municipalities where the reference hospital changed over time. In 1999, hospitals started organizing into hospital centers with two to four small hospitals located in neighborhood municipalities [122,123]. This reorganization aimed to address the geographical disparities [93] and it was able to improve accessibility, especially from those communities on the outskirts of the municipalities that were closer to another hospital. However, in 2011 there were municipalities that were not assigned to the closest hospital and the difference in the population-weighted driving time was significatively high (more than 15 min). These municipalities are closer to small social hospitals that do not have enough human and technological resources to provide healthcare for people outside their catchment area.

Finally, the demographic changes between regions (from inland to littoral) and within municipalities (from rural to urban) is partially responsible for changes in population mobility, affecting almost three quarters of the population. The population living in inland municipalities decreased (some by more than 10%), in opposition to the municipalities along the littoral [134] where most hospitals are concentrated. Additionally, within most municipalities, the population is leaving the rural areas and becoming concentrated in cities and villages—namely young adults. Note that, in 1991, less than a half of the population was living in urban settlements with more than 2000 inhabitants (48%). In 2011, 61% of the population was living in urban settlements [135]. Nonetheless, although population living in urban areas is increasing in Portugal, the share of the population living in rural areas is still high compared to other European Countries, and more than half lives in remote areas [136]. Therefore, Portugal remains a polarized country whose littoral is characterized by high accessibility, urban development and higher population density, in contrast with the municipalities located inland, revealing low-density and increasingly vulnerability to depopulation and ageing. Notice that the population that lives in inland municipalities from the Norte (North) and Centro (Central) Regions face challenges due to the sharp hilly terrain and those from Alentejo and Algarve face issues with the low density of the road network.

4.2. Municipalities Requiring Higher Attention

Geographical access models have enormous potential for informing local decision-makers on how to achieve social equity on hospital accessibility [111]. They offer critical information suitable for planning and service provision as it allows for the identification of areas with lower (or higher) access to healthcare resources, the assessment of spatial and social inequalities in access, and the identification of underserved populations [18,95,111].

Focusing on the results of the population-weighted driving time results, this study highlights the less empowered municipalities facing barriers to access and requiring intervention to improve geographical access to a hospital: municipalities (1) with a population-weighted driving time exceeding 30 min to reach healthcare services; (2) closer the border; (3) with a high rate of older population; (4) with a higher rate of premature mortality.

First, our results stress that 7.2% of the population live in municipalities whose population-weighted driving time is higher than 30 min and more than 50 thousand inhabitants live in municipalities with an average driving time higher than 60 min. Those communities are located in municipalities that are mainly rural, inland and from the Alentejo region where population density is lower and distances between communities are longer as the road network is not so developed.

Second, the municipalities closer to the Spanish border have the worst accessibility, as also stated by other authors [27]. Border regions are often seen as poorly connected, and with reduced accessibility, relative to the central regions [137,138]. The lack of accessible health services is one of the major issues explaining the depopulation process in these areas [128].

Third, access to hospitals is particularly relevant for the elderly population with limited mobility and revenue. However, higher rates of elderly people are found in municipalities with worse access to hospitals; namely those living on the north–south central axis that crosses Portugal. As previously noted, this is due to the demographic changes occurring in Portugal. Younger populations often present higher mobility than older ones, mainly due to the former's search for employment. The metropolitan areas, as well as the municipalities on the littoral, are those attracting younger people. Thus, some municipalities are simultaneously presenting both a loss of younger people and an ageing population. Previous studies have already identified this phenomenon: regions with the lowest levels of accessibility are often regions with the biggest share of the elderly population [27,66,98]. Moreover, the elderly were already identified as one of the most vulnerable groups accessing health [128,139], especially during the economic crisis [44], and access to healthcare is associated with old-age survival [140]. According to Padeiro [5], in ageing societies, the time and distance to healthcare services require a better match between location policies and demand for services. This issue is even more problematic in Portugal due to the high dependency on cars for daily journeys, combined with the fact that most of the older population no longer holds a driving license (2016; 63,6%). According to Comber and Colleagues [16], non-car ownership is a significant predictor of difficulty in accessing critical infrastructure, such as hospitals, and it is even more significant than geographical distance with respect to utilization.

The lack of accessibility does not only affect the elderly. Premature mortality, an indicator that accounts for deaths before the age of 75, is also a constant concern in some municipalities with a population-weighted driving time higher than 30 min, both on the border with Spain and in the central axis across Portugal. Previous studies already highlighted increasing mortality in Portugal in the context of decreasing health services [128]. This reveals that primary care is not able to bridge the gap in access and that there is an urgent need to increase the number of contacts with healthcare and provide preventable and specialized care. It is known that remote access to healthcare structures constitute a barrier that discourages healthcare consumption [141], so it is important to improve access.

Since it is not possible to build a multi-specialized hospital in every municipality, results reveal where it is important to act and the importance of designing public policies at local level and promoting interventions able to overcome the lack of geographical accessibility to the hospital.

Municipalities with the worst geographical access might promote the organization of services into Local Health Units, namely in the center of the Centro region and in the Alentejo region. Those whose services are already organized in this type of structure might enhance communication between services to promote better access to specialized care. According to our results, seven out the eight Local Health Units available in Portugal are in areas with average to bad geographical accessibility, located closer to the Spanish border. These units integrate local hospitals and related primary care centers into a unique provider entity, based partly on geographical proximity and partly on the balance of specialties and availability of an emergency department [142]. These units can also help to overcome a major barrier to access healthcare in Portugal, by improving the lack of coordination or communication between services [44,93] and improving access for those living far from the hospital and closer to a primary health care center.

Municipalities located near the border with Spain might assist in the establishment of agreements with Spanish healthcare services located near the border. The Euroregions, a transnational co-operation structure between contiguous territories located in different European countries, are intended to help reduce the disadvantages of the border regions, promote their integrated development and improve the living conditions of the population in these areas [143] so they represent an excellent tool for promoting access to health. There are four official Euroregions joining Portuguese and Spanish municipalities. However, only two of them have established health as a priority, although information about the type of partnerships [138,144,145] was unavailable. Besides these, some regions are implementing some initiatives. For instance, the Centro (PT) and Castille and Léon (ES) regions have implemented a cross-border innovation network for the early diagnosis of leukaemia, and the Local Health Unit of Guarda (PT) and the University Hospital of Salamanca (ES) set a protocol that helps the Portuguese unit to request support with surgical interventions and medical examinations or clinical support from human resources in those specialties [146]. Local decision-makers with closer healthcare services on the other side of the border (e.g., hospitals located in Vigo, Badajoz and Huelva), should promote these types of partnerships and seek fundraising for the implementation of projects that can bring added value to both sides of the border.

Finally, municipalities with a high rate of elderly people and/or high rates of premature mortality might also consider telehealth as a viable solution to overcome the distance to the hospital and provide the early detection of some pathologies. According to the literature, when compared to face-to-face consultations, telehealth affords doctors the ability to see a higher volume of patients, a broader geographical reach, a shorter waiting time and a more effective way to reduce avoidable hospitalizations [147]. Still, in order to achieve these benefits, it is important that primary care has adequate technology to support the examinations and communicate the results, and that doctors and other health professionals receive training on how to use those technologies [148]. Municipalities can act on both issues and, thus, provide improved access to healthcare.

The reasons behind poor accessibility are complex and some territories will require more than one solution. Successful implementation will rely on excellent digital communication infrastructure, cooperation between services and adequate information about the new solutions for both health professionals and the general public.

4.3. Relevance of the Population-Weighted Driving Time Indicator

To date, there is no consensus on a standard measure, accurate representation and adequate way to communicate geographical accessibility [16,27,31,105,149], so most authors defend the use of simpler accessibility measures [150]. Still, the population-weighted driving time indicator revealed to be the adequate method to measure geographical accessibility from the Portuguese municipalities to the reference hospital. Considering the five parameters previously discussed, this indicator deploys on the census tract delimitation (the definition of the residential area), the number of inhabitants on the census tract (the aggregation method), the time to the hospital (the measurement of geographical accessibility between demand and supply), the distance based on a network (the type of distance) and the outcome revealed in minutes (the unit of measurement).

Three main reasons explain the relevance of this indicator to measure geographic access to healthcare.

The first one concerns the spatial resolution of the data. Portugal has very different administrative units in terms of area: the North has much smaller administrative units when compared to the administrative units in the South. The geographic variation in the dimension in area of the administrative units poses a problem of bias in the results of calculating accessibility weighted by the population when using the municipality centroid or the parish. For this reason, the centroid of the census tract (thinner spatial unit) was used to calculate the travel time and to use the population value (weight) that this census tract contains. The increase in the spatial resolution of the data increases the quality of the population and the travel time. In fact, this had already been addressed by some authors [117,151] as a problem that influences the quality of spatial data collection. The results achieved with this indicator have greater accuracy and are more useful to policy makers because they better reveal local problems (very fine scale) of accessibility to hospitals.

The second one concerns the scale. Small-area is the most adequate to capture the right level of areal differentiation and to avoid estimation errors [77,95,98,100,115,118]. However, it is less relevant for decision-makers since it does not adequately fit their needs. Displaying results in units of analysis that are significant to decision-makers will increase the likelihood that such results will be embedded in policy [15,77,112]. Therefore, finding the scale that better fits the evaluation and decision is not easy, as well as the balance between accuracy and relevance that might compromise further action. With this method, it is possible to move from a small-area level geographic accessibility indicator to a local one without falling into a statistical bias that may lead to different conclusions and policies [115,152]. Population-weighted accessibility metrics minimizes those errors since they account for the uneven population distribution within a study area and integrate the power and flexibility of the spatial interaction model-based approach [29]. Therefore, these measures fit better in studies where geographical accessibility is included as a dimension of the territory to investigate the association with health outcomes [98]. Thus, the characteristics of this metric make it easily applied to any administrative level and a useful tool for decision-makers, contributing to the design of policies and intervention programs. For example, it can be used to identify the extent to which people living in different locations may "gain or lose" from the applications of those planning policies or programs. This way, it is a decision-making support tool with the capacity to improve evaluation and, at the same time, decision-making at local, regional and national levels.

The last reason is based on the outcome result. The population-weighted driving time results are presented as time, measured in minutes. Since it is a universal measure directly interpretable in absolute units, as such it does not require any comparison with other values to be understandable. Thus, population-weighted driving time significantly enhances understanding of access to healthcare services by providing legible information that raises awareness and promotes evidence-based governance and contributes towards a productive discourse on future directions for healthcare planning.

Hence, the population-weighted driving time approach: (1) is much easier to use; (2) is sensitive to locally low areas of accessibility where populations live; (3) considers the population distribution at small-area level; (4) provides prompt awareness of priority interventions to national and local decision-makers regarding which regions require interventions. Moreover, the population-weighted bottom-up approach provides great flexibility in generating geographical accessibility measures at any geographic level that could be linked with population health outcomes of interest [29]. Therefore, it is valuable for policymakers to optimize current service provision and organization, which may lead to improved efficiency and reduced inequality, and for researchers to gain a better understanding of the mechanisms underlying inequality in care. The relevance of the calculation of potential geographical access to health equipment is fundamental for the pursuit of the policies of service providers, given that there is a constant need to monitor compliance with national guidelines on equity, to ensure full coverage of the provision healthcare services and their operational management and to contribute to the consolidation of future planning policies at the national, regional and local level.

4.4. Limitations and Future Developments of the Indicator

From our knowledge this is the first study in Portugal considering geographical accessibility based on the catchment area of the hospitals. Most studies published to date consider the closest hospital to evaluate geographical accessibility in Portugal [27,105,106,127]. This was due to some instability in the delimitation of the hospital catchment areas and the constant changes in the hierarchical organization. Moreover, it is the first study that provides evidence on the inappropriateness of considering the centroid of the municipality to account for the whole of the population in Portugal, ignoring the spatial distribution of the population inside the municipality, especially in rural areas where census tracts mostly have lower population densities and where land use is largely non-residential.

Nonetheless, the methodology presents some limitations requiring awareness. First, geographical accessibility is modelled as a static concept with no consideration of temporal variations in services and transportation provision across the diurnal cycle and week. Second, the method considers ideal travel conditions for all individuals, without considering issues, such as road congestion and means of transportation. Third, population-weighted driving times only account for spatial aspects of accessibility and do not take into account the fact that healthcare services are different between them and are spatially and temporally linked in chains or even consider the financial, social or economic constraints in the access to the hospital [76,153]. Fourth, the grained scale could be even smaller by considering the building block where the population lives. Finally, this metric is dependent on the census survey since there are no projections of population by census tract, so updating it is only possible every ten years.

Further enhancements can be introduced on future studies to improve the detail obtained by this metric. For example, other studies might consider different data regarding the health services (e.g., integrate the Spanish hospitals closer to the border, evaluate geographical accessibility to the closest hospital, consider the hospital capacity or other types of health services), the transportation mode (e.g., calculate the time by public transportation according to the main transportation mode used by the population or using the average travel speed on the road) and the population (e.g., taking into account the age of the population and its potential use in health services annually and the temporal fluctuations in population or applying a distance decay based on real utilization of the services).

5. Conclusions

This study provides evidence that, although geographical access has improved over the years, municipalities still present considerable differences in terms of the time it takes to reach the reference hospital. The results highlight that inequalities are still visible, especially in municipalities with a high share of older population, a population-weighted time greater than 30 min and border communities that require higher attention.

By reflecting the current status of the geographical accessibility of the Portuguese municipalities, these findings can contribute to the decision-making process, both local and national, in terms of directing the current and future efforts to reduce disparities between municipalities. Notice that municipalities with weak geographical accessibility have been spotted, explained, discussed and suggestions have been put forward for policy-makers.

The value of using this approach has also been demonstrated and contributes to the field of healthcare planning, population health, public health and probably to other human services. Although this study focuses on a European Union' peripheric country, such as Portugal, the methodology illustrates possibilities for future research to inform local, regional and national healthcare planning and implementation elsewhere. These results exhibit that it is possible to bring the detail of small-area level information to a larger administrative level by producing an indicator that is directly interpretable in absolute units and is, therefore, easily communicable to and readily understood by policy makers and civil society. This advantage is a direct outcome of the spatial resolution and of the aggregation method this research has achieved. Thus, this method is a step forward in terms of measuring and communicating geographical accessibility.

Author Contributions: Cláudia Costa: Conceptualization, Methodology, Investigation, Writing—Original Draft Preparation, Writing—Review and Editing; José António Tenedório: Methodology, Writing—Review and Editing, Supervision; Paula Santana: Writing—Review and Editing, Funding Acquisition, Supervision. All authors have read and agreed to the published version of the manuscript.

Funding: This research was supported by a Research fellow from the Portuguese Science and Technology Foundation (SFRH/BD/132218/2017), the project GeoHealthS—"Geography of Health Status. An application of a Population Health Index in the last 20 Years" (PTDC/CS-GEO/122566/2010), the project GRAMPCITY—Moving towards accessible and inclusive urban environments for our elders (PTDC/GES-TRA/32121/2017), and received support from the Centre of Studies in Geography and Spatial Planning (CEGOT), funded by national funds through the Foundation for Science and Technology (FCT) under the reference UIDB/04084/2020.

Acknowledgments: The researchers would like to thank to ESRI—Portugal, Statistics Portugal and the Central Administration of the Health Ministry for providing access to the data. The researchers would also like to thank Adriana Loureiro, Ricardo Almendra, Ângela Freitas, Iwa Stefanik and Joaquim Patriarca for assistance with the analysis and to Karen Bennett, Scott M. Culp and Linda Naughton for reviewing the manuscript.

Conflicts of Interest: The authors declare no conflict of interest.

References

1. Santana, P.; Almendra, R. The health of the Portuguese over the last four decades. *Méditerranée* **2018**. [CrossRef]
2. Yang, D.-H.H.; Goerge, R.; Mullner, R. Comparing GIS-Based Methods of Measuring Spatial Accessibility to Health Services. *J. Med. Syst.* **2006**, *30*, 23–32. [CrossRef]
3. Gu, X.; Zhang, L.; Tao, S.; Xie, B. Spatial accessibility to healthcare services in metropolitan suburbs: The case of qingpu, Shanghai. *Int. J. Environ. Res. Public Health* **2019**, *16*, 225. [CrossRef]
4. Yenisetty, P.T.; Bahadure, P. Measuring Accessibility to Various ASFs from Public Transit using Spatial Distance Measures in Indian Cities. *ISPRS Int. J. Geo-Inf.* **2020**, *9*, 446. [CrossRef]
5. Padeiro, M. Comparing alternative methods to measuring pedestrian access to community pharmacies. *Health Serv. Outcomes Res. Methodol.* **2018**, *18*, 1–16. [CrossRef]
6. European Commission. *Delivering the Sustainable Development Goals at Local and Regional Level*; European Commission: Brussels, Belgium, 2018.
7. Zaucha, J.; Komornicki, T.; Böhme, K.; Świątek, D.; Zuber, P. Territorial Keys for Bringing Closer the Territorial Agenda of the EU and Europe 2020. *Eur. Plan. Stud.* **2014**. [CrossRef]
8. Murad, A. Using GIS for Determining Variations in Health Access in Jeddah City, Saudi Arabia. *ISPRS Int. J. Geo-Inf.* **2018**, *7*, 254. [CrossRef]
9. Khakh, A.K.; Fast, V.; Shahid, R. Spatial accessibility to primary healthcare services by multimodal means of travel: Synthesis and case study in the city of calgary. *Int. J. Environ. Res. Public Health* **2019**, *16*, 270. [CrossRef]
10. El-Geneidy, A.M.; Levinson, D.M. *Access to Destinations: Development of Accessibility Measures*; Minnesota Department of Transportation Research Services Section: Minneapolis, MN, USA, 2006.
11. Penchansky, R.; Thomas, J.W. The concept of access: Definition and relationship to consumer satisfaction. *Med. Care* **1981**, *19*, 127–140. [CrossRef] [PubMed]
12. Gulzar, L. Access to health care. *J. Nurs. Scholarsh.* **1999**. [CrossRef] [PubMed]
13. Joseph, A.E.; Phillips, D.R. *Accessibility and Utilization: Geographical Perspectives on Health Care Delivery*; Harper & Row: London, UK, 1984; ISBN 0063182769.
14. Guagliardo, M.F. Spatial accessibility of primary care: Concepts, methods and challenges. *Int. J. Health Geogr.* **2004**, *3*, 3. [CrossRef] [PubMed]

15. Geurs, K.T.; van Wee, B. Accessibility evaluation of land-use and transport strategies: Review and research directions. *J. Transp. Geogr.* **2004**. [CrossRef]
16. Comber, A.J.; Brunsdon, C.; Radburn, R. A spatial analysis of variations in health access: Linking geography, socio-economic status and access perceptions. *Int. J. Health Geogr.* **2011**, *10*. [CrossRef]
17. Joseph, A.E.; Bantock, P.R. Measuring potential physical accessibility to general practitioners in rural areas: A method and case study. *Soc. Sci. Med.* **1982**, *16*, 85–90. [CrossRef]
18. Ni, J.; Liang, M.; Lin, Y.; Wu, Y.; Wang, C. Multi-Mode Two-Step Floating Catchment Area (2SFCA) Method to Measure the Potential Spatial Accessibility of Healthcare Services. *ISPRS Int. J. Geo-Inf.* **2019**, *8*, 236. [CrossRef]
19. Mizen, A.; Fry, R.; Grinnell, D.; Rodgers, S.E. Quantifying the Error Associated with Alternative GIS-based Techniques to Measure Access to Health Care Services. *AIMS Public Health* **2015**, *2*, 746–761. [CrossRef] [PubMed]
20. Zhou, X.; Yu, Z.; Yuan, L.; Wang, L.; Wu, C. Measuring Accessibility of Healthcare Facilities for Populations with Multiple Transportation Modes Considering Residential Transportation Mode Choice. *ISPRS Int. J. Geo-Inf.* **2020**, *9*, 394. [CrossRef]
21. Lee Deborah, O.M.; Lung Chiu, M.Y.; Cao, K. Geographical accessibility of community health assist system general practitioners for the elderly population in singapore: A case study on the elderly living in housing development board flats. *Int. J. Environ. Res. Public Health* **2018**, *15*, 1988. [CrossRef]
22. Geurs, K.T.; Ritsema van Eck, J. *Accessibility Measures: Review and Applications*; Rijksinstituut voor Volksgezondheid en Milieu: Utrecht, The Netherlands, 2001; Volume 787. Available online: wwww.rivm.nl/bibliotheek/rapporten/408505006.html (accessed on 6 April 2020).
23. Santana, P.; Freitas, A.; Costa, C.; Vaz, A.; Freitas, Â.; Costa, C.; Vaz, A. Evaluating Population Health: The selection of main Dimensions and Indicators through a participatory approach. *Eur. J. Geogr.* **2015**, *6*, 51–63.
24. McGrail, M.R. Spatial accessibility of primary health care utilising the two step floating catchment area method: An assessment of recent improvements. *Int. J. Health Geogr.* **2012**, *11*, 50. [CrossRef]
25. Santana, P. *Acessibilidade e Utilização dos Serviços de Saúde. Ensaio Metodológico em Geografia da Saúde*; CCDR-Centro/ARSCentro: Coimbra, Portugal, 1995.
26. McLafferty, S.L. GIS and health care. *Annu. Rev. Public Health* **2003**, *24*, 25–42. [CrossRef] [PubMed]
27. Sá Marques, T.; Saraiva, M.; Ribeiro, D.; Amante, A.; Silva, D.; Melo, P. Accessibility to services of general interest in polycentric urban system planning: The case of Portugal. *Eur. Plan. Stud.* **2020**. [CrossRef]
28. Maheswaran, R.; Pearson, T.; Jordan, H.; Black, D. Socioeconomic deprivation, travel distance, location of service, and uptake of breast cancer screening in North Derbyshire, UK. *J. Epidemiol. Community Health* **2006**, *60*, 208. [CrossRef]
29. Lu, H.; Zhang, X.; Holt, J.B.; Kanny, D.; Croft, J.B. Quantifying spatial accessibility in public health practice and research: An application to on-premise alcohol outlets, United States, 2013. *Int. J. Health Geogr.* **2018**, *17*, 23. [CrossRef]
30. Apparicio, P.; Cloutier, M.S.; Shearmur, R. The case of Montréal's missing food deserts: Evaluation of accessibility to food supermarkets. *Int. J. Health Geogr.* **2007**. [CrossRef] [PubMed]
31. Neutens, T. Accessibility, equity and health care: Review and research directions for transport geographers. *J. Transp. Geogr.* **2015**, *43*, 14–27. [CrossRef]
32. Pearce, J.; Witten, K.; Hiscock, R.; Blakely, T. Are socially disadvantaged neighbourhoods deprived of health-related community resources? *Int. J. Epidemiol.* **2007**, *36*, 348–355. [CrossRef]
33. Kelly, C.; Hulme, C.; Farragher, T.; Clarke, G. Are differences in travel time or distance to healthcare for adults in global north countries associated with an impact on health outcomes? A systematic review. *BMJ Open* **2016**, *6*. [CrossRef]
34. Bissonnette, L.; Wilson, K.; Bell, S.; Shah, T.I. Neighbourhoods and potential access to health care: The role of spatial and aspatial factors. *Health Place* **2012**. [CrossRef]
35. Rosero-Bixby, L. Spatial access to health care in Costa Rica and its equity: A GIS-based study. *Soc. Sci. Med.* **2004**, *58*, 1271–1284. [CrossRef]
36. Wang, F.; McLafferty, S.; Escamilla, V.; Luo, L. Late-stage breast cancer diagnosis and health care access in Illinois. *Prof. Geogr.* **2008**. [CrossRef] [PubMed]
37. Hsia, R.Y.J.; Shen, Y.C. Rising closures of hospital trauma centers disproportionately Burden vulnerable populations. *Health Aff.* **2011**. [CrossRef] [PubMed]

38. Fayet, Y.; Coindre, J.M.; Dalban, C.; Gouin, F.; De Pinieux, G.; Farsi, F.; Ducimetière, F.; Chemin-Airiau, C.; Jean-Denis, M.; Chabaud, S.; et al. Geographical accessibility of the referral networks in france. Intermediate results from the IGéAS research program. *Int. J. Environ. Res. Public Health* **2018**, *15*, 2204. [CrossRef] [PubMed]
39. Baird, G.; Flynn, R.; Baxter, G.; Donnelly, M.; Lawrence, J. Travel time and cancer care: An example of the inverse care law? *Rural Remote Health* **2008**. [CrossRef]
40. Onega, T.; Duell, E.J.; Shi, X.; Wang, D.; Demidenko, E.; Goodman, D. Geographic access to cancer care in the U.S. *Cancer* **2008**. [CrossRef]
41. Blais, S.; Dejardin, O.; Boutreux, S.; Launoy, G. Social determinants of access to reference care centres for patients with colorectal cancer–A multilevel analysis. *Eur. J. Cancer* **2006**. [CrossRef]
42. Wu, H.C.; Tseng, M.H. Evaluating disparities in elderly community care resources: Using a geographic accessibility and inequality index. *Int. J. Environ. Res. Public Health* **2018**, *15*, 1353. [CrossRef]
43. Buchmueller, T.C.; Jacobson, M.; Wold, C. How far to the hospital? The effect of hospital closures on access to care. *J. Health Econ.* **2006**. [CrossRef]
44. Doetsch, J.; Pilot, E.; Santana, P.; Krafft, T. Potential barriers in healthcare access of the elderly population influenced by the economic crisis and the troika agreement: A qualitative case study in Lisbon, Portugal. *Int. J. Equity Health* **2017**, *16*, 184. [CrossRef]
45. Arcury, T.A.; Gesler, W.M.; Preisser, J.S.; Sherman, J.; Spencer, J.; Perin, J. The effects of geography and spatial behavior on health care utilization among the residents of a rural region. *Health Serv. Res.* **2005**, *40*, 135–155. [CrossRef]
46. Syed, S.T.; Gerber, B.S.; Sharp, L.K. Traveling towards disease: Transportation barriers to health care access. *J. Community Health* **2013**, *38*, 976–993. [CrossRef] [PubMed]
47. Pierce, R.P.; Williamson, H.A.; Kruse, R.L. Distance, use of resources, and mortality among rural Missouri residents with acute myocardial infarction. *J. Rural Health* **1998**. [CrossRef]
48. Friedman, J.M.; Hagander, L.; Hughes, C.D.; Nash, K.A.; Linden, A.F.; Blossom, J.; Meara, J.G. Distance to hospital and utilization of surgical services in Haiti: Do children, delivering mothers, and patients with emergent surgical conditions experience greater geographical barriers to surgical care? *Int. J. Health Plan. Manag.* **2013**. [CrossRef] [PubMed]
49. Brual, J.; Gravely-Witte, S.; Suskin, N.; Stewart, D.E.; Macpherson, A.; Grace, S.L. Drive time to cardiac rehabilitation: At what point does it affect utilization? *Int. J. Health Geogr.* **2010**, *9*, 1–11. [CrossRef] [PubMed]
50. Målqvist, M.; Sohel, N.; Do, T.T.; Eriksson, L.; Persson, L.Å. Distance decay in delivery care utilisation associated with neonatal mortality. A case referent study in northern Vietnam. *BMC Public Health* **2010**. [CrossRef]
51. Monnet, E.; Ramée, C.; Minello, A.; Jooste, V.; Carel, D.; Di Martino, V. Socioeconomic context, distance to primary care and detection of hepatitis C: A French population-based study. *Soc. Sci. Med.* **2008**. [CrossRef]
52. De Souza, V.C.; Strachan, D.P. Relationship between travel time to the nearest hospital and survival from ruptured abdominal aortic aneurysms: Record linkage study. *J. Public Health* **2005**. [CrossRef]
53. Wei, L.; Lang, C.C.; Sullivan, F.M.; Boyle, P.; Wang, J.; Pringle, S.D.; MacDonald, T.M. Impact on mortality following first acute myocardial infarction of distance between home and hospital: Cohort study. *Heart* **2008**. [CrossRef]
54. Lyon, R.M.; Cobbe, S.M.; Bradley, J.M.; Grubb, N.R. Surviving out of hospital cardiac arrest at home: A postcode lottery? *Emerg. Med. J.* **2004**, *21*, 619–624. [CrossRef]
55. Jones, A.P.; Haynes, R.; Sauerzapf, V.; Crawford, S.M.; Zhao, H.; Forman, D. Travel times to health care and survival from cancers in Northern England. *Eur. J. Cancer* **2008**, *44*, 269–274. [CrossRef]
56. Campbell, N.C.; Elliott, A.M.; Sharp, L.; Ritchie, L.D.; Cassidy, J.; Little, J. Rural and urban differences in stage at diagnosis of colorectal and lung cancers. *Br. J. Cancer* **2001**. [CrossRef] [PubMed]
57. Jones, A.P.; Haynes, R.; Sauerzapf, V.; Crawford, S.M.; Zhao, H.; Forman, D. Travel time to hospital and treatment for breast, colon, rectum, lung, ovary and prostate cancer. *Eur. J. Cancer* **2008**, *44*, 992–999. [CrossRef]
58. Jones, A.P.; Bentham, G.; Horwell, C. Health service accessibility and deaths from asthma. *Int. J. Epidemiol.* **1999**. [CrossRef] [PubMed]

59. Combier, E.; Charreire, H.; Le Vaillant, M.; Michaut, F.; Ferdynus, C.; Amat-Roze, J.M.; Gouyon, J.B.; Quantin, C.; Zeitlin, J. Perinatal health inequalities and accessibility of maternity services in a rural French region: Closing maternity units in Burgundy. *Health Place* **2013**, *24*, 225–233. [CrossRef] [PubMed]
60. Ravelli, A.; Jager, K.; de Groot, M.; Erwich, J.; Rijninks-van Driel, G.; Tromp, M.; Eskes, M.; Abu-Hanna, A.; Mol, B. Travel time from home to hospital and adverse perinatal outcomes in women at term in the Netherlands. *BJOG Int. J. Obstet. Gynaecol.* **2011**, *118*, 457–465. [CrossRef]
61. Campbell, N.C.; Elliott, A.M.; Sharp, L.; Ritchie, L.D.; Cassidy, J.; Little, J. Rural factors and survival from cancer: Analysis of Scottish cancer registrations. *Br. J. Cancer* **2000**. [CrossRef]
62. McCoy, C.E.; Menchine, M.; Sampson, S.; Anderson, C.; Kahn, C. Emergency medical services out-of-hospital scene and transport times and their association with mortality in trauma patients presenting to an urban level i trauma center. *Ann. Emerg. Med.* **2013**, *61*, 167–174. [CrossRef]
63. Clarke, J.R.; Trooskin, S.Z.; Doshi, P.J.; Greenwald, L.; Mode, C.J. Time to laparotomy for intra-abdominal bleeding from trauma does affect survival for delays up to 90 min. *J. Trauma* **2002**. [CrossRef]
64. Taylor, A.; Pettit, C. Are Health Services in New South Wales Available Where They are Needed? Using AURIN to Understand the Equity of Service Distribution and Future Demand. *Appl. Spat. Anal. Policy* **2020**. [CrossRef]
65. Braveman, P. What are Health Disparities and Health Equity? We Need to Be Clear. *Public Health Rep.* **2014**, *129*, 5–8. [CrossRef]
66. Ruiz, V.; Veneri, P. *Measuring the Access to Public Services: The Case of Public Hospitals*; OECD Working Party on Territorial Indicators: Paris, France, 2012.
67. Braveman, P. *Monitoring Equity in Health: A Policy-Oriented Approach in Low-And Middle-Income Countries (WHO/CHS/HSS/98.1)*; World Health Organization: Geneva, Switzerland, 1998.
68. Shen, Y.-C.; Hsia, R.Y. Changes in Emergency Department Access Between 2001 and 2005 Among General and Vulnerable Populations. *Am. J. Public Health* **2010**, *100*, 1462–1469. [CrossRef] [PubMed]
69. Casas, I.; Delmelle, E.; Varela, A. A Space-Time Approach to Diffusion of Health Service Provision Information. *Int. Reg. Sci. Rev.* **2010**, *33*, 134–156. [CrossRef]
70. Alcaraz, K.I.; Kreuter, M.W.; Bryan, R.P. Use of GIS to identify optimal settings for cancer prevention and control in African American communities. *Prev. Med.* **2009**, *49*, 54–57. [CrossRef] [PubMed]
71. Al-Taiar, A.; Clark, A.; Longenecker, J.C.; Whitty, C.J. Physical accessibility and utilization of health services in Yemen. *Int. J. Health Geogr.* **2010**, *9*, 38. [CrossRef] [PubMed]
72. Polo, G.; Acosta, C.M.; Ferreira, F.; Dias, R.A. Location-Allocation and Accessibility Models for Improving the Spatial Planning of Public Health Services. *PLoS ONE* **2015**, *10*, e0119190. [CrossRef]
73. Costa, C. *Localização Óptima do Futuro Hospital de Sintra: Aplicação de Modelos de Location-Allocation no Planeamento de Cuidados de Saúde*; NOVA Information Management School: Lisboa, Portugal, 2011.
74. Schuurman, N.; Fiedler, R.S.; Grzybowski, S.C.W.; Grund, D. Defining rational hospital catchments for non-urban areas based on travel-time. *Int. J. Health Geogr.* **2006**, *5*, 43. [CrossRef]
75. Patel, A.B.; Waters, N.M.; Ghali, W.A. Determining geographic areas and populations with timely access to cardiac catheterization facilities for acute myocardial infarction care in Alberta, Canada. *Int. J. Health Geogr.* **2007**, *6*, 47. [CrossRef]
76. Wan, N.; Zhan, F.B.; Zou, B.; Chow, E. A relative spatial access assessment approach for analyzing potential spatial access to colorectal cancer services in Texas. *Appl. Geogr.* **2012**, *32*, 291–299. [CrossRef]
77. Bell, S.; Wilson, K.; Bissonnette, L.; Shah, T. Access to Primary Health Care: Does Neighborhood of Residence Matter? *Ann. Assoc. Am. Geogr.* **2013**, *103*, 85–105. [CrossRef]
78. Ray, N.; Ebener, S. AccessMod 3.0: Computing geographic coverage and accessibility to health care services using anisotropic movement of patients. *Int. J. Health Geogr.* **2008**, *7*, 63. [CrossRef]
79. Braveman, P.; Gottlieb, L. The social determinants of health: It's time to consider the causes of the causes. *Public Health Rep.* **2014**, *129*, 19–31. [CrossRef] [PubMed]
80. Walsh, S.J.; Page, P.H.; Gesler, W.M. Normative models and healthcare planning: Network-based simulations within a geographic information system environment. *Health Serv. Res.* **1997**, *32*, 243. [PubMed]
81. Cai, E.; Liu, Y.; Jing, Y.; Zhang, L.; Li, J.; Yin, C. Assessing spatial accessibility of public and private residential aged care facilities: A case study in Wuhan, Central China. *ISPRS Int. J. Geo-Inf.* **2017**, *6*, 304. [CrossRef]
82. Hu, S.; Song, W.; Li, C.; Lu, J. The spatial equity of nursing homes in Changchun: A multi-trip modes analysis. *ISPRS Int. J. Geo-Inf.* **2019**, *8*, 223. [CrossRef]

83. Frew, R.; Higgs, G.; Harding, J.; Langford, M. Investigating geospatial data usability from a health geography perspective using sensitivity analysis: The example of potential accessibility to primary healthcare. *J. Transp. Health* **2017**, *6*, 128–142. [CrossRef]
84. Rodrigues, A.; Santana, P.; Santos, R.; Nogueira, H. Optimization of the Urgency-Emergency Network in Mainland Portugal: A methodology for the spatial reorganization of the existing capacity. In *Proceedings of the 47th Congress of European Regional Science Association "Local Governance and Sustainable Development"*; European Regional Science Association: Paris, France, 2007.
85. Shah, T.I.; Bell, S.; Wilson, K. Spatial accessibility to health care services: Identifying under-serviced neighbourhoods in Canadian urban areas. *PLoS ONE* **2016**, *11*, e0168208. [CrossRef]
86. Parker, E.B.; Campbell, J.L. Measuring access to primary medical care: Some examples of the use of geographical information systems. *Health Place* **1998**. [CrossRef]
87. Sasaki, S.; Comber, A.J.; Suzuki, H.; Brunsdon, C. Using genetic algorithms to optimise current and future health planning–the example of ambulance locations. *Int. J. Health Geogr.* **2010**. [CrossRef]
88. Baeten, R.; Spasova, S.; Vanhercke, B.; Coster, S. *Inequalities in Access to Healthcare. A study of National Policies 2018*; European Commission: Brussels, Belgium, 2018.
89. OECD/European Observatory on Health Systems and Policies. *Portugal: Country Health Profile 2017, State of Health in the EU*; OECD Publishing: Brussels, Belgium, 2017.
90. Santana, P. Utilização dos cuidados hospitalares: Uma abordagem da geografia da saúde. In *As Reformas dos Sistemas de Saúde*; Vaz, A., Ramos, F., Pereira, J., Eds.; APES: Lisboa, Portugal, 1996; pp. 182–208.
91. Vaz, S.; Ramos, P.; Santana, P. Distance effects on the accessibility to emergency departments in Portugal. *Saúde e Soc.* **2014**. [CrossRef]
92. Costa, C.; Tenedório, J.A.; Santana, P. Amenable mortality and the geographic accessibility to healthcare in Portugal. In Proceedings of the 3rd Congresso Internacional de Saúde do IPLeiria, Leiria, Portugal, 1 July 2016; Volume 16.
93. Perista, P. *ESPN Thematic Report on Inequalities in Access to Healthcare–Portugal*; European Commission: Brussels, Belgium, 2018.
94. Assembleia da República Lei-Quadro da Transferência de Competências para as Autarquias Locais e para as Entidades Intermunicipais. Available online: https://dre.pt/application/conteudo/116068877 (accessed on 10 June 2020).
95. Hewko, J.; Smoyer-Tomic, K.E.; Hodgson, M.J. Measuring neighbourhood spatial accessibility to urban amenities: Does aggregation error matter? *Environ. Plan. A* **2002**, *34*, 1185–1206. [CrossRef]
96. Apparicio, P.; Shearmur, R.G.; Brochu, M.; Dussault, G. The measure of distance in a social science policy context: Advantages and costs of using network distances in eight canadians metropolitan areas. *J. Geogr. Inf. Decis. Anal.* **2003**, *7*, I05–I31.
97. Handy, S.L.; Niemeier, D.A. Measuring Accessibility: An Exploration of Issues and Alternatives. *Environ. Plan. A Econ. Sp.* **1997**, *29*, 1175–1194. [CrossRef]
98. Apparicio, P.; Abdelmajid, M.; Riva, M.; Shearmur, R. Comparing alternative approaches to measuring the geographical accessibility of urban health services: Distance types and aggregation-error issues. *Int. J. Health Geogr.* **2008**, *7*, 7. [CrossRef] [PubMed]
99. Roquette, R.; Nunes, B.; Painho, M. The relevance of spatial aggregation level and of applied methods in the analysis of geographical distribution of cancer mortality in mainland Portugal (2009–2013). *Popul. Health Metr.* **2018**, *16*, 6. [CrossRef]
100. Apparicio, P.; Gelb, J.; Dubé, A.S.; Kingham, S.; Gauvin, L.; Robitaille, É. The approaches to measuring the potential spatial access to urban health services revisited: Distance types and aggregation-error issues. *Int. J. Health Geogr.* **2017**. [CrossRef]
101. Delamater, P.L.; Messina, J.P.; Shortridge, A.M.; Grady, S.C. Measuring geographic access to health care: Raster and network-based methods. *Int. J. Health Geogr.* **2012**, *11*, 15. [CrossRef]
102. Dewulf, B.; Neutens, T.; De Weerdt, Y.; Van De Weghe, N. Accessibility to primary health care in Belgium: An evaluation of policies awarding financial assistance in shortage areas. *BMC Fam. Pract.* **2013**. [CrossRef]
103. Luo, W.; Wang, F. Measures of spatial accessibility to health care in a GIS environment: Synthesis and a case study in the Chicago region. *Environ. Plan. B Plan. Des.* **2003**, *30*, 865–884. [CrossRef]
104. Boisjoly, G.; El-Geneidy, A. Daily fluctuations in transit and job availability: A comparative assessment of time-sensitive accessibility measures. *J. Transp. Geogr.* **2016**. [CrossRef]

105. Freiria, S.; Tavares, A.O.; Julião, R.P. The benefits of a link-based assessment of health services accessibility: Unveiling gaps in Central Region of Portugal. *Land Use Policy* **2019**, *87*, 104034. [CrossRef]
106. Polzin, P.; Borges, J.; Coelho, A. An extended kernel density two-step floating catchment area method to analyze access to health care. *Environ. Plan. B Plan. Des.* **2014**. [CrossRef]
107. Langford, M.; Higgs, G.; Jones, S. Understanding Spatial Variations in Accessibility to Banks Using Variable Floating Catchment Area Techniques. *Appl. Spat. Anal. Policy* **2020**, 1–24. [CrossRef]
108. Zhu, L.; Zhong, S.; Tu, W.; Zheng, J.; He, S.; Bao, J.; Huang, C. Assessing spatial accessibility to medical resources at the community level in shenzhen, China. *Int. J. Environ. Res. Public Health* **2019**, *16*, 242. [CrossRef] [PubMed]
109. Jamtsho, S.; Corner, R.; Dewan, A. Spatio-temporal analysis of spatial accessibility to primary health care in Bhutan. *ISPRS Int. J. Geo-Inf.* **2015**, *4*, 1584–1604. [CrossRef]
110. Padeiro, M. Geographical accessibility to community pharmacies by the elderly in metropolitan Lisbon. *Res. Soc. Adm. Pharm.* **2018**, *14*, 653–662. [CrossRef] [PubMed]
111. Brabyn, L.; Skelly, C. Modeling population access to New Zealand public hospitals. *Int. J. Health Geogr.* **2002**. [CrossRef]
112. Schuurman, N.; Bérubé, M.; Crooks, V.A. Measuring potential spatial access to primary health care physicians using a modified gravity model. *Can. Geogr./Le Géographe Can.* **2010**, *54*, 29–45. [CrossRef]
113. Bhat, C.; Handy, S.; Kockelman, K.; Mahmassani, H.; Chen, Q.; Weston, L.L.; Handy, S.; Mahmassani, H.; Weston, L.L. *Urban Accessibility Index: Literature Review*; The University of Texas at Austin: Austin, TX, USA, 2000.
114. Tenkanen, H.; Saarsalmi, P.; Järv, O.; Salonen, M.; Toivonen, T. Health research needs more comprehensive accessibility measures: Integrating time and transport modes from open data. *Int. J. Health Geogr.* **2016**, *15*, 23. [CrossRef] [PubMed]
115. Openshaw, S. *The Modifiable Areal Unit Problem. Concepts and Techniques in Modern Geography*; Geobooks: Norwich, UK, 1984.
116. Zhang, X.; Lu, H.; Holt, J.B. Modeling spatial accessibility to parks: A national study. *Int. J. Health Geogr.* **2011**, *10*, 31. [CrossRef]
117. Rodrigues, A.M.; Tenedório, J.A. Sensitivity analysis of spatial autocorrelation using distinct geometrical settings: Guidelines for the quantitative geographer. *Int. J. Agric. Environ. Inf. Syst.* **2016**. [CrossRef]
118. Diez Roux, A.V. Investigating neighborhood and area effects on health. *Am. J. Public Health* **2001**, *91*, 1783–1789. [CrossRef] [PubMed]
119. Almendra, R.; Santana, P.; Vasconcelos, J. Evidence of social deprivation on the spatial patterns of excess winter mortality. *Int. J. Public Health* **2017**, *62*, 849–856. [CrossRef] [PubMed]
120. Santana, P.; Costa, C.; Loureiro, A.; Raposo, J.; Boavida, J.M. The geography of Diabetes Mellitus in Portugal: How context influence the risk of dying. *Acta Med. Port.* **2014**, *27*, 309–317. [CrossRef] [PubMed]
121. Santana, P.; Costa, C.; Cardoso, G.; Loureiro, A.; Ferrão, J. Suicide in Portugal: Spatial determinants in a context of economic crisis. *Health Place* **2015**, *35*, 85–94. [CrossRef]
122. de Almeida Simoes, J.; Augusto, G.F.; Fronteira, I.; Hernandez-Quevedo, C. Portugal: Health System Review. *Health Syst. Transit.* **2017**, *19*, 1–184.
123. Santana, P. *A Geografia da Saúde da População. Evolução nos Últimos 20 anos em Portugal Continental*; Centro de Estudos de Geografia e Ordenamento do Território (CEGOT)–Universidade de Coimbra, Ed.; Universidade de Coimbra: Coimbra, Portugal, 2015.
124. Dimitrovová, K.; Perelman, J.; Serrano-Alarcón, M. Effect of a national primary care reform on avoidable hospital admissions (2000–2015): A difference-in-difference analysis. *Soc. Sci. Med.* **2020**, *252*, 112908. [CrossRef]
125. Rego, G.; Nunes, R.; Costa, J. The challenge of corporatisation: The experience of Portuguese public hospitals. *Eur. J. Health Econ.* **2010**, *11*, 367–381. [CrossRef]
126. OECD. OECD Review of Policy Indicators for Portugal. 2015. Available online: https://www.fct.pt/gabestudosestrategia/OCDE/docs/OECD_Policy_Indicators_for_Portugal_report.pdf. (accessed on 10 June 2020).
127. Lopes, H.S.; Ribeiro, V.; Remoaldo, P.C. Spatial Accessibility and Social Inclusion: The Impact of Portugal's Last Health Reform. *GeoHealth* **2019**. [CrossRef]

128. Vidal, D.G.; Pontes, M.; Barreira, E.; Oliveira, G.M.; Maia, R.L. Differential mortality and inequalities in health services access in Mainland Portugal. *Finisterra* **2018**, *53*, 53–70. [CrossRef]
129. Ferrão, J. Portugal, três geografias em recombinação: Espacialidades, mapas cognitivos e identidades territoriais. *Lusotopie* **2002**, *2*, 151–158.
130. Lopes, H.; Remoaldo, P. Acessibilidade espacial aos serviços de saúde em Portugal Continental. In *Proceedings of the XV Colóquio Ibérico de Geografia*; Associação Portuguesa de Geógrafos: Porto, Portugal, 2016.
131. European Commission. *Directorate General XVI. Thematic Study of Transport: Country Report Portugal*; European Commission (EC): Brussels, Belgium, 2000.
132. Pereira Rosmaninho, G. *The Regulation of Road Infrastructure Operators in Portugal*; Technical University of Lisbon: Lisbon, Portugal, 2010.
133. Santana, P. Os ganhos em saúde e no acesso aos serviços de saúde. In *30 anos do Serviço Nacional de Saúde: Um Percurso Comentado*; Simões, J., Ed.; Editora Almedina: Coimbra, Portugal, 2010.
134. Nicolau, R.; David, J.; Caetano, M.; Pereira, J.M.C. Ratio of land consumption rate to population growth rate-analysis of different formulations applied to mainland Portugal. *ISPRS Int. J. Geo-Inf.* **2019**, *8*, 10. [CrossRef]
135. Statistics National Institute. Censos 2011. Available online: https://www.ine.pt/xportal/xmain?xpid=INE&xpgid=ine_publicacoes&PUBLICACOESpub_boui=73212469&PUBLICACOESmodo=2 (accessed on 9 June 2020).
136. OECD. *OECD Regions and Cities at a Glance 2018*; OECD Regions and Cities at a Glance; OECD: Paris, France, 2018.
137. Condeço-Melhorado, A.; Christidis, P. Road Accessibility in Border Regions: A Joint Approach. *Netw. Spat. Econ.* **2018**. [CrossRef]
138. Vulevic, A.; Castanho, R.A.; Gómez, J.M.N.; Loures, L.; Cabezas, J.; Fernández-Pozo, L.; Gallardo, J.M.; Naranjo Gómez, J.M.; Loures, L.; Cabezas, J.; et al. Accessibility dynamics and regional cross-border cooperation (cbc) perspectives in the Portuguese-Spanish Borderland. *Sustainability* **2020**, *12*, 1978. [CrossRef]
139. Crisp, L.N.; Berwick, D.; Kickbusch, I.; Antunes, J.L.; Barros, P.P.; Soares, J. Um Futuro para a Saúde–Todos Temos um Papel a Desempenhar; Lisbon. Available online: https://content.gulbenkian.pt/wp-content/uploads/2016/03/30003652/PGIS_BrochuraRelatorioCompletoHealthPortugues.pdf (accessed on 9 June 2020).
140. Ribeiro, A.I.; Krainski, E.T.; Carvalho, M.S.; de Pina, M.D.F. The influence of socioeconomic deprivation, access to healthcare and physical environment on old-age survival in Portugal. *Geospat. Health* **2017**, *12*, 252–263. [CrossRef] [PubMed]
141. Andersen, R.M. Revisiting the behavioral model and access to medical care: Does it matter? *J. Health Soc. Behav.* **1995**. [CrossRef]
142. Pita, P.; Sara, B.; Machado, R.; De, J.; Simões, A. Health Systems in Transition. Available online: http://https://www.euro.who.int/__data/assets/pdf_file/0007/337471/HiT-Portugal.pdf?ua=1 (accessed on 4 July 2020).
143. Brand, H.; Hollederer, A.; Wolf, U.; Brand, A. Cross-border health activities in the Euregios: Good practice for better health. *Health Policy* **2008**, *86*, 245–254. [CrossRef] [PubMed]
144. Ferreira, V. Cross-border cooperation in the galicia-northern Portugal euroregion. *JANUS. NET* **2019**, *10*, 143–151. [CrossRef]
145. Durà, A.; Camonita, F.; Berzi, M.; Noferini, A. *Euroregions, Excellence and Innovation across EU Borders. A Catalogue of Good Practices.|FUTURIUM|European Commission*; Barcelona; Department of Geography: Abu Dhabi, UAE, 2018.
146. Regions for Health Network. *The Healthacross Initiative: How Lower Austria Is Boosting Cross-Border Collaboration in Health*; World Health Organization: Copenhagen, Denmark, 2018.
147. Lillicrap, L.; Hunter, C.; Goldswain, P. Improving geriatric care and reducing hospitalisations in regional and remote areas: The benefits of telehealth. *J. Telemed. Telecare* **2019**. [CrossRef] [PubMed]
148. Ferreira, D. Papel da Telesaúde em Tempos de Pandemia COVID-19: Para Grandes Males, Grandes Remédios The Role of Telehealth in the COVID-19 Era: Great Ills Require Great Remedies. *Med. Interna* **2020**, 1–5. [CrossRef]
149. Langford, M.; Fry, R.; Higgs, G. Measuring transit system accessibility using a modified two-step floating catchment technique. *Int. J. Geogr. Inf. Sci.* **2012**. [CrossRef]
150. Vandenbulcke, G.; Steenberghen, T.; Thomas, I. Mapping accessibility in Belgium: A tool for land-use and transport planning? *J. Transp. Geogr.* **2009**, *17*, 39–53. [CrossRef]

151. Tatem, A.J.; Adamo, S.; Bharti, N.; Burgert, C.R.; Castro, M.; Dorelien, A.; Fink, G.; Linard, C.; John, M.; Montana, L.; et al. Mapping populations at risk: Improving spatial demographic data for infectious disease modeling and metric derivation. *Popul. Health Metr.* **2012**. [CrossRef] [PubMed]
152. Costa, C.; Santana, P.; Santos, R.; Loureiro, A. Pre-School Facilities and Catchment Area Profiling: A Planning Support Method. In *Geospatial Thinking. Lecture Notes in Geoinformation and Cartography*; Paínho, M., Santos, M., Pundt, H., Eds.; Springer: Berlin/Heidelberg, Germany, 2010; pp. 97–117.
153. Neutens, T.; Delafontaine, M.; Scott, D.M.; De Maeyer, P. A GIS-based method to identify spatiotemporal gaps in public service delivery. *Appl. Geogr.* **2012**, *32*, 253–264. [CrossRef]

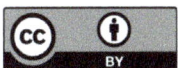 © 2020 by the authors. Licensee MDPI, Basel, Switzerland. This article is an open access article distributed under the terms and conditions of the Creative Commons Attribution (CC BY) license (http://creativecommons.org/licenses/by/4.0/).

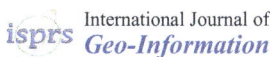

Article

Development of a Novel Framework to Propose New Strategies for Automated External Defibrillators Deployment Targeting Residential Out-Of-Hospital Cardiac Arrests: Application to the City of Milan

Gianquintieri Lorenzo [1], Brovelli Maria Antonia [2], Brambilla Piero Maria [3], Pagliosa Andrea [3], Villa Guido Francesco [3] and Caiani Enrico Gianluca [1,4,*]

[1] Electronics, Information and Biomedical Engineering dpt, Politecnico di Milano, 20133 Milano, Italy; lorenzo.gianquintieri@polimi.it
[2] Civil and Environmental Engineering dpt, Politecnico di Milano, 20133 Milano, Italy; maria.brovelli@polimi.it
[3] Azienda Regionale Emergenza Urgenza (AREU), 20124 Milano, Italy; p.brambilla@areu.lombardia.it (B.P.M.); a.pagliosa@areu.lombardia.it (P.A.); g.villa@areu.lombardia.it (V.G.F.)
[4] Consiglio Nazionale delle Ricerche, Istituto di Elettronica e di Ingegneria dell'Informazione e delle Telecomunicazioni, 20133 Milan, Italy
* Correspondence: enrico.caiani@polimi.it; Tel.: +39-02-2399-3390

Received: 7 July 2020; Accepted: 10 August 2020; Published: 17 August 2020

Abstract: Public Access Defibrillation (PAD) is the leading strategy in reducing time to first defibrillation in cases of Out-Of-Hospital Cardiac Arrest (OHCA), but PAD programs are underperforming considering their potentiality. Our aim was to develop an analysis and optimization framework, exploiting georeferenced information processed with Geographic Information Systems (GISs), specifically targeting residential OHCAs. The framework, based on an historical database of OHCAs, location of Automated External Defibrillators (AEDs), topographic and demographic information, proposes new strategies for AED deployment focusing on residential OHCAs, where performance assessment was evaluated using AEDs "catchment area" (area that can be reached within 6 min walk along streets). The proposed framework was applied to the city of Milan, Lombardy (Italy), considering the OHCA database of four years (2015–2018), including 8152 OHCA, of which 7179 (88.06%) occurred in residential locations. The proposed strategy for AEDs deployment resulted more effective compared to the existing distribution, with a significant improvement (from 41.77% to 73.33%) in OHCAs' spatial coverage. Further improvements were simulated with different cost scenarios, resulting in more cost-efficient solutions. Results suggest that PAD programs, either in brand-new territories or in further improvements, could significantly benefit from a comprehensive planning, based on mathematical models for risk mapping and on geographical tools.

Keywords: automated external defibrillator; public access defibrillation; out-of-hospital cardiac arrest; resuscitation; geographic information system; risk mapping

1. Introduction

The American Heart Association (AHA) defines Out–Of–Hospital Cardiac Arrest (OHCA) as the cessation of mechanical cardiac activity outside of a medical care setting [1]. Survival is strongly correlated with the time between OHCA occurrence and first defibrillation [2–5], with 6 min considered as the time limit for an effective intervention [6], as the survival probability declines by 7–12% for every minute of delay in the treatment [7–9]. To address the need for a fast emergency response, the leading strategy is constituted by Public Access Defibrillation (PAD), based on the placement of publicly accessible Automated External Defibrillators (AEDs, fully automatic devices composed by two electrodes to be placed on the patient, and a main body, which records the ECG signal and delivers electric shock if potentially necessary to restore the physiological rhythm) over the cities' territory [10], on the training of lay rescuers on how to perform Cardio-Pulmonary Resuscitation (CPR) and how to use AED, and on campaigns for awareness raising.

PAD programs are nowadays diffused worldwide [11,12], but it is recognized that they are underperforming, considering their potential [13–16]. In an attempt of improvement, recent research is focusing on the development of analysis and optimization frameworks [9,17–20], but, whereas current guidelines focus on public places with a significant flow of people during daytime, multiple statistical analyses revealed that 60%–80% of OHCAs usually occur in residential locations [18,21–25]. For example, in Sondergaard et al. [25], in a study aimed at assessing the impact of location of OHCA on rescue intervention timing and clinical outcome, it was shown that, from a database of 25,505 OHCA records that occurred in Denmark between 2001 and 2014, 26.4% of them occurred in public places, whereas 73.6% were in residential locations. Moreover, different studies [22,26,27] found out that residential OHCA is characterized by higher mortality when compared with OHCA in public places. This included the study by Folke et al. [22], in which, with the aim of identifying residential areas suitable for AED installation, from a database of 4828 OHCA records that occurred in Copenhagen from 1994 to 2005, it resulted that OHCA survival rates were 13.9% and 3.2% for public and residential locations, respectively. Although the likelihood of use of a publicly accessible AED is significantly lower in residential events when compared to public ones [28], recent studies highlighted, as a priority, the development of new strategies to reduce the mortality in residential areas by early defibrillation [22,25,29–31].

The frameworks proposed in previous studies for optimization of AED deployment are usually characterized by three main processes:

1. Efficiency analysis of the current distribution of AEDs, based on the area where AEDs can be used within the scientifically assessed time limit for an effective and beneficial use, hence there is no standard in how to convert this time limit into a spatial measure.
2. Mapping of OHCA occurrence risk by development of a geographic risk function using different approaches: purely statistical (simulation of events based on retrospective data or application of distribution models, such as Poisson regression or Kernel density analysis) or more sophisticated ones (modelling of explicative factors, relevant to demography, socio-economic conditions, and land-use). Given the intrinsic randomness of the phenomenon, both predictive performance and generalization of the proposed methods are uncertain.
3. Identification of new AED spatial distributions, based on the optimization of a target function, and assessment of the related performance by a validation procedure. Whereas the proposed mathematical optimizations of target functions are detailed and successful, their conversion into PAD performance improvement is hard to validate.

Recent research has identified Geographic Information Systems (GISs, a set of tools for capturing, storing, checking, manipulating, analyzing and displaying spatially georeferenced data [32]) as a key tool addressing the problem of optimizing PAD [33–35]. For example, in Ringh et al. [35], a study aimed at discussing existing evidence of Public Access Defibrillation and knowledge gaps and future directions to improve outcomes for OHCA, the use of GIS in planning deployment of AED is listed among the eight key actions to improve PAD results. We hypothesized that a GIS-based deployment strategy could be more successful in targeting residential OHCAs, as encouraged by multiple studies [22,25,29–31], including Rea T. [30], who encourages a "paradigm" shift for PAD towards an "all-access defibrillation" beyond the conventional public setting use, and cites the use of "advanced mapping techniques" as a potential source of improvement.

Accordingly, our aim was to develop an analysis and optimization framework exploiting georeferenced information from a historical database of OHCAs, known AED locations, and topographic and demographic information, to define a geographic risk function and propose new strategies for AED deployment specifically targeting residential OHCAs. This framework was applied and validated on the city of Milan, Lombardy (Italy), counting 1,372,810 residents (as of 31 July 2017) over a surface of 181.67 km^2.

2. Materials and Methods

2.1. Data Sources and Pre-Processing

Four different data sources were utilized:

1. Georeferenced database of OHCAs (collected and made available for this research by AREU, Azienda Regionale Emergenza/Urgenza, responsible for the 112 emergency number service and Emergency Medical Services (EMS) provider for Lombardy region): it includes records of all OHCAs that occurred in Lombardy from 2015 to 2018 for a total of 45,043 records. In this timeframe, 8152 OHCAs occurred in the city of Milan, of which 7179 (88.06%) in residential locations. The anonymized database contains, as fields, the geolocation of each event, its date and time, time-to-intervention, information related to CPR and AED use, and more.
2. Georeferenced database of AED (from AREU): it includes geo-reference (geographic coordinates), location (description of the AED's installation place), and accessibility of known publicly accessible AEDs in Lombardy as of 31 December 2018 (10,023 devices, 1001 in the city of Milan).
3. Milan City Topographic Database (open data at https://geoportale.comune.milano.it/sit/): Geographic information about residential buildings, roads, subdivision of the city into 88 districts (Local Identity Nuclei, LINs: an administrative subdivision of the city based on traditional areas of the city and history of urban development).
4. Demography (open data at http://dati.comune.milano.it/): demographic and socioeconomic information about the resident population specifically for each LIN (gender, age, and nationality).

All georeferenced information was converted to the World Geodetic System 84 (WGS 84)–UTM (Universal Transverse Mercator) 32 North coordinates system and imported into an open source and free-to-use under the GNU GPL license GIS software (QGIS, http://www.qgis.org), to be visualized as separate layers in the same map. Figure 1 shows an example of this visualization, with the georeferenced records in the OHCA database filtered for the city of Milan.

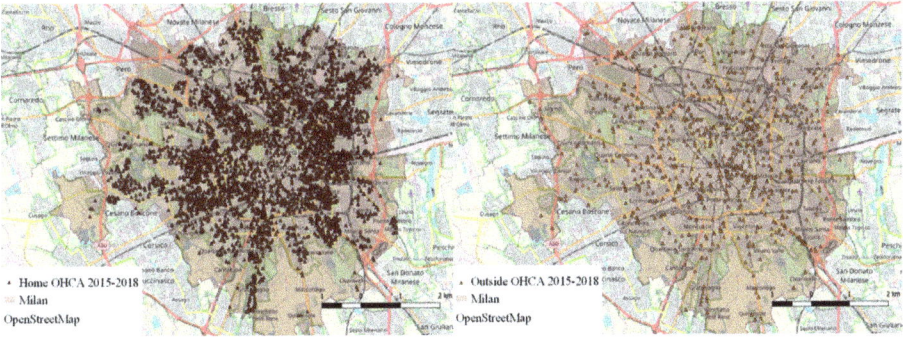

Figure 1. Distribution of georeferenced Out-Of-Hospital Cardiac Arrests (OHCAs), over the territory of the city of Milan from 2015 to 2018, that occurred at residential location (left panel) and outside of residential locations (right panel).

Routing issues were managed through pgRouting (https://pgrouting.org/) and PostGIS, open source SQL libraries run on PostgreSQL (http://www.postgresql.org), available on OSGeo, an operative system developed by the Open Source Geospatial Foundation (https://www.osgeo.org/). Processing of metadata and the optimization algorithm were implemented using the programming platform MATLAB (https://www.mathworks.com/products/matlab.html).

Figure 2 reports the schematic of the proposed framework (data sources highlighted in the gray box). The first step (right side) is represented by the evaluation of the current distribution of AEDs, based on the computation of the catchment areas of currently placed devices (area where they can be effectively used within the time limit, see next paragraph for implementation details), and a model for estimation of the distribution of the resident population. This output is exploited (left side) by the development of a geographic risk function to estimate the risk of residential OHCA occurrence along the territory, and by the final optimization defining a new geographical distribution for AEDs, that is subsequently evaluated with the same approach applied to the current deployment.

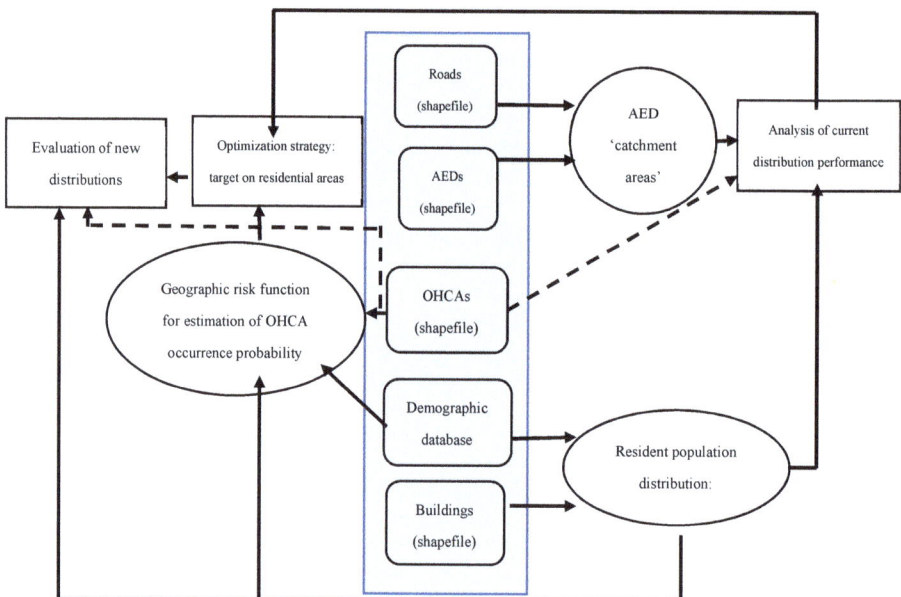

Figure 2. Schematic representation of the proposed framework, with data sources highlighted in the gray box. See text for further details.

2.2. AED "Catchment Areas"

In order to assess the performance of AEDs, a "catchment area" was defined as the area that can be reached from the position of each AED within the set time limit (portion of territory potentially covered by the AED presence). Guidelines from AHA [36] suggest a time of 3 min as the limit (thus allowing back and forth within 6 min), but the conversion of this time limit into a space indication is not established [19,24,37]. In most of the previous studies, catchment areas were computed as 100 m radius circles [17,20,22,34,38,39]. For example, in the study by Sun et al. [39], a paper that studied if optimized AED locations improved coverage of OHCA, results showed an increase in estimation between 50% and 100%, where 100 m circular buffers were used as the measurement of device catchment areas. However, other studies, such as Deakin et al. [24], where the impact of AED accessibility and locations on the clinical outcome is investigated, and Bonnet et al. [9] where a platform for planning of optimal AED deployment in urban environments is developed and validated, suggested the use of realistic topography-based catchment areas. This second approach was followed in our research by computing them considering the reachable distance moving along the streets network (not through Euclidian distance), thus resulting in very different mapping results [24,28], especially when considering OHCA coverage (i.e., when studying the whole territory of Lombardy region from 2015 to 2018, we reported a 15.35% OHCA coverage considering 200 m realistic areas against 9.43% considering 100 m circular buffers [40]). The computation resulted successful for 929 of the 1001 AEDs (92.8%), whereas for the remaining 72 (7.2%), the computation failed due to limitations in mapping quality, specifically in relation to open spaces such as parks, squares and large facilities, where the walkable paths are not clearly reported, and it is not possible to exclude the presence of obstacles. In these cases, the traditional 100 m circular buffer was considered, being the approach that better estimates the spatial coverage in cases where roads mapping is insufficient, resulting in a comparable mean surface of the catchment area [40]. Setting a 1.5 m/s walking speed (that is relatively low, in order to correct for the human factor and delays due to non-trained bystanders), 3 min correspond to a distance of 270 m centered on each AED. However, considering the time needed to reach the ground level from residential locations at higher floors, a non-negligible issue in the urban environment of Milan, the path length for computation of the catchment areas was reduced by a variable distance factor (max 70 m, down to a min final measure of 200 m) based on the mean height of the buildings in an outer 100 m portion of territory (between 150 and 250 m from the location of the AED) and weighting each building according to its estimated resident population. Details about this adjustment are reported in Appendix A.

2.3. Geographic Risk Function

A geographic risk function, developed from retrospective data, expressing the expected probability of residential OHCA occurrence, was computed on 200 × 200 m squared cells obtained gridding the city territory; the cell dimension was set as a first conservative estimate for the possible presence of an AED catchment area, with the AED to be installed at the center of the cell. The amount of resident population in the area constituted the main factor; since a high level of granularity is required, a model for the estimation of the amount of residents building-by-building was developed for the whole city, as this information was not directly available. The estimate was derived as:

$$building\_pop = \frac{building\_vol}{vol\_u_d} = \frac{building\_vol * tot\_pop_d}{tot\_vol_d} \quad (1)$$

where *building_pop* is the estimated number of residents for each building, *building_vol* the building volume; vol_u_d the LIN-specific residential volume available for each resident person, computed as tot_vol_d/tot_pop_d, with tot_vol_d representing the total residential volume in each LIN; and tot_pop_d the total resident population in each LIN.

However, aiming at a more accurate risk function definition, a purely geographic factor unbound from the absolute number of residents was developed using supervised machine learning, where the target variable (set as a geographic risk estimator) was constituted by the percentage incidence of residential OHCA in the resident population. As previously stated, the whole territory was divided into 200 × 200 m cells; those with < 200 inhabitants were discarded as they were considered statistically meaningless, since the random noise component of the measured phenomenon (the percentage incidence of residential OHCA in the population) is prevalent within these records. This operation resulted in a final set composed of 2124 items. Each item was characterized by 35 attributes (three cell-specific, 32 LIN-specific) considering relevant factors with respect to OHCA occurrence probability [41], including age and gender of the resident population, percentage of foreign citizens (divided by ethnicity), resident population density, mean price of the properties in the district (considered as a socioeconomic indicator), percentage of edified surface in the area, and more. Attributes were reduced by applying Principal Components Analysis [42] separately on demography, ethnicity, and socio-economical subsets of attributes, and maintaining resulting attributes until the total explained variance was > 95% for each category, leading to a total of eight attributes; only these resulting eight attributes are used in the following steps of the algorithm. Outliers were identified through z-index (defined as $z_i^{ind} = \frac{x_i - \bar{\mu}}{\bar{\sigma}}$ where x_i is the value of record i, $\bar{\mu}$ is the sample mean and $\bar{\sigma}$ is the sample standard deviation) with threshold set to 5 [42] and then removed. The third-degree polynomial interpolation (four estimated coefficients) for each of the right attributes with the target variable was computed (32 total coefficients). The final predictor was calculated as a weighted average among all the eight estimators (results of the interpolation for each attribute):

$$\hat{p}_i = \frac{\sum_{j=1}^{n} w_j \left(c_{1,j} v_{i,j}^3 + c_{2,j} v_{i,j}^2 + c_{3,j} v_{i,j} + c_{4,j} \right)}{\sum_{j=1}^{n} w_j} \qquad (2)$$

with:

$\hat{p}_i$: Target variable predictor (*i*-th item), estimate for the purely geographic risk function;
n: Attributes number;
$c_{x,j}$: Coefficients for polynomial third degree interpolation (*j*-th attribute);
$v_{i,j}$: Value of the *j*-th attribute for the *i*-th item;
w_j: $\frac{1}{\overline{r}_j}$, where $\overline{r}_j$ is the absolute value of the mean of residuals for the estimator from interpolation of *j*-th attribute.

Figure 3 shows a schematization of the procedure: the model output values (geographic risk function, represented by the target variable estimate) were rescaled in the [0,1] range and applied as a weight to the number of resident population in the cell, providing the final risk level:

$$R_i = \hat{p}_i\big|_{0-1} * pop_i \qquad (3)$$

with:

R_i: Final risk level (*i*-th cell);
$\hat{p}_i\big|_{0-1}$: Predictor of OHCA percentage incidence (*i*-th cell, rescaled [0,1]), representing the estimate of the purely geographic risk function;
pop_i: Estimated resident population (*i*-th cell);

The implemented risk function was validated through a Receiving Operating Characteristic (ROC) curve: the cells where at least one OHCA occurred in a biennium (repeated on 2015–2016, 2016–2017, and 2017–2018) were considered "positive", otherwise they were considered "negative". Setting a threshold risk value ("alpha" threshold) separating "positive" and "negative" test outputs allowed the computation of true positives (TPs), false positives (FPs), true negatives (TNs), and false negatives (FNs). ROC curve was obtained plotting the sensitivity ($\frac{TP}{TP+FN}$) on y axis and 1-specificity ($1 - \frac{TN}{TN+FP}$) on x axis for different values of alpha threshold (ranging 0–1).

2.4. Optimization Strategy

An algorithm was implemented for the priority-ranked identification of cells where the installation of an AED is required, according to the user-defined figure of merit, which can be budget constraint, or the achievement of a target performance (in terms of coverage of final risk level, territory, resident population, or retrospective OHCAs: in this latter case, the performance was estimated on the basis of the coverage provided by the 200 × 200 m cell, set to be the a first rough and conservative estimate of the possible presence of a catchment area). The optimization algorithm has as inputs:

- AEDs database, each weighted by an efficiency score (coverage of final risk level through its catchment area), and by a time-accessibility score (ts) ranged 0 to 1, with 1 assigned to AEDs accessible 24/7.
- dataset of 200 × 200 m cells not covered by an AED, where each cell has a priority score expressed by the final risk level.

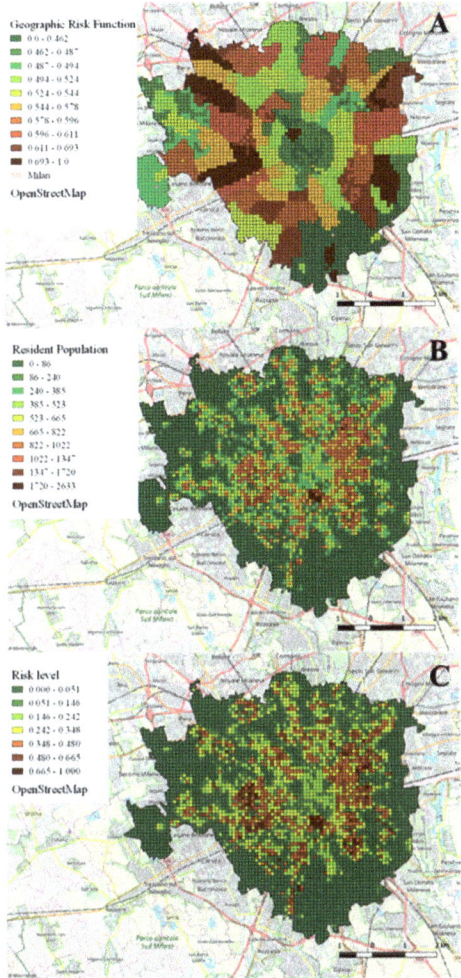

Figure 3. Schematization of the implementation of the geographic risk function. **Panel A**: The purely geographic risk estimator (scaled in the range 0 to 1) is computed for each 200 × 200 m cell in which the city territory was divided. **Panel B**: Number of estimated residents for each cell. **Panel C**: Their product, where the geographic risk estimator was applied as a weight, providing a final risk function estimating Out-of-Hospital Cardiac Arrest (OHCA) occurrence probability (scaled in the range 0 to 1).

The algorithm proceeds iteratively, identifying at each step the cell with the highest risk and the least efficient AED (i.e., considering only AEDs in whose catchment areas where no OHCA occurred in the last four years), choosing between the installation of a new AED or the repositioning of a pre-existing one, considering the ratio between performance gain (coverage of final risk level) and implementation cost (accordingly to AREU, 2500 € for a new installation and 500 € for a re-displacement), until the user-defined objective was reached.

The outputs of the algorithm consist in:

1. Identification of all the cells where an AED should be positioned according to the selected goal, with priority ranking, as a new installation or a re-displacement;
2. Identification of the currently located AEDs that should be repositioned.

To assess efficiency (benefits/costs), a dedicated score (CE, Cost-Efficiency figure of merit) was calculated:

$$CE(\%) = \frac{\Delta Tp}{Tc/10^6} \quad (4)$$

where:

- ΔTp represents the increase in percentage of covered OHCAs from the baseline: when evaluating the current AED distribution, the baseline value is assumed as 0%, whereas when evaluating new distributions, the baseline represents the percentage of OHCAs covered through the pre-existing deployment. As an example, a new simulated deployment covering 60% of retrospective events could results in ΔTp = 60 if representing a new distribution starting from blank (i.e., no AED on the territory); otherwise in case of a coverage of 41.77% provided by the current distribution, it results in ΔTp = 60 − 41.77 = 18.23, thus representing further processing of the currently implemented deployment.
- Tc is the cost for the implementation of such distribution, expressed in M€.

3. Results

From the analysis of the age distribution of the observed 7179 (88.06%) OHCAs in residential locations (recorded from 2015 to 2018 in the city of Milan), most of the victims were older than 60 years (61–80 years old = 32.9%; >80 years old = 53.21%), where 46–60 years old accounted for 9.21%, 30–45 years old for 2.87%, <30 years old for 1.06%, while 0.74% of the records did not report the victim's age. Median time (25th, 75th) to arrival of EMS was 8 min 44 sec (6 min 55 s, 11 min), and in only 143 cases (1.99%) of home OHCA the use of a public AED was reported. In Figure 4, in a zoomed portion of Milan, the position of each AED currently installed, with its realistic catchment area, and of each residential OHCA are shown.

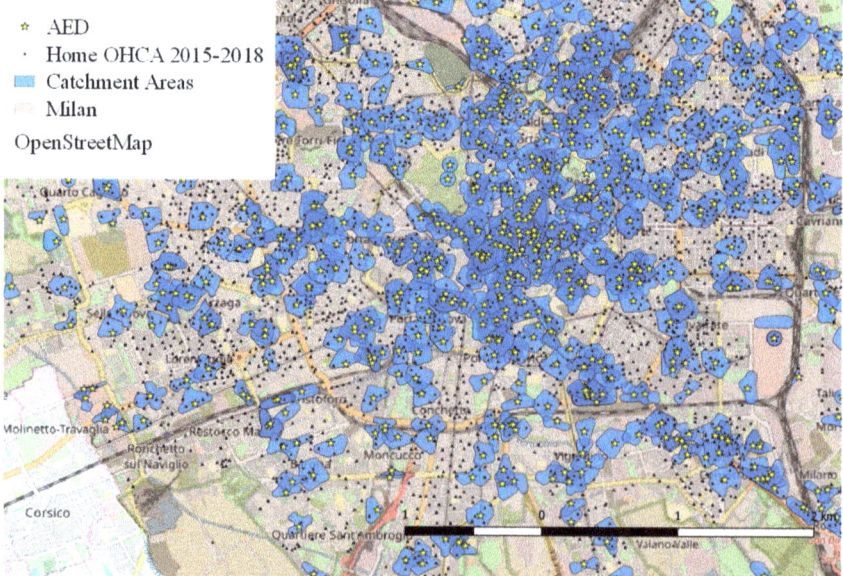

Figure 4. A zoomed portion of the city of Milan, with the position of each Automated External Defibrillator (AED, yellow stars) and its realistic catchment area, and the position of each residential Out-of-Hospital Cardiac Arrest (OHCA) in the period 2015–2018 (black dot).

3.1. Performance of Current AEDs Distribution

Table 1 reports the results of performance analysis of the current distribution of AEDs for the OHCA database for the city of Milan. The sub-optimal coverage both of territory (23.14%) and resident population (40%) was noticeable. Moreover, a high overlapping of catchment areas (39.28% of the total catchment area of AEDs) was observed, where its elimination alone could provide a 9% increase in coverage of city territory. The 41.77% of total OHCAs occurred within a catchment area (cost-efficiency parameter CE = 16.69%), of which 50.46% for "outside" OHCAs, and 40.59% for residential OHCAs, with a lowering the overall performance, as residential events represented almost the 90% of the total. The 41.77% actual coverage was considered as the baseline to compute the cost-efficiency CE parameter in new distributions.

Table 1. Results of performance analysis of the initial distribution of Automated External Defibrillators (AEDs). Out-of-Hospital Cardiac Arrest (OHCA) coverage values are reported separately for residential events ('Home'), non-residential ones ('Out') and aggregated ('Tot', enlightened in bold).

Territory	Coverage on Milan City Area (%)			Overlapping (%)			Overlapped Coverage on Milan City Area (%)		
	23.14%			39.28%			9.09%		
Population	Covered Population (%)			Percentage of Covered Population in Overlap			Total Population in Overlap (%)		
	40.02%			40.3%			16.13%		
OHCAs Coverage	2015–2016			2017–2018			Overall (2015–2018)		
	Home	Out	Tot	Home	Out	Tot	Home	Out	Tot
#	1387	222	1609	1527	269	1796	2914	491	3405
% on Total	39.56%	47.54%	40.5%	41.57%	53.16%	42.98%	40.59%	50.46%	41.77%
# in overlapping	484	113	597	559	149	708	1043	262	1305
% in overl. on cov	34.9%	50.9%	37.1%	36.61%	55.39%	39.42%	35.79%	53.36%	38.33%
% in overl. on tot	13.8%	24.2%	15.03%	15.22%	29.45%	16.94%	14.53%	26.93%	16.01%

The correlation between common GIS attributes relevant to LIN and the use of AED in presence of residential OHCA was analyzed. Interestingly, higher levels of use were associated with a lower resident population (1720 [1119; 2587.5] vs. 2005 [1412; 2617.25]) with larger residential volume/person available (219.6 [176.4; 265.73] vs. 190.44 [172.85; 256.38] m^3/person), thus evidencing wealthier areas, and with less prevalence of residents > 60 years old (27.5 [25.5; 30.1] vs. 28.2 [26.1; 30.7] %).

3.2. Validation of the Geographic Risk Function

Despite the actual prediction of OHCA incidence being impossible (due to the strong randomness observed in the occurrence of OHCA), the small variations of the target value were considered representative of the relative difference in the risk distribution.

The area of the obtained ROC curve was 0.887 for 2015–2016 (best "alpha" threshold at 0.037, with 95% sensitivity and 68.2% specificity), 0.886 for 2016–2017 (best "alpha" threshold at 0.0317, with 95% sensitivity and 67.8% specificity), 0.884 for 2017–2018 (best "alpha" threshold at 0.0263, with 95% sensitivity and 67% specificity), confirming the reliability of the computed geographic risk function.

3.3. Performance of the Optimized Distribution of AEDs

First, the optimization algorithm was applied to a scenario that replicated the number of currently available AEDs, to test for possible improved configurations achievable if the proposed model would have been used to assist in the decision about where to put each AED, as suggested by Sun et al. [39]. As expected, a better performance achievable in respect to the current one was evidenced, estimating an increase in spatial coverage of all OHCAs of +31.56% (from 41.77% to 73.33%), with a CE parameter increasing from 16.69% to 29.3% (+12.61%). Detailed results are reported in Table 2.

Table 2. Detailed results of performance analysis where a model-based distribution of the same number of Automated External Defibrillators (AEDs) that are currently deployed is simulated.

Coverages	OHCAs (Home, Outside)	Geographic Risk Function	Area	Resident Population	Cost-Efficiency Parameter CE
Current deployment	41.77% (40.59%, 50.46%)	39.51%	23.14%	40.02%	16.69%
Model-based simulated deployment (% Δ)	73.33% (+31.56%) (75.65%, 56.22%) (+35.06%, +5.76%)	65.27% (+25.76%)	29.07% (+5.93%)	70.15% (+30.13%)	29.3% (+12.61%)

In order to evaluate the potential improvements, starting from the current situation, four additional scenarios were simulated:

1. Displacements only (no new AED is installed, some of the currently located AEDs are re-displaced): the algorithm suggested the re-displacement of 373 (37.26% of the total) AEDs, providing an expected increase of covered OHCAs between 2015 and 2018 of 23.06% (from 41.77% to 64.83%), with a CE of 123.65% (resulting very high due to the low cost of re-displacements).

2. Installation of fixed number (N = 100) of new AEDs and re-displacement of existing ones: a total of 366 re-displacements (36.56%) were suggested in addition to the installation of 100 new devices, potentially covering the 68.69% of OHCAs between 2015 and 2018, with a CE of 62.4%.

3. Doubling the current risk coverage (from 39.51% to 79.03%): this scenario resulted in an increase, hence not a doubling, in total covered OHCAs from 41.77% to 74.9%, with a +33.13%, associated to a remarkable coverage level, and with a CE which is twice that of the current deployment (from 16.69% to 36.17%, +19.48%).

4. Doubling the initial investment relevant to the current distribution (estimated as 2,502,500 €, based on the cost of installation of 1001 AED): results of this scenario showed the re-displacement of 293 (29.27%) AEDs together with 942 new installations, obtaining a risk function coverage close to the total (98.79%), accounting for the 88% of all the OHCAs, with a CE slightly higher than the initial level (18.47%).

In Table 3, the detailed results of performance analysis for the simulated scenarios are presented.

Table 3. Detailed results of performance analysis of the simulated scenarios for new distributions of Automated External Defibrillators (AEDs); signed values within brackets represent the delta in respect to the corresponding value in the current placement (first column).

	Current Placement	Displacements Only	100 New AEDs	Risk Coverage Doubling	Budget Doubling
Final AEDs N°	1001	1001 (=)	1101 (+100)	1396 (+295)	1943 (+942)
N° of re-displaced AEDs (%)	/	373 (37.26%)	366 (36.56%)	357 (35.66%)	293 (29.27%)
Total Cost (€) (% of initial estimated investment)	2,502,500	186,500 (7.45%)	433,000 (17.3%)	916,000 (36.6%)	2,501,500 (99.96%)
Covered Risk	39.51%	64.52% (+25.01%)	69.96% (+30.45%)	79.03% (+39.52%)	98.79% (+59.28%)
Covered Area	23.14%	17.94% (-5.2%)	19.98% (-3.16%)	23.91% (+0.77%)	36.43% (+13.29%)
Covered Resident Population	40.02%	59.49% (+19.47%)	64.08% (+24.06%)	71.66% (+31.64%)	88.75% (+48.73%)
Covered home OHCAs 2015–2016	39.56%	65.43% (+25.87%)	69.91% (+30.35%)	76.41% (+36.85%)	89.45% (+49.89%)
Covered home OHCAs 2017–2018	41.57%	64.69% (+23.12%)	68.69% (+27.12%)	74.93% (+33.36%)	89.14% (+47.57%)
Covered home OHCAs 2015–2018	40.59%	65.05% (+24.46%)	69.29% (+28.7%)	75.65% (+35.06%)	89.29% (+48.7%)
Covered outside OHCAs 2015–2018	50.46%	63.21% (+12.75%)	65.15% (+14.69%)	69.37% (+18.91%)	78.52% (+28.06%)

Table 3. *Cont.*

Total Covered OHCAs 2015–2018	41.77%	64.83% (+23.06%)	68.79% (+27.02%)	74.9% (+33.13%)	88% (+46.23%)
Cost-efficiency (% coverage improvement over baseline/M€)	16.69%	123.65% (+106.96%)	62.4% (+45.71%)	36.17% (+19.48%)	18.47% (+16.78%)

It should be noticed that the estimation of the expected performance is strongly conservative, as the catchment areas of hypothetical new AED installations are 200 × 200 m cells (and not referring to a potential distance of 270 m), which is therefore an estimate by default.

Figure 5 reports a graphical representation of the output, where the algorithm returns currently located AEDs that should be re-positioned and identifies cells where the installation of a new device is suggested.

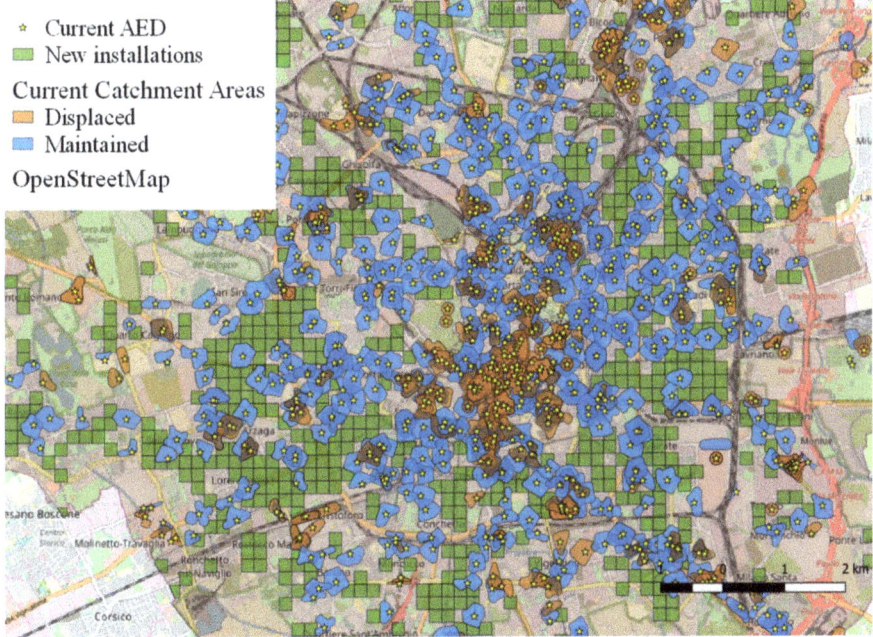

Figure 5. Example of the graphical representation of the output of the optimization strategy. Among currently available Automated External Defibrillators (AEDs), those that should be re-displaced (orange catchment areas) or not (blue catchment areas) are indicated, while the cells where the installation of a new device is suggested are depicted in green.

4. Discussion

In the context of deployment strategy of AEDs for improving spatial coverage of residential OHCAs, several unsolved issues relevant to optimization frameworks in PAD programs were addressed:

- Dimensioning of the catchment areas: the proposed computation considers realistic areas, based on the reachable distance within 3 min (allowing back and forth within 6 min) at 1.5 m/s velocity (270 m), reduced by a variable quantity (max 70 m) depending on the mean height of the surrounding buildings. This solution constitutes a possible improvement in matching a real-world scenario, compared to previous literature (100 m circular area [17,20,22,34,38,39]).

- Development of the risk function: the main innovation was to focus on OHCAs occurring inside residential locations constituting the majority of the events (almost 90% in the considered dataset), characterized by higher mortality. Differently from previous studies [9,20,39], a supervised learning approach inspecting the relation between geographic risk (target) and attributes related to demography, socio-economic conditions and land-use was applied.
- Applicability as a decision-making support tool: in literature, only one example [9] of an interactive interface for the optimization framework with the possibility for the user to modify the initial parameters as a decision-making support was present. The novelty (and main potentiality) of the proposed framework is related to its generalization and application to any new territory where the input data (AEDs and past OHCAs geolocation, streets network, demography) are available, although with variable accuracy to be determined according to the provided information (both regarding quantity and quality). Moreover, the proposed framework also considers the possibility to re-displace current devices (as suggested by Tierney et al. [38]) and allows the user to set the target constraints for optimization, choosing among a wider number of different criteria including area, population or risk coverage, not just limited to budget or number of devices.

As a result, in the context of its application to the case study of the city of Milan, the proposed strategy for AEDs deployment resulted more effective compared to the existing distribution. The initial spatial coverage of OHCAs (41.77%) was significantly lower than that estimated to be achieved by the new distribution (73.33%), resulting in a higher cost-efficiency parameter CE (from 16.69% OHCAs coverage increase for 1 M € invested, up to 29.3%).

Based on the results of this study, AEDs placement should be directed by the public authority according to a predefined plan, which is in line with results from similar studies [19,39]. Although private funding is a primary source for the development of PAD programs, and should always be encouraged, a centralized management of every initiative relevant to the installation of an AED would result in a more efficient exploitation of the allocated resources, which is enlightened as a primary objective by Deakin et al. [24].

This main conclusion is in line with Folke et al. [33], that examined cost-effectiveness of covering OHCA in public places in the city of Copenhagen (Denmark) and concluded that strategic placement of AEDs based on historical occurrence was economically acceptable, whereas unguided initiatives lead to AEDs being placed inappropriately. Similarly, the use of geographical information together with mathematical modelling helped in identifying such high-risk areas for the city of Toronto (Canada), thus proving that strategic placement of AEDs in a limited number of sites may result in an increase in public OHCA coverage in a large urban center [34]. When combined with community responder programs, the proportion of OHCA in public settings treated by AED in the Seattle area increased every year, from 1.56% in 1999 to 5.23% in 2002, with no adverse outcome from AED application in non-arrest events, and with 25% survival for OHCA in residential settings [43].

In addition, it is worth noting that the resulting AEDs distributions in this study scenario focused on residential events were not worsening (and actually improving, from 50.46% to 56.22%) the coverage of OHCAs in outdoor locations, by globally covering a higher portion of territory. This relevant finding suggests that a home-OHCA-based strategy does not impact negatively on the possibility of receiving assistance by a bystander in case of outdoor OHCA. Whereas, on the contrary, policies focused on optimizing AEDs distribution to cover outdoor OHCAs will have no or minimal impact in increasing the coverage of residential OHCAs, resulting in a lower level of use of AEDs in residential locations with respect to public places, as confirmed by recent studies [23,28].

Considering the performed simulations of further improvements in AEDs deployment (even though results should be considered conservative, because catchment areas of new hypothetical devices were estimated covering a 200 × 200 m area, instead of a realistic one), all new computed distributions are more cost-efficient from the point of view of spatial coverage when compared with the current deployment, including the most demanding simulated scenario ("budget doubling"), where the expected coverage of OHCAs reached 88%.

The relationship between risk coverage and OHCAs coverage is non-linear due to the random component of the phenomenon, which cannot be modelled; therefore, high levels of covered risk (as percentage of the total) correspond to a lower percentage of covered OHCAs (e.g., in the "budget doubling" scenario a 98.79% of covered risk corresponds to a 88% coverage of OHCAs). However, the overall trend of the results in the different scenarios is coherent: an increase in risk coverage does correspond to an increase in OHCAs and resident population coverages, although with a decreasing ratio when approaching higher levels, implying a reduction in cost-efficiency. Despite the model being targeted on residential OHCAs, the coverage of events happening outside the residential location was increased too, although with lower ratios.

Main limitations concerning the utilized methodology were:

- Data quality: topographic and demographic open data, not specifically collected for scientific purposes, were used for the development of the risk function. Moreover, the topographic mapping information was not complete and prevented the computation of realistic catchment areas for 72 (7.2%) of the considered devices, for which the use of the traditional (yet inefficient in terms of OHCA coverage [40]) 100 m circular buffer was implemented. However, due to the limited number of affected AED and their location (parks, squares and large facilities), which is not relevant in addressing residential events (i.e., the main focus of this study), we considered the resulting approximation as acceptable.
- AED placement spot: the algorithm identifies squared cells where an installation is considered necessary (according to specifications), but no output is provided about the exact spot within the cell where the AED should be placed, which means that the resulting coverage area might not be the most efficient. A future development could address the identification of these spots, with a following phase of fine-tuning positioning for each cell.
- Follow-up survival data not available: due to Italian legislation and separate database system between the EMS provider and the hospitals, the assessment of the rescue outcome, neither in short-term (as EMS crew often does not include a physician, so death could not be declared until body arrival to the hospital) nor in long-term survival, was not available. This prevented a possible comparison of the rate of AED use and successful resuscitation between cases of home-OHCA, which occurred within the actual public AED catchment areas, versus those that occurred outside. Although timely interventions on OHCA with a public AED do increase survival probability [4,5], and the likelihood of such interventions is higher when the distance between the OHCA location and the AED is shorter [28], the proposed increase in spatial coverage provided by public AEDs, which is the target of this study, could be evaluated from an efficiency point of view (e.g., by computing the results in terms of Quality-Adjusted Life Years, QALYs). This is only if correlating more frequent uses of AED in events occurring within their catchment areas with higher survival rates and better medical outcomes, of which were not available in this study. However, Sondergaard et al. [28] reported a higher likelihood of use of public AEDs when placed closer to OHCA locations, while Sun et al. [39] demonstrated, exploiting the Utstein-based outcome prediction, that the increase in spatial coverage provided by AEDs is correlated with higher survival chances and better neurological outcome. In addition, the report remarked that this kind of "in-silico" trial "can be used to identify promising interventions based on objective performance criteria and inform trial design in a data-driven manner, potentially saving significant time and money".

As the risk function was computed considering all OHCA etiologies, with both shockable rhythms and pulseless electrical activity, a further improvement could be to limit the risk function computation on OHCA with shockable rhythms only, in order to potentially maximize cost-effectiveness of AED distribution. However, this was not possible with the available data, where 5963 records (73.15%) had missing information for this field, and only in 352 records (4.32%) a shockable rhythm was reported, also due to the result of the time-dependent deterioration of ventricular fibrillation to asystole [44], considering that the median time to arrival of EMS was larger than the recommended 6 min.

Moreover, by expanding the spatial-temporal sample and having more records where a publicly accessible AED is used, the correlation between territorial attributes (routing, environment etc.) and the level (and quality) of public AEDs use could be further inspected, as well as possible correlations with the medical outcome.

Finally, it is worth noticing that the actual use of public AEDs is still very low, in line with data from other countries [37], with 227 reported uses in the 8152 total OHCA, accounting for 2.78% of the cases, of which 143 were related to a home OHCA, also due to a 45.46% of missing data in the available database. While increasing geographic coverage and spatial accessibility does not ensure by itself an increase in the use of public AEDs (although Sondergaard et al. [28] enlightened a correlation between AED-to-OHCA proximity and AED use), providing policy makers with methods for increasing AED spatial accessibility represents a first step towards increasing their utilization and survival probability, particularly if accompanied by public campaigns for awareness raising. The HAT trial [21], despite not finding differences in terms of mortality between the patients in the control group (conventional response) and those to which a personal AED was given at home, confirmed that the use of AED at home on loved ones or neighbors by lay users with minimal training was feasible, risk free, and resulted in overall survival after cardiac arrest at home of 12% (18.3% for witnessed events), better than the 2% previously reported [45].

Therefore, even if a more accurate distribution of the devices could improve PAD performance, the first and key resource where more efforts should be invested are the final users. Campaigns for awareness raising and citizens training [46], together with the inclusion of this kind of resource in the EMS [25,47,48] (e.g., via smartphone app [49]), could positively improve PAD performance regardless to the optimality of the deployment of the devices. These improvements in the usage model could also provide AEDs retriever with the exact location and potentially with the faster routing, significantly reducing the time to retrieval. Moreover, despite the assessed safeness of AED use from untrained people, legal restrictions are still negatively impacting use level of AEDs from bystanders, especially in Italy [16]. In other countries too, where willingness of bystanders to initiate resuscitation is higher, usage is still low, at least to some extent due to the reduced accessibility [25,37].

5. Conclusions

The proposed framework for PAD, considering realistic catchment areas, showed that, in the city of Milan, the current distribution of publicly accessible AEDs, based on the current guidelines and use practice, is sub-optimal, both regarding the coverage of territory, of OHCA events, and of resident population. The following optimization, exploiting a geographic risk function for estimation of OHCA occurrence probability, could provide a highly valuable decision-making support for policy makers, from which new installations or re-displacement of existing AEDs could result in effective improvement in the spatial accessibility of publicly accessible AEDs.

Based on the results of this study, AEDs placement should be directed by the public authority according to a predefined plan both concerning public and private initiatives, as stated in similar studies [19,39]. The focus on residential OHCAs, following recent suggestions encouraging this approach [22,25,29–31], revealed that, from a spatial point of view, targeting residential areas is more effective in increasing coverage of both in-home and public OHCA.

The obtained findings could be considered as a relevant starting point for a real field application of the proposed framework, which can be implemented for any territory in which the required information is available. If including medical follow up of OHCA outcome, it could provide definite data for policy makers on performance of algorithms for the most cost-effective placement of AEDs, leading to a more effective definition of PAD programs guidelines. However, in line with conclusions by Sun et al. [39], the proposed approach could already be considered valuable in guiding AED placements in order to increase spatial coverage, which is likely to result in better clinical outcome for victims of OHCA.

Author Contributions: Conceptualization: Gianquintieri Lorenzo, Brovelli Maria Antonia and Caiani Enrico Gianluca Methodology: Gianquintieri Lorenzo, Brovelli Maria Antonia and Caiani Enrico Gianluca. Software: Gianquintieri Lorenzo Validation: Gianquintieri Lorenzo Formal Analysis: Gianquintieri Lorenzo, Brovelli Maria Antonia and CAIANI ENRICO GIANLUCA Investigation: Brambilla Piero Maria, Pagliosa Andrea and Villa Guido Francesco Resources: Brambilla Piero Maria, Pagliosa Andrea, Villa Guido Francesco and Caiani Enrico Gianluca Data Curation: Gianquintieri Lorenzo, Brambilla Piero Maria, Pagliosa Andrea and Villa Guido Francesco Writing-Original Draft Preparation: Gianquintieri Lorenzo, Brovelli Maria Antonia and Caiani Enrico Gianluca Writing-Review & Editing: Gianquintieri Lorenzo, Brovelli Maria Antonia and Caiani Enrico Gianluca Visualization: Gianquintieri Lorenzo, Brovelli Maria Antonia and Caiani Enrico Gianluca Supervision: Caiani Enrico Gianluca Project Administration: Caiani Enrico Gianluca. All authors have read and agreed to the published version of the manuscript.

Funding: This research received no external funding.

Acknowledgments: We acknowledge the support of AREU in sharing the historical data on OHCAs for the city of Milan.

Conflicts of Interest: No actual or potential conflict of interest declared.

Appendix A

Adjustment of catchment areas dimensions considering buildings height.

1. Computation of a realistic catchment area with a target path dimension of 150 m, considered to be the minimal distance after which the effect of building height could prevent the possibility to reach the OHCA location within the time limit of 6 min (back and forth).

2. Computation of a realistic catchment area with a target path dimension of 250 m, considered to be the maximal distance in which the OHCA location can be reached within the time limit of 6 min (back and forth) even when considering buildings height.

3. Computation of the portion of the territory included within the realistic catchment areas with 150 and 250 m target path, considered to be the area in which buildings height could have an impact and should be evaluated.

4. Identification of all the buildings in the territory included within the 150 and 250 m realistic catchment areas, considered to be the buildings potentially impacting reaching the OHCA locations in due time.

5. Computation of the weighted (on the base of estimated hosted resident population) mean height m_{wh} of buildings in the territory within the 150 and 250 m realistic catchment areas:

$$m_{wh} = \frac{\sum_i h_i * pop_i}{\sum_i pop_i}$$

where h_i is the height of the i-th building in the interest area, pop_i is the estimated resident population living in the i-th building in the interest area (with the estimation method previously described).

6. Reduction of the dimension of the catchment area: The vertical movement speed is considered to be 1.5 m/s, therefore the reduction dimension is computed as $m_{wh} * 1.5$, where m_{wh} is the weighted mean height [m] of the buildings in the interest area (step 3).

$$lr = m_{wh} * 1.5 = \frac{\sum_i h_i * pop_i}{\sum_i pop_i} * 1.5$$

References

1. Roger, V.L.; Go, A.S.; Lloyd-Jones, D.M.; Adams, R.J.; Berry, J.D.; Brown, T.M.; Carnethon, M.R.; Dai, S.; Simone, D.G.; Ford, E.S.; et al. Heart Disease and Stroke Statistics—2011 Update: A Report From the American Heart Association. *Circulation* **2011**, *123*, 18–209. [CrossRef] [PubMed]

2. Priori, S.G.; Blomstrom-Lundqvist, C.; Mazzanti, A.; Blom, N.; Borggrefe, M.; Camm, J.; Elliott, P.M.; Fitzsimons, D.; Hatala, R.; Hindricks, G.; et al. 2015 ESC Guidelines for the management of patients with ventricular arrhythmias and the prevention of sudden cardiac Death. The Task Force for the Management of Patients with Ventricular Arrhythmias and the Prevention of Sudden Cardiac Death of the European Society of Cardiology (ESC). *Eur. Heart J.* **2015**, *36*, 2793–2867. [PubMed]
3. Wellens, H.J.; Lindemans, F.W.; Houben, R.P.; Gorgels, A.; Volders, P.G.; Bekke, R.M.; Crijns, H.J. Improving survival after out-of-hospital cardiac arrest requires new tools. *Eur. Heart J.* **2016**, *37*, 1499–1503. [CrossRef] [PubMed]
4. Holmberg, M.J.; Vognsen, M.; Andersen, M.S.; Donnino, M.W.; Andersen, L.W. Bystander automated external defibrillator use and clinical outcomes after out-of-hospital cardiac arrest: A systematic review and meta-analysis. *Resuscitation* **2017**, *120*, 77–87. [CrossRef]
5. Kiyohara, K.; Nishiyama, C.; Kitamura, T.; Matsuyama, T.; Sado, J.; Shimamoto, T.; Kobayashi, D.; Kiguchi, T.; Okabayashi, S.; Kawamura, T.; et al. The association between public access defibrillation and outcome in witnessed out-of-hospital cardiac arrest with shockable rhythm. *Resuscitation* **2019**, *140*, 93–97. [CrossRef]
6. Zulli, L. La Morte Cardiaca Improvvisa—L'arresto Cardiocircolatorio—La Rianimazione Cardiopolmonare. Available online: http://internetsfn.asl-rme.it/file_allegati/morte_improvvisa.pdf (accessed on 10 September 2019).
7. Jost, D.; Degrange, H.; Verret, C.; Hersan, O.; Banville, I.L.; Chapman, F.W.; Lank, P.; Petit, J.L.; Fuilla, C.; Migliani, R.; et al. DEFI 2005: A randomized controlled trial of the effect of automated external defibrillator cardiopulmonary resuscitation protocol on outcome from out-of-hospital cardiac arrest. *Circulation* **2010**, *121*, 1614–1622. [CrossRef]
8. Perkins, G.D.; Handley, A.J.; Koster, R.W.; Castren, M.; Smyth, M.; Olasveengen, T.; Monsieurs, K.G.; Raffay, V.; Gräsner, J.-T.; Wenzel, V.; et al. European Resuscitation Council Guidelines for Resuscitation 2015: Section 2. Adult basic life support and automated external defibrillation. *Resuscitation* **2015**, *95*, 81–99. [CrossRef]
9. Bonnet, B.; Dessavre, D.G.; Kraus, K.; Ramirez-Marquez, J.E. Optimal placement of public-access AEDs in urban environments. *Comput. Ind. Eng.* **2015**, *90*, 269–280. [CrossRef]
10. Weisfeldt, M.L.; Kreber, R.E.; McGoldrick, R.P.; Moss, A.J.; Nichol, G.; Ornato, J.P.; Palmer, D.G.; Reigel, B.; Smith, S.C. Public Access Defibrillation A Statement for Healthcare Professionals From the American Heart Association Task Force on Automatic External Defibrillation. *Circulation* **1995**, *92*, 2763. [CrossRef]
11. Mauri, R.; Burkart, R.; Benvenuti, C.; Caputo, M.L.; Moccetti, T.; Bufalo, D.A.; Gallino, A.; Casso, C.; Anselmi, L.; Cassina, T.; et al. Better management of out-ofhospital cardiac arrest increases survival rate and improves neurological outcome in the Swiss Canton Ticino. *Europace* **2016**, *18*, 398–404. [CrossRef]
12. Smith, C.M.; Wilson, M.H.; Hartley-Sharpe, C.; Gwinnutt, C.; Dicker, B.; Perkins, G.D. The use of trained volunteers in the response to out-of-hospital cardiac arrest—The GoodSAM experience. *Resuscitation* **2017**, *121*, 123–126. [CrossRef] [PubMed]
13. Weisfeldt, M.L.; Sitlani, C.M.; Ornato, J.P.; Rea, T.; Aufderheide, T.P.; Davis, D.; Dreyer, J.; Hess, E.P.; Jui, J.; Maloney, J.; et al. Survival after application of automatic external defibrillators before arrival of the emergency medical system: Evaluation in the resuscitation outcomes consortium population of 21 million. *J. Am. Coll. Cardiol.* **2010**, *55*, 1713–1720. [CrossRef] [PubMed]
14. Deakin, C.D.; Shewry, E.; Gray, H.H. Public access defibrillation remains out of reach for most victims of out-of-hospital sudden cardiac arrest. *Heart* **2014**, *100*, 619–623. [CrossRef] [PubMed]
15. Mao, R.D.; Ong, M.E.H. Public access defibrillation: Improving accessibility and outcomes. *Br. Med. Bull.* **2016**, *118*, 25–32. [CrossRef] [PubMed]
16. Baldi, E.; Savastano, S. AED use before EMS arrival: When survival becomes a matter of law and system in Italy, which can be improved. *Eur. Heart J.* **2018**, *39*, 1664. [CrossRef]
17. Sun, C.L.F.; Demirtas, D.; Brooks, S.; Morrison, L.J.; Chan, T.C. Overcoming Spatial and Temporal Barriers to Public Access Defibrillators Via Optimization. *J. Am. Coll. Cardiol.* **2016**, *68*, 836–845. [CrossRef]
18. Lin, B.-C.; Chen, C.-W.; Chen, C.-C.; Kuo, C.-L.; Fan, I.-C.; Ho, C.-K.; Liu, I.-C.; Chan, T.-C. Spatial decision on allocating automated external defibrillators (AED) in communities by multi-criterion two-step floating catchment area (MC2SFCA). *Int. J. Health Geogr.* **2016**, *15*, 17. [CrossRef]

19. Chrisinger, B.; Grossestreuer, A.V.; Laguna, M.C.; Griffis, H.M.; Branas, C.C.; Wiebe, U.J.; Merchant, R.M. Characteristics of automated external defibrillator coverage in Philadelphia, PA, based on land use and estimated risk. *Resuscitation* **2016**, *109*, 9–15. [CrossRef]
20. Chan, T.C.; Demirtas, D.; Kwon, R.H. Optimizing the Deployment of Public Access Defibrillators. *Manag. Sci.* **2017**, *62*, 3617–3635. [CrossRef]
21. Bardy, G.H.; Lee, K.L.; Mark, D.B.; Poole, J.E.; Toff, W.; Tonkin, A.M.; Smith, W.; Dorian, P.; Packer, U.L.; White, R.D.; et al. Home Use of Automated External Defibrillators for Sudden Cardiac Arrest. *N. Engl. J. Med.* **2008**, *358*, 1793–1804. [CrossRef]
22. Folke, F.; Gislason, G.H.; Lippert, F.; Nielsen, S.L.; Weeke, P.; Hansen, M.L.; Fosbøl, E.L.; Andersen, S.S.; Rasmussen, S.; Schramm, T.K.; et al. Differences Between Out-of-Hospital Cardiac Arrest in Residential and Public Locations and Implications for Public-Access Defibrillation. *Circulation* **2010**, *122*, 623–630. [CrossRef] [PubMed]
23. Hansen, S.M.; Hansen, C.M.; Folke, F.; Rajan, S.; Kragholm, K.; Ejlskov, L.; Gislason, G.; Køber, L.; Gerds, T.A.; Hjortshøj, S.; et al. Bystander Defibrillation for Out-of-Hospital Cardiac Arrest in Public vs Residential Locations. *JAMA Cardiol.* **2017**, *2*, 507–514. [CrossRef] [PubMed]
24. Deakin, C.D.; Anfield, S.A.; Hodgetts, G. Underutilisation of public access defibrillation is related to retrieval distance and time-dependent availability. *Heart* **2018**, *104*, 1339–1343. [CrossRef] [PubMed]
25. Sondergaard, K.B.; Wissenberg, M.; Gerds, T.A.; Rajan, S.; Karlsson, L.; Kragholm, K.; Pape, M.; Lippert, F.; Gislason, G.; Folke, F.; et al. Bystander cardiopulmonary resuscitation and long-term outcomes in out-of-hospital cardiac arrest according to location of arrest. *Eur. Heart J.* **2019**, *40*, 309–318. [CrossRef]
26. Iwami, T.; Hiraide, A.; Nakanishi, N.; Hayashi, Y.; Nishiuchi, T.; Uejima, T.; Morita, H.; Shigemoto, T.; Ikeuchi, H.; Matsusaka, M.; et al. Outcome and characteristics of out-of-hospital cardiac arrest according to location of arrest: A report from a large-scale, population-based study in Osaka, Japan. *Resuscitation* **2006**, *69*, 221–228. [CrossRef]
27. Weisfeldt, M.L.; Everson-Stewart, S.; Sitlani, C.; Rea, T.; Aufderheide, T.P.; Atkins, D.L.; Bigham, B.; Brooks, S.; Foerster, C.; Gray, R.; et al. Ventricular Tachyarrhythmias after Cardiac Arrest in Public versus at Home. *N. Engl. J. Med.* **2011**, *364*, 313–321. [CrossRef]
28. Sondergaard, K.B.; Hansen, S.M.; Pallisgaard, J.L.; Gerds, T.A.; Wissenberg, M.; Karlsson, L.; Lippert, F.; Gislason, G.H.; Madelaire, C.; Folke, F. Out-of-hospital cardiac arrest: Probability of bystander defibrillation relative to distance to nearest automated external defibrillator. *Resuscitation* **2018**, *124*, 138–144. [CrossRef]
29. Giacoppo, D. Impact of bystander-initiated cardiopulmonary resuscitation for out-of-hospital cardiac arrest: Where would you be happy to have a cardiac arrest? *Eur. Heart J.* **2019**, *40*, 319–321. [CrossRef]
30. Rea, T. Paradigm shift: Changing public access to all-access defibrillation. *Heart* **2018**, *104*, 1311–1312. [CrossRef]
31. Blackwood, J.; Eisenberg, M.; Jorgenson, D.; Nania, J.; Howard, B.; Collins, B.; Connell, P.; Day, T.; Rohrbach, C.; Rea, T.D. Strategy to Address Private Location Cardiac Arrest: A Public Safety Survey. *Prehospital Emerg. Care* **2018**, *22*, 784–787. [CrossRef]
32. Open Geospatial Consortium. Glossary of Terms. Available online: https://www.opengeospatial.org/ogc/glossary/g (accessed on 10 August 2020).
33. Folke, F.; Knudsen Lippert, F.; Nielsen, S.L.; Gislason, G.H.; Hansen, M.L.; Schramm, T.K.; Sorensen, R.; Loldrup Fosbol, E.; Andresen, S.S.; Rasmussen, S.; et al. Location of cardiac arrest in a city centre strategic placement of automated external defibrillators in public locations. *Circulation* **2009**, *120*, 510–517. [CrossRef] [PubMed]
34. Chan, T.C.; Li, H.; Lebovic, G.; Tang, S.K.; Chan, J.Y.; Cheng, H.C.; Morrison, L.J.; Brooks, S. Identifying Locations for Public Access Defibrillators Using Mathematical Optimization. *Circulation* **2013**, *127*, 1801–1809. [CrossRef] [PubMed]
35. Ringh, M.; Hollenberg, J.; Møller, T.P.; Svensson, L.; Rosenqvist, M.; Lippert, F.; Wissenberg, M.; Hansen, C.M.; Claessen, A.; Viereck, S.; et al. The challenges and possibilities of public access defibrillation. *J. Intern. Med.* **2018**, *283*, 238–256. [CrossRef] [PubMed]
36. American Heart Association. Implementing an AED Program, DS13398 5/18. Available online: https://cpr.heart.org/idc/groups/ahaecc-public/@wcm/@ecc/documents/downloadable/ucm_501521.pdf (accessed on 10 August 2020).

37. Smith, C.M.; Keung, S.N.L.C.; Khan, M.O.; Arvanitis, T.N.; Fothergill, R.; Hartley-Sharpe, C.; Wilson, M.; Perkins, G.D. Barriers and facilitators to public access defibrillation in out-of-hospital cardiac arrest: A systematic review. *Eur. Heart J. Qual. Care Clin. Outcomes* **2017**, *3*, 264–273. [CrossRef]
38. Tierney, N.J.; Reinhold, H.; Mira, A.; Weiser, M.; Burkart, R.; Benvenuti, C.; Auricchio, A. Novel relocation methods for automatic external defibrillator improve out-of-hospital cardiac arrest coverage under limited resources. *Resuscitation* **2018**, *125*, 83–89. [CrossRef]
39. Sun, C.L.; Karlsson, L.; Torp-Pedersen, C.; Morrison, L.J.; Brooks, S.; Folke, F.; Chan, T.C. In Silico Trial of Optimized Versus Actual Public Defibrillator Locations. *J. Am. Coll. Cardiol.* **2019**, *74*, 1557–1567. [CrossRef]
40. Gianquintieri, L.; Caiani, E.G.; Brambilla, P.; Pagliosa, A.; Villa, G.F.; Brovelli, M.A. Open Data in Health-Geomatics: Mapping and Evaluating Publicly Accessible Defibrillators. *Isprs Archives* **2019**, *XLII-4/W14*, 63–70. [CrossRef]
41. Dicker, B.; Garrett, N.; Wong, S.; McKenzie, H.; McCarthy, J.; Jenkin, G.; Smith, T.; Skinner, J.R.; Pegg, T.; Devlin, G.; et al. Relationship between socioeconomic factors, distribution of public access defibrillators and incidence of out-of-hospital cardiac arrest. *Resuscitation* **2019**, *138*, 53–58. [CrossRef]
42. Vercellis, C. *Business Intelligence Modelli Matematici e Sistemi per le Decisioni*, 1st ed.; McGraw-Hill: Milano, Italy, 2006; pp. 77–79, 83–88.
43. Culley, L.L.; Rea, T.D.; Murray, J.A.; Welles, B.; Fahrenbruch, C.E.; Olsufka, M.; Eisenberg, M.S.; Copass, M.K. Public Access Defibrillation in Out-of-Hospital Cardiac Arrest. *Circulation* **2004**, *109*, 1859–1863. [CrossRef]
44. Holmberg, M.; Holmberg, S.; Herlitz, J. Incidence, duration and survival of ventricular fibrillation in out-of-hospital cardiac arrest patients in sweden. *Resuscitation* **2000**, *44*, 7–17. [CrossRef]
45. Norris, R.M.; UK Heart Attack Study (UKHAS) Collaborative Group. Circumstances of out of hospital cardiac arrest in patients with ischaemic heart disease. *Heart* **2005**, *91*, 1537–1540. [CrossRef] [PubMed]
46. Nehme, Z.; Andrew, E.; Bernard, S.; Patsamanis, H.; Cameron, P.; Bray, J.; Meredith, I.T.; Smith, K. Impact of a public awareness campaign on out-of-hospital cardiac arrest incidence and mortality rates. *Eur. Heart J.* **2017**, *38*, 1666–1673. [CrossRef] [PubMed]
47. Nordberg, P.; Hollenberg, J.; Rosenqvist, M.; Herlitz, J.; Jonsson, M.; Järnbert-Petterson, H.; Forsberg, S.; Dahlqvist, T.; Ringh, M.; Svensson, L. The implementation of a dual dispatch system in out-of-hospital cardiac arrest is associated with improved short and long term survival. *Eur. Heart J. Acute Cardiovasc. Care* **2014**, *3*, 293–303. [CrossRef] [PubMed]
48. Pijls, R.W.; Nelemans, P.J.; Rahel, B.M.; Gorgels, A.P. Factors modifying performance of a novel citizen text message alert system in improving survival of out-of-hospital cardiac arrest. *Eur. Heart J. Acute Cardiovasc. Care* **2018**, *7*, 397–404. [CrossRef] [PubMed]
49. Caputo, M.L.; Muschietti, S.; Burkart, R.; Benvenuti, C.; Conte, G.; Regoli, F.; Mauri, R.; Klersy, C.; Moccetti, T.; Auricchio, A.; et al. Lay persons alerted by mobile application system initiate earlier cardio-pulmonary resuscitation: A comparison with SMS-based system notification. *Resuscitation* **2018**, *114*, 73–78. [CrossRef]

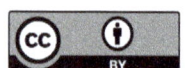

© 2020 by the authors. Licensee MDPI, Basel, Switzerland. This article is an open access article distributed under the terms and conditions of the Creative Commons Attribution (CC BY) license (http://creativecommons.org/licenses/by/4.0/).

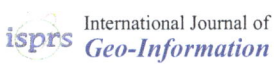

Article

Exploring Urban Spatial Features of COVID-19 Transmission in Wuhan Based on Social Media Data

Zhenghong Peng [1], Ru Wang [1], Lingbo Liu [2] and Hao Wu [1,*]

[1] Department of Graphics and Digital Technology, School of Urban Design, Wuhan University, Wuhan 430072, China; pengzhenghong@whu.edu.cn (Z.P.); wang_ru@whu.edu.cn (R.W.)
[2] Department of Urban Planning, School of Urban Design, Wuhan University, Wuhan 430072, China; lingbo.liu@whu.edu.cn
* Correspondence: wh79@whu.edu.cn; Tel.: +86-27-6877-3062

Received: 24 April 2020; Accepted: 15 June 2020; Published: 19 June 2020

Abstract: During the early stage of the COVID-19 outbreak in Wuhan, there was a short run of medical resources, and Sina Weibo, a social media platform in China, built a channel for novel coronavirus pneumonia patients to seek help. Based on the geo-tagging Sina Weibo data from February 3rd to 12th, 2020, this paper analyzes the spatiotemporal distribution of COVID-19 cases in the main urban area of Wuhan and explores the urban spatial features of COVID-19 transmission in Wuhan. The results show that the elderly population accounts for more than half of the total number of Weibo help seekers, and a close correlation between them has also been found in terms of spatial distribution features, which confirms that the elderly population is the group of high-risk and high-prevalence in the COVID-19 outbreak, needing more attention of public health and epidemic prevention policies. On the other hand, the early transmission of COVID-19 in Wuhan could be divide into three phrases: Scattered infection, community spread, and full-scale outbreak. This paper can help to understand the spatial transmission of COVID-19 in Wuhan, so as to propose an effective public health preventive strategy for urban space optimization.

Keywords: COVID-19; social media data; sina weibo; spatiotemporal characteristics

1. Introduction

In January 2020, the novel coronavirus pneumonia, COVID-19, broke out in Wuhan, the capital of Hubei province in China and the development of the epidemic has been a rising worldwide concern [1]. In order to slow down and block the spread of the virus, Wuhan announced a shutdown on January 23rd, 2020 to suspend the city's public transportation and imposed an unprecedented restriction on personal mobility. The effect of contact limitation gradually appeared after one month, which proves that for cities with high population density, severe restrictions on population movement can play a positive role in suppressing the spread of infectious diseases [2].

The existing researches include the spatial-temporal dynamics study of COVID-19 on the country level [3–5], with the deficiency of the detail reveal of the characteristics in the early stage in the urban space, which is critical for the development of prevention and control work in the city during the epidemic. The outbreak of COVID-19 verifies that epidemic prevention in public health is an essential part of urban planning and governance [6,7]. It is important to understand the heterogeneity of urban space in terms of social space and geographic space in the city [8], to identify susceptible people [9,10] and disease-prone spaces, and to grasp the dynamic spread of infectious diseases in urban spaces [11]. Thus, preventive control nodes can deploy corresponding measures for specific groups and spaces [12,13].

With the rapid development of information and communications technology (ICT), big data has been widely used in the field of public health [14,15] in recent years. Social media data such as Twitter and Weibo data were used to study the public attention [16,17], to predict epidemic outbreak [18–20], and to make research on human sentiments [21,22] during the COVID-19 epidemic. Compared with traditional cases data, there are unique advantages such as the wider population sample coverage, the easier accessibility, and the accurate geographic information. Such big data in epidemic studies can improve the understanding of the epidemic in time and space and will play an important role in formulating targeted urban prevention and control strategies.

In the early days of the lockdown, Wuhan, as the epidemic center, faced great challenges. The panic caused by COVID-19 outbreak stimulated a large number of people to enter the hospital, leading to a short-term collapse of medical system. Such a squeeze on medical resources also prevented many diagnosed and suspected people of having COVID-19 from receiving timely treatment. More than 1000 families in Wuhan posted help information on Sina Weibo, a Chinese social media platform, seeking immediate medical treatments. Most information was posted from February fourth to eighth, and then decreased rapidly, when the policy that "Guarantee that all suspected and confirmed cases should be collected and cured" was released on February fifth and a series of measures were taken by the government to quickly supplement medical resources, including increase the number of medical beds and medical staff supporting Wuhan (Figure 1).

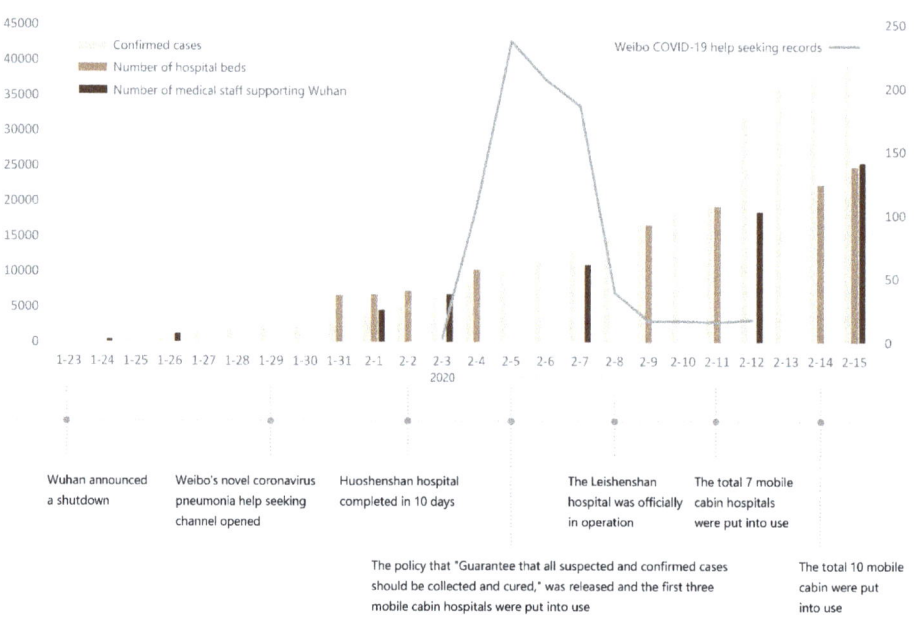

Figure 1. Time-series change histogram in the early stage of the epidemic.

The geotagged Weibo data can reflect the spatial distribution of COVID-19 infectors and provided an accessible sample data reflecting the spatiotemporal characteristics of the epidemic development. On the other hand, mobile phone data with age tag may help to characterize the spatial distribution of the elderly population in the study area. This article aims to analyze the spatial distribution of COVID-19 transmission based on geographic information system (GIS) visualization [23,24] with Weibo COVID-19 help-seekers data from February 3rd to February 12th, to explore the correlation between the spatial characteristics of the epidemic distribution and aged population, and to analyze the spatiotemporal features of epidemic spread. The analysis of the detailed characteristics of the epidemic in urban space can help cities that may have or have had outbreak to better understand the mechanism of disease transmission and it is of great significance to improve citizens' awareness of protection and provide certain policy references for government departments.

2. Study Area

Wuhan, as the capital of Hubei Province, (Figure 2a) was the earliest COVID-19 outbreak area in China. There was a short medical run period between the lockdown on January 23rd, 2020 and the increase in the number of medical beds and medical staff supporting Wuhan, leading to 99% of Weibo help seeking patients being in Wuhan (Figure 3). Wuhan is located in the east of Jianghan Plain and the middle reaches of the Yangtze River. The Yangtze River and its largest tributary, the Han River, run across the center of the city, dividing the central urban area of Wuhan into three regions of Wuchang, Hankou, and Hanyang, standing across the river (Figure 2b). Wuhan's main urban area (MUA) is the main concentration of urban function area, overlapped with the administration boundary of sub-districts.

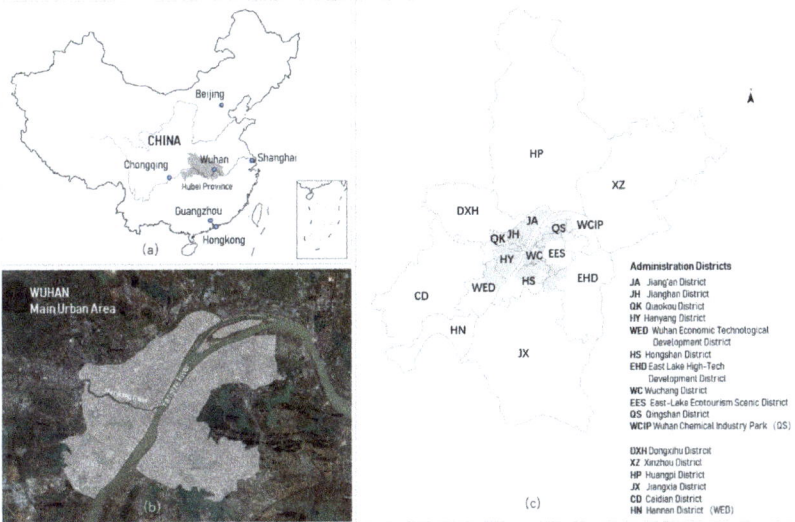

Figure 2. Map of the study area in Wuhan, China: (**a**) the geographic location of the Wuhan, China; (**b**) the main urban area of Wuhan (MUA); and (**c**) administrative districts of Wuhan.

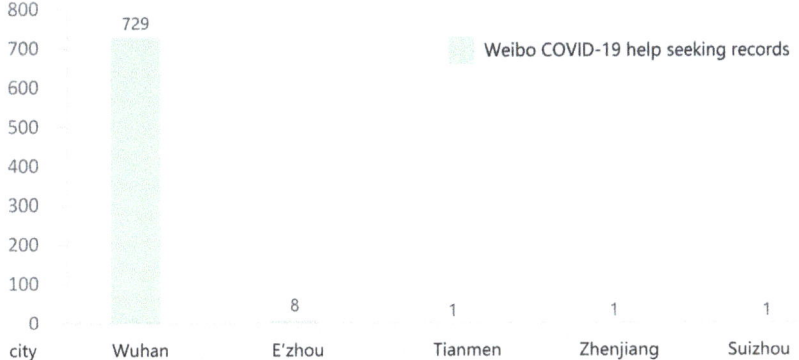

Figure 3. The distribution of Weibo COVID-19 help seeking records.

Wuhan contains seventeen sub-districts, which concludes Jiang'an (JA), Jianghan (JH), Qiaokou (QK), Hanyang (HY), Wuhan Economic Technological Development District (WED), Hongshan (HS), East Lake High-Tech Development District (EHD), Wuchang (WC), East-Lake Ecotourism Scenic District (EES), Qingshan (QS), Wuhan Chemical Industry Park (WCIP), Dongxihu (DXH), Xinzhou

(XZ), Huangpi (HP), Jiangxia (JX), Caidian (CD), and Hannan (HN) (Figure 2c). Wherein, WCIP and HN usually statistically belong to QS and WED, respectively.

According to the epidemic data of June 11th, 2020, about 76.327% of the total cumulative cases in Wuhan were in the MUA (Table 1), which is also the relatively concentrated area for early Weibo help seekers.

Table 1. Case statistics of Wuhan. (As of June 11th, 2020 source: Wuhan Municipal Commission of Health).

Districts	Cumulative Confirmed Case	Proportion
Jiang'an (MUA)	6563	13.037%
Jianghan(MUA)	5242	10.413%
Qiaokou(MUA)	6854	13.616%
Hanyang(MUA)	4691	9.319%
Wuchang(MUA)	7551	15.000%
Qingshan(MUA)	2804	5.570%
Hongshan(MUA)	4718	9.372%
Dongxihu	2478	4.923%
Caidian	1424	2.829%
Jiangxia	860	1.708%
Huangpi	2117	4.205%
Xinzhou	1071	2.128%
East Lake Ecotourism Scenic District	483	0.959%
East Lake High-Tech Development District	2173	4.317%
Wuhan Economic Technological Development District	1088	2.161%
Other places	223	0.443%
Total	50340	100.00%

3. Materials and Methods

3.1. Data and Preprocessing

3.1.1. Weibo Data

Sina Weibo is one of the most influential social media platforms in China. It had 486 million monthly active users by the end of June, 2019 [25]. In the early stage of the COVD-19 epidemic, due to the short-term collapse of medical system, Weibo opened the novel coronavirus pneumonia help seeking channel [26] to help patients who could not get timely treatment. The help seeking records were mainly from February 3rd to February 12th, 2020. The study collected about 1200 Weibo records under the topic of "novel coronavirus pneumonia help-seeking" and considered valid information including name, age, home address, time of illness, and number of people infected (Figure 4). As such, 740 records of valid information were finally obtained after data cleaning, wherein 729 records were in Wuhan (Figure 3).

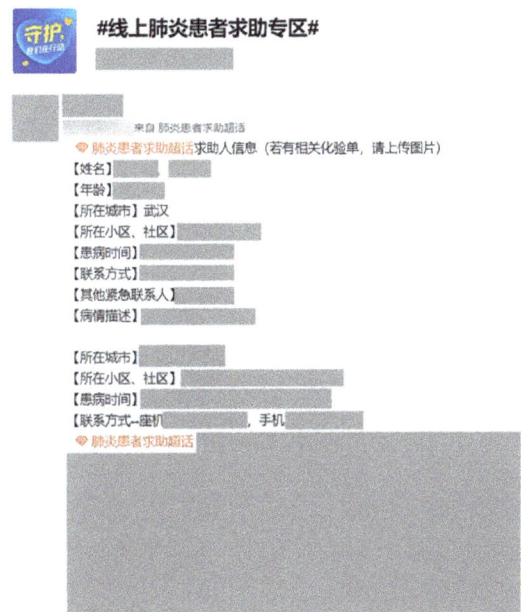

Figure 4. An example of Weibo help-seeking information.

The spatial distribution of help seekers is obtained by geocoding (Figure 5). The data shows that a large number of help seekers were concentrated in the main urban area of Wuhan, and a small number of records were outside.

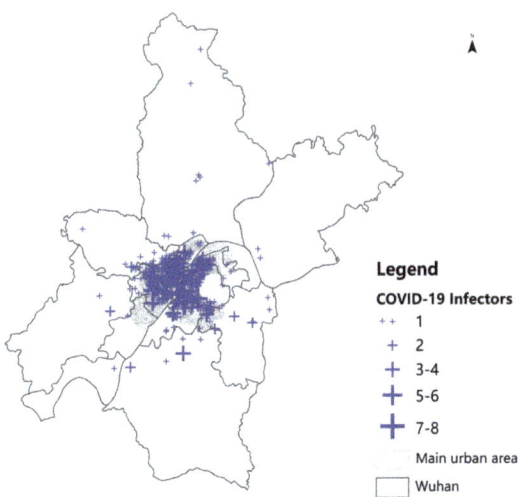

Figure 5. Spatial distribution of Wuhan Weibo help-seeking data.

3.1.2. Mobile Phone Data

Wuhan city's March 2017 call detail record (CDR) data with age tags was used in this study and the spatial distribution of base stations is shown in Figure 6. The steps were as follows to obtain the spatial distribution of the mobile phone population and the elderly population.

- We matched the mobile phone number and the user ID to eliminate all private information, and then removed the invalid and noise data.
- We counted the base stations with the highest call frequency of users, matching the base station code and the user ID, and summarized the number of users that the base station served.

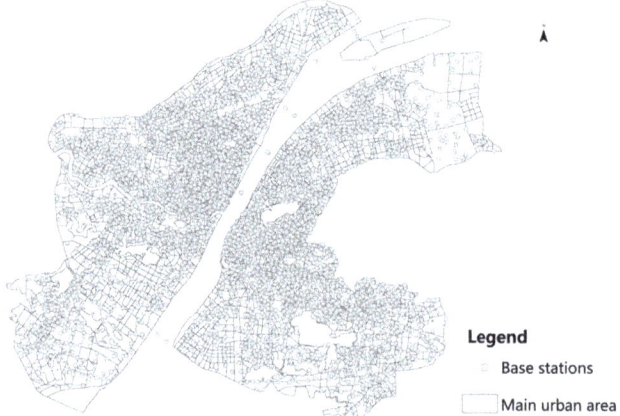

Figure 6. Spatial distribution of base stations in the main urban area of Wuhan.

3.2. Research Methods

3.2.1. Kernel Density Analysis

The Kernel density method was applied since the Weibo data could be seen as a sample data from total COVID-19 infectors. Kernel density analysis is capable to calculate the unit density of the measured values of points and line elements within a specified neighborhood, intuitively reflecting the distribution of discrete measured values in the continuous area. The result is the smooth surface with a large median value and a small peripheral value. The grid value is the unit density, which is reduced to 0 at the boundary of the neighborhood. Kernel density analysis can be used for service facility accessibility [27], crime prediction [28], business analysis, etc. Its function expression is as follows:

$$\hat{f}_h(x) = \frac{1}{nh} \sum_{i=1}^{n} K\left(\frac{x - x_i}{h}\right) \tag{1}$$

where K is the kernel (a non-negative function), $h > 0$ is a smoothing parameter called the bandwidth, x_i is the sample point.

3.2.2. Ordinary Least Square Regression

Based on Kernel density method, the average value of each space unit is calculated. The regression models, using the interpolation of infected people from Weibo data, the interpolation of population, and the elderly population generated by mobile phone data in community units in the main urban area were then constructed. The covariant explanatory variables were checked by the variance inflation factor (VIF) parameter, and the explanatory variables passing the P value of 1% significance level test were obtained. The function expression are as follows:

$$Y = \beta_m + \beta_1 x_1 + \varepsilon_1 \tag{2}$$

$$Y = \beta_n + \beta_2 x_2 + \varepsilon_2 \tag{3}$$

where Y is the interpolation of Weibo infected people in the community unit, x_1 is the interpolation of population derived from mobile phone data in the community unit, x_2 is the interpolation of the elderly population derived from mobile phone data in the community unit, β_m and β_n are intercepts, β_1 and β_2 are regression coefficients of factors, and ε_1 and ε_2 are random errors.

4. Results

4.1. Preliminary Analysis on COVID-19 Cases of Weibo Data

4.1.1. Demographic Statistics

There are 691 records containing age tags, wherein the maximum age was 95 and the minimum was 11-months. Among them, the proportion of infectors between 30 and 69 was 69.47%, which was lower than the corresponding proportion of 77.2% in the whole sample of Wuhan till February 11th, 2020 [29], and the proportion of infectors over 60 was 57.02%, which was higher than the corresponding proportion of 44.1% in the whole sample of Wuhan, showing that the susceptible population of novel coronavirus was mainly the middle-aged and the elderly groups. Moreover, the elderly who suffer from basic diseases are more likely to develop into critical patients, making the elderly patients become the group that accounted for more than half of Weibo help seekers (Figure 7).

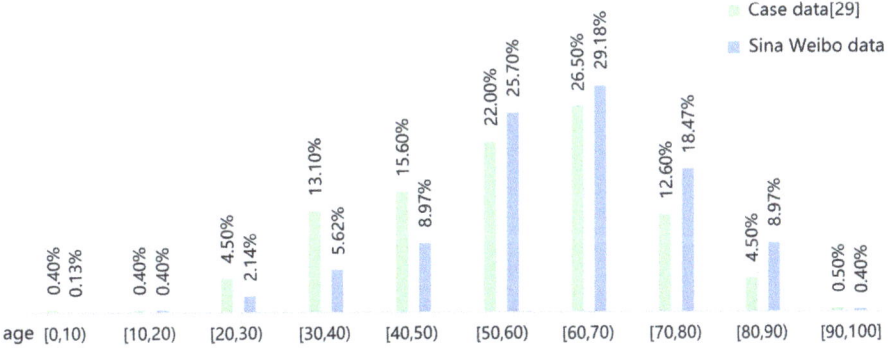

Figure 7. Histogram of patient age distribution of case data and Weibo data.

4.1.2. Spatial Distribution

According to the statistics of the number of household infectors reported in each single record, most records reported one to two infections, with the highest number of eight, reflecting the severity of clustered infections in families (Figure 8). The spatial distribution of COVID-19 cases of Weibo data in MUA showed relatively concentrated regional patterns in Hankou, northern Hanyang, and Wuchang (Figure 9).

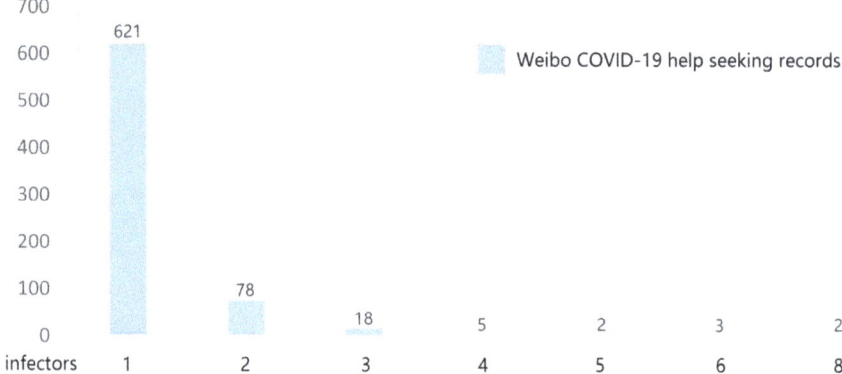

Figure 8. The number of infectors reported in each of the Weibo records.

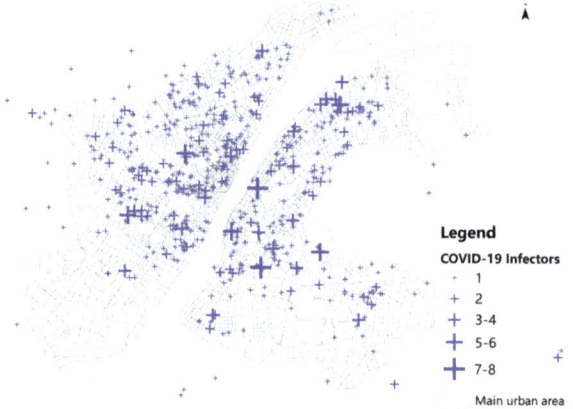

Figure 9. Spatial distribution of Weibo help seekers in the main urban area of Wuhan.

4.1.3. Time Series Statistics

Based on the number of COVID-19 infection of Weibo records and total infector reported, the corresponding change curve by onset time from December 20th, 2019 to February 10th, 2020 was obtained (Figure 10). It can be clearly seen that as time goes on, the absolute value of the difference between the two increased gradually, reaching the maximum when the epidemic was in full outbreak, around January 23rd, 2020, and then a general downward trend. It reflected that during the period of rapid growth of the infectors from December 22nd, 2020, the isolation control measures such as traffic restrictions and the improvement of medical facilities reduced the number of household infections effectively.

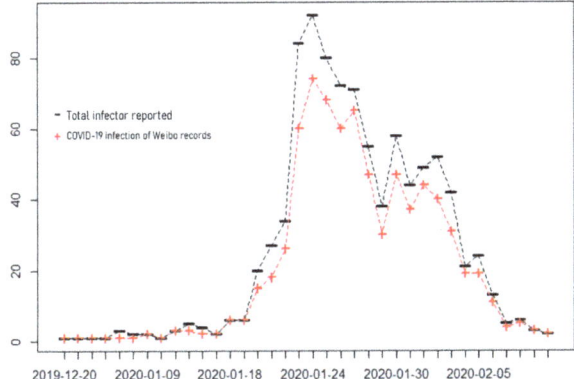

Figure 10. Timing chart of COVID-19 infection of Weibo records and total infector reported

4.2. Spatial Correlation Between COVID-19 Cases and Population Density

4.2.1. Kernel Density Analysis

The spatial features of COVID-19 cases and population density were visualized and compared, with the weight of the number of infections, population, and the elderly population, respectively, according to the Kernel density method. As is shown in Figure 11, COVID-19 cases of Weibo data were mainly concentrated in the central area along the Yangtze river, which is similar to the spatial distribution of population density, especially of the elderly population (Figure 11).

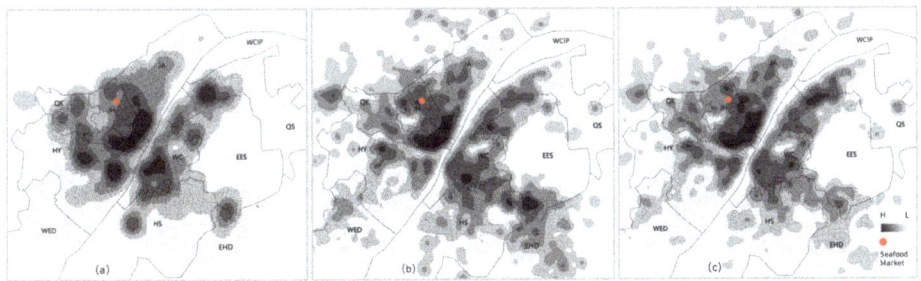

Figure 11. Kernel density analysis: (**a**) COVID-19 cases by Weibo data; (**b**) population density; and (**c**) the elderly population density generated by mobile phone data.

Interestingly, the Huanan Seafood Market, regarded as the origin point of the outbreak, had not been the geographic center of epidemic outbreak. This may be explained by the medium population density and low density of elderly population.

4.2.2. Ordinary Least Squares (OLS) Regression

According to the urban arterial roads, traffic analysis zone (TAZ) [30], the spatial statistical unit for urban population commuting characteristics analysis, was divided by the traffic management department. Since there was collinearity between the population and the elderly population in the study, the OLS model was established based on the TAZ level, using the interpolation of help seekers from Weibo data, with the interpolation of the population and the elderly population generated by mobile phone data, respectively. The results further verify that the distribution of the elderly population was significantly related to the infectors, with higher adjusted R-Squared of 0.7038 (Table 2).

Table 2. OLS diagnostics.

Variable	Coefficient	Stand Error	*p*-Value	Intercept	R-Squared	Adjusted R-Squared
The elderly	39.8216	0.5408	0.0000	7212.6697	0.7039	0.7038
population	3.2416	0.0576	0.0000	7265.7562	0.5811	0.5809

4.3. Spatiotemporal Features of COVID-19 Transmission

This paper further explored the early spatiotemporal characteristics of the epidemic transmission based on the infection time of COVID-19 cases provided by Weibo data. Wherein, the hot spots can be regarded as the initial pathogen transmission, and the areas with the highest density levels in each period can be regarded as the areas with the fastest transmission of infection. The COVID-19 transmission map of Weibo data shows a clear process of three stages: Scattered infection, community spread, and full-scale outbreak.

In the COVID-19 data of Weibo, only 3 infectors had been reported before 2020, and 25 infectors were from January 1st to 18th, 2020. The earliest infected spots already covered all the outbreak areas except hotspots in Hongshan district (Figure 12a), which began to appear in the second period (Figure 12b). The result shows that before the lockdown of Wuhan on January 23rd, cases mainly existed in the Jiang'an, Jianghan, Qiaokou, Hanyang, Wuchang, Hongshan, and Qingshan districts in the early stage (Figure 12).

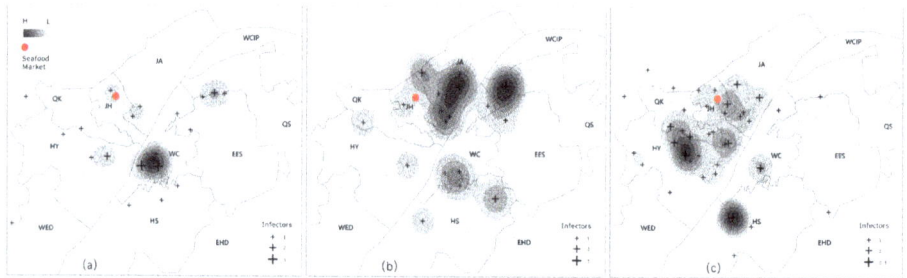

Figure 12. Spatial distribution of help seekers from December 20th, 2019 to January 22nd, 2020: (**a**) before January 18th, 2020; (**b**) from January 19th to 20th, 2020; and (**c**) from January 21st to 22nd, 2020.

The epidemic peak appeared around January 23rd, 2020 (Figure 13a). There had been multiple outbreak centers, and the higher ones were the hotspots in Qiaokou, Jiang'an, Wuchang, Hongshan, and Qingshan. It was found that the epidemic outbreak areas were all high-density residential areas, representing the entering stage of community transmission (Figure 13).

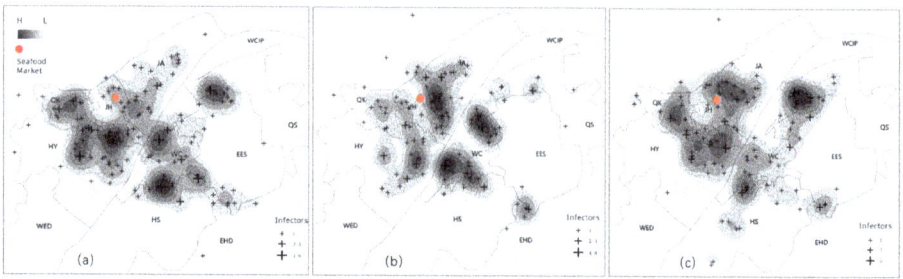

Figure 13. Spatial distribution of help seekers from January 23rd to 28th, 2020: (**a**) from January 23rd to 24th, 2020; (**b**) from January 25th to 26th, 2020; and (**c**) from January 27th to 28th, 2020.

From January 29th, 2020 to February 3rd, 2020, it was the sub peak in several periods (Figure 14a–c). The distribution of cases was in an average trend in all regions, with the hotspots concentrated in Jiang'an, Jianghan, Wuchang, and Qingshan districts, being still basically within the initial range. The number of the core density regions decreased while the range of transmission further expanded from February 4th to February 7th, 2020 (Figure 14d,e). By February 10th, 2020, the number of patients had been trending to single digit, and the spatial distribution characteristics were no longer typical in terms of sampling coverage (Figure 14f).

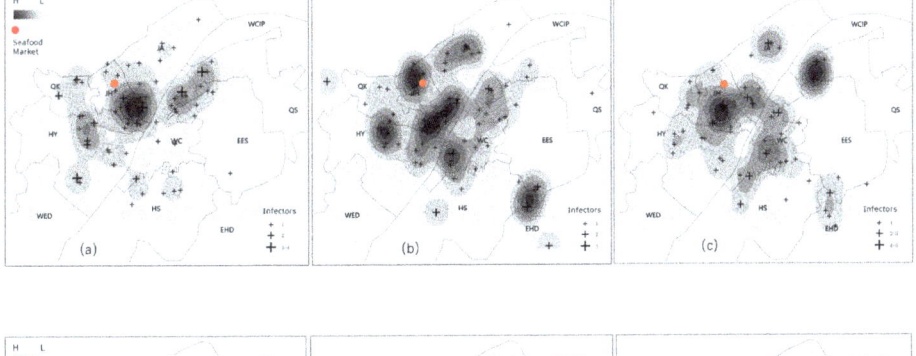

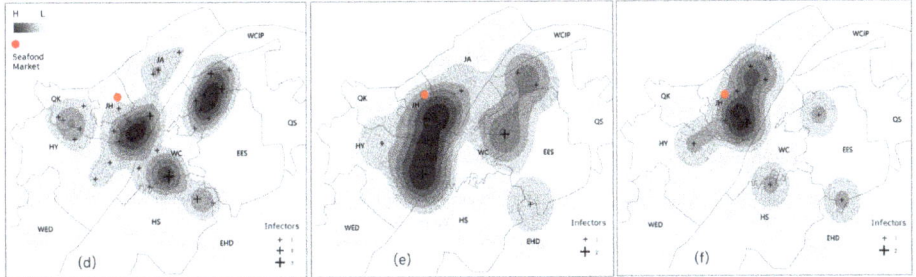

Figure 14. Spatial distribution of help seekers from January 29th to February 10th, 2020: (**a**) from January 29th to 30th, 2020; (**b**) from January 31st to February 1st, 2020; (**c**) from February 2nd to 3rd, 2020; (**d**) from February 4th to 5th, 2020; (**e**) from February 6th to 7th, 2020; and (**f**) from February 8th to 10th, 2020.

5. Discussion

The spatial distribution of COVID-19 cases extracted by Weibo data is highly correlated with the density of population, especially of the elderly population. As the first region of the outbreak in China, Wuhan entered the community transmission stage earlier. Therefore, it can be inferred that after the epidemic development for a period of time, the regeneration index R0 of each district tended to be consistent, leading to a strong correlation between the case and population. The closer relationship between the cases and the elderly population confirms that the elderly population is the high-risk group, consistent with the current medical observations [29,31]. Consequently, the study proposes that the elderly, as the susceptible population with high incidence and high risk of the COVID-19, should be the key target for active response in the epidemic prevention.

Compared with the traditional cases data, spatiotemporal data such as social media data, is more available, more time-sensitive. Differing from the previous study in the data sources [32], the study proposes social media data and mobile phone data to explore spatial features of novel coronavirus transmission. Weibo data is of great significance to identify the spatial distribution of infectors and mobile phone provides fine-scale population with age tags.

The results indicate that:

(1) When the capita medical resources were extremely scarce, the incidence rates in urban areas tended to be the same after entering the community transmission period. The spatial distribution of help seekers was related to the regional population density. Since the elderly are more likely to convert severe groups, the space distribution of help seekers had a higher correlation with the density of the elderly population.

(2) The new coronavirus epidemic showed the obvious spatiotemporal characteristic of scattered infection, community spread, and full-scale outbreak in the early stage, which was specifically manifested in the process of mobile diffusion centered on the early cases found in Jiang'an, Jianghan, Qiaokou, Wuchang, Hongshan, and Hanyang districts before January 23rd, the interior spread of each community that forming the polycentric structure after January 23rd, and the explosion process in which the density core area further spread later.

Compared with the research on the country level l [3–5], the spatiotemporal characteristics of the epidemic in emerging city can help us understand the detail inter-regional interactions in the urban space, and help other cities that are likely to have outbreaks or have had outbreaks to better understand the mechanism of disease transmission and the relationship between urban governance and public health epidemic prevention, so as to take appropriate protective measures in each stage, respectively.

During the epidemic period, countries have different principles for the use of privacy data in the general policy of epidemic prevention and control. When the detailed disease data that involves privacy issues is difficult to obtain, the spontaneous data provided by the media can be used as an effective means to provide a certain degree of reference information for the public and government departments. Meanwhile, due to the inaccessibility of data, we used the call detail record data of March 2017 in Wuhan city. The inconsistency of data on the time profile may lead to a certain difference in results, while we consider that such a time period will not change greatly in terms of macroscopic characteristics.

The release time of Weibo help information was mainly from February 3rd to February 12th. With the gradual completion of medical resources, help information tended to be no update. It can be seen from the spatial correlation analysis that the help seeking data in the period had good spatial coverage, consequently, the study believes that it can reflect the early three stages of disease transmission in Wuhan urban space from December 20th, 2019 to February 10th, 2020 to a certain extent. It should also be noted that, due to the small sample size of Weibo cases and the onset time were mostly after 2020, in spite of the good sample coverage, there was still missing information. The significance of our research is to make such an attempt on limited data, to carry out a retrospective analysis of the development of the epidemic situation, and to analyze the possible laws of the spread of disease in space and time, with a certain degree of verification. Therefore, if the detailed spatial distribution information of early patients can be obtained, a complete retrospective deduction of the spatial transmission path of the entire early epidemic can be obtained in a similar way.

Furthermore, the study can be expanded in the following aspects: (1) the further exploration of the influencing factors of epidemic to better understand the transmission mechanism and (2) combined with more detailed flow data to build agent model for further simulation and analysis.

6. Conclusions

In the context of the outbreak of the COVID-19 in Wuhan, the spatiotemporal mapping is of vital importance to understand the spatial features of the new coronavirus transmission mechanism. This study contributes to propose the combination of Weibo help seeking data and mobile phone data to achieve the quantitative study of the new coronavirus epidemic. Help seeking mapping can reflect the actual spatial distribution of the infectors who could not get timely treatment in the epidemic city under the condition of the short run of medical resources in Wuhan, and help us to identify the obvious transmission characteristics of epidemic development, which is specifically manifested in the earlier scattered infection, community spread, and full-scale outbreak process on the whole. Simultaneously, the population derived from mobile phone data enables to find the high-similarity of distribution patterns between Weibo COVID-19 cases and the elderly population, which is verified by the result of the OLS model. Consequently, it can be used as the evidence for the elderly population groups being the susceptible population of the new coronavirus pneumonia. Moreover, the study proposes that elderly population should be the key target for active response in the epidemic prevention while corresponding measures should be deployed.

In general, the study based on the usage of Weibo data, mobile phone data, and other spatial big data resources can clearly identify the susceptible people and disease-prone spaces, and explore the process of the spatiotemporal dynamic spread of the new coronavirus, which is helpful to provide decision-making basis for disease prevention and control to a certain extent.

Author Contributions: Lingbo Liu and Ru Wang conceived and designed the experiments; Zhenghong Peng and Hao Wu acquired and analyzed the data; Hao Wu and Ru Wang contributed analysis tools; Lingbo Liu and Ru Wang wrote the paper. All authors have read and agreed to the published version of the manuscript.

Funding: The study was funded by National Natural Science Foundation of China (No. 51978535); Humanities and Social Science Project of the Ministry of Education (No. 19YJCZH187); Wuhan University Experiment Technology Project Funding.

Acknowledgments: The authors acknowledge the contribution of all the anonymous reviewers that improved the quality of the paper.

Conflicts of Interest: The authors declare no conflict of interest.

References

1. Wu, F.; Zhao, S.; Yu, B.; Chen, Y.M.; Wang, W.; Song, Z.G.; Hu, Y.; Tao, Z.W.; Tian, J.H.; Pei, Y.Y.; et al. A new coronavirus associated with human respiratory disease in China. *Nature* **2020**, *579*, 265–269. [CrossRef] [PubMed]
2. Tian, H.; Liu, Y.; Li, Y.; Wu, C.-H.; Chen, B.; Kraemer, M.U.; Li, B.; Cai, J.; Xu, B.; Yang, Q. An investigation of transmission control measures during the first 50 days of the COVID-19 epidemic in China. *Science* **2020**, *368*, 638–642. [CrossRef] [PubMed]
3. Gao, S.; Rao, J.; Kang, Y.; Liang, Y.; Kruse, J. Mapping county-level mobility pattern changes in the United States in response to COVID-19. *Sigspatial Spec.* **2020**, *12*, 16–26. [CrossRef]
4. Huang, R.; Liu, M.; Ding, Y. Spatial-temporal distribution of COVID-19 in China and its prediction: A data-driven modeling analysis. *J. Infect. Dev. Ctries.* **2020**, *14*, 246–253. [CrossRef] [PubMed]
5. Kang, D.; Choi, H.; Kim, J.-H.; Choi, J. Spatial epidemic dynamics of the COVID-19 outbreak in China. *Int. J. Infect. Dis.* **2020**, *94*, 96–102. [CrossRef]
6. Keil, R.; Ali, H. Governing the sick city: Urban governance in the age of emerging infectious disease. *Antipode* **2007**, *39*, 846–873. [CrossRef]
7. Neiderud, C.-J. How urbanization affects the epidemiology of emerging infectious diseases. *Infect. Ecol. Epidemiol.* **2015**, *5*, 27060. [CrossRef]
8. Jaglin, S. Rethinking urban heterogeneity. In *The Routledge Handbook on Cities of the Global South*; Routledge: Abingdon, UK, 2014; pp. 434–446.
9. Breiman, R.F.; Cosmas, L.; Njenga, M.K.; Williamson, J.; Mott, J.A.; Katz, M.A.; Erdman, D.D.; Schneider, E.; Oberste, M.S.; Neatherlin, J.C. Severe acute respiratory infection in children in a densely populated urban slum in Kenya, 2007–2011. *BMC Infect. Dis.* **2015**, *15*, 95. [CrossRef]
10. Huang, C.; Xu, X.; Cai, Y.; Ge, Q.; Zeng, G.; Li, X.; Zhang, W.; Ji, C.; Yang, L. Mining the Characteristics of COVID-19 Patients in China: Analysis of Social Media Posts. *J. Med. Internet Res.* **2020**, *22*, e19087. [CrossRef]
11. Penrose, K.; de Castro, M.C.; Werema, J.; Ryan, E.T. Informal urban settlements and cholera risk in Dar es Salaam, Tanzania. *PLoS Negl. Trop. Dis.* **2010**, *4*. [CrossRef]
12. Li, Q.; Guan, X.; Wu, P.; Wang, X.; Zhou, L.; Tong, Y.; Ren, R.; Leung, K.S.M.; Lau, E.H.Y.; Wong, J.Y.; et al. Early Transmission Dynamics in Wuhan, China, of Novel Coronavirus-Infected Pneumonia. *N. Engl. J. Med.* **2020**, *382*, 1199–1207. [CrossRef] [PubMed]
13. Perlman, S. Another decade, another coronavirus. *Mass. Med. Soc.* **2020**. [CrossRef] [PubMed]

14. Bansal, S.; Chowell, G.; Simonsen, L.; Vespignani, A.; Viboud, C. Big data for infectious disease surveillance and modeling. *J. Infect. Dis.* **2016**, *214*, S375–S379. [CrossRef] [PubMed]
15. Lee, E.C.; Asher, J.M.; Goldlust, S.; Kraemer, J.D.; Lawson, A.B.; Bansal, S. Mind the scales: Harnessing spatial big data for infectious disease surveillance and inference. *J. Infect. Dis.* **2016**, *214*, S409–S413. [CrossRef] [PubMed]
16. Li, L.; Zhang, Q.; Wang, X.; Zhang, J.; Wang, T.; Gao, T.-L.; Duan, W.; Tsoi, K.K.-f.; Wang, F.-Y. Characterizing the Propagation of Situational Information in Social Media During COVID-19 Epidemic: A Case Study on Weibo. *IEEE Trans. Comput. Soc. Syst.* **2020**, *7*, 556–562. [CrossRef]
17. Zhao, Y.; Xu, H. Chinese public attention to COVID-19 epidemic: Based on social media. *medRxiv* **2020**. [CrossRef]
18. Li, J.; Xu, Q.; Cuomo, R.; Purushothaman, V.; Mackey, T. Data Mining and Content Analysis of the Chinese Social Media Platform Weibo During the Early COVID-19 Outbreak: Retrospective Observational Infoveillance Study. *Jmir Public Health Surveill* **2020**, *6*, e18700. [CrossRef]
19. Prabhakar Kaila, D.; Prasad, D.A. Informational flow on Twitter–Corona virus outbreak–topic modelling approach. *Int. J. Adv. Res. Eng. Technol.* **2020**, *11*, 128–134.
20. Jahanbin, K.; Rahmanian, V. Using Twitter and web news mining to predict COVID-19 outbreak. *Asian Pac. J. Trop. Med.* **2020**, *13*. [CrossRef]
21. Schild, L.; Ling, C.; Blackburn, J.; Stringhini, G.; Zhang, Y.; Zannettou, S. "Go eat a bat, Chang!": An Early Look on the Emergence of Sinophobic Behavior on Web Communities in the Face of COVID-19. *arXiv* **2020**, arXiv:2004.04046.
22. Li, S.; Wang, Y.; Xue, J.; Zhao, N.; Zhu, T. The Impact of COVID-19 Epidemic Declaration on Psychological Consequences: A Study on Active Weibo Users. *Int. J. Env. Res. Public Health* **2020**, *17*, 2032. [CrossRef] [PubMed]
23. Carroll, L.N.; Au, A.P.; Detwiler, L.T.; Fu, T.-c.; Painter, I.S.; Abernethy, N.F. Visualization and analytics tools for infectious disease epidemiology: A systematic review. *J. Biomed. Inform.* **2014**, *51*, 287–298. [CrossRef] [PubMed]
24. Cromley, E.K.; McLafferty, S.L. *GIS and Public Health*; Guilford Press: New York, NY, USA, 2011.
25. Weibo Reports Robust Q2 User Growth. Available online: http://www.xinhuanet.com/english/2019-08/20/c_138323288.htm (accessed on 1 June 2020).
26. Weibo Novel Coronavirus Pneumonia Help Seeking Channel. Available online: https://s.weibo.com/weibo?q=%23%E7%BA%BF%E4%B8%8A%E8%82%BA%E7%82%8E%E6%82%A3%E8%80%85%E6%B1%82%E5%8A%A9%E4%B8%93%E5%8C%BA%23 (accessed on 13 February 2020).
27. Spencer, J.; Angeles, G. Kernel density estimation as a technique for assessing availability of health services in Nicaragua. *Health Serv. Outcomes Res. Methodol.* **2007**, *7*, 145–157. [CrossRef]
28. Gerber, M.S. Predicting crime using Twitter and kernel density estimation. *Decis. Support Syst.* **2014**, *61*, 115–125. [CrossRef]
29. Response, E.W.G.f.N.E. The epidemiological characteristics of an outbreak of 2019 novel coronavirus diseases (COVID-19) in China. *Chin. J. Epidemiol.* **2020**, *41*, 145–151.
30. Miller, H.J.; Shaw, S.-L. *Geographic Information Systems for Transportation: Principles and Applications*; Oxford University Press: London, UK, 2001.
31. Huang, C.; Wang, Y.; Li, X.; Ren, L.; Zhao, J.; Hu, Y.; Zhang, L.; Fan, G.; Xu, J.; Gu, X. Clinical features of patients infected with 2019 novel coronavirus in Wuhan, China. *Lancet* **2020**, *395*, 497–506. [CrossRef]
32. Wesolowski, A.; Buckee, C.O.; Engø-Monsen, K.; Metcalf, C.J.E. Connecting mobility to infectious diseases: The promise and limits of mobile phone data. *J. Infect. Dis.* **2016**, *214*, S414–S420. [CrossRef]

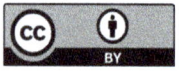

© 2020 by the authors. Licensee MDPI, Basel, Switzerland. This article is an open access article distributed under the terms and conditions of the Creative Commons Attribution (CC BY) license (http://creativecommons.org/licenses/by/4.0/).

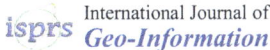

Article

Interdependent Healthcare Critical Infrastructure Analysis in a Spatiotemporal Environment: A Case Study

Nivedita Nukavarapu * and Surya Durbha

Centre of Studies in Resources Engineering, Indian Institute of Technology Bombay, Powai, Mumbai 400076, India; sdurbha@iitb.ac.in
* Correspondence: nnivedita@iitb.ac.in

Received: 3 April 2020; Accepted: 16 May 2020; Published: 11 June 2020

Abstract: During an urban flooding scenario, Healthcare Critical Infrastructure (HCI) represents a critical and essential resource. As the flood levels rise and the existing HCI facilities struggle to keep up with the pace, the under-preparedness of most urban cities to address this challenge becomes evident. Due to the disruptions in the interdependent Critical Infrastructures (CI) network (i.e., water supply, communications, electricity, transportation, etc.), during an urban flooding event, the operations at the healthcare CI facilities are inevitably affected. Hence, there is a need to identify cascading CI failure scenarios to visualize the propagation of failure of one CI facility to another CI, which can impact vast geographical areas. The goal of this work is to develop an interdependent HCI simulation model in a spatiotemporal environment to understand the dynamics in real-time and model the propagation of cascading CI failures in an interdependent HCI network. The model is developed based on a real-world cascading CI failure case study on an interdependent HCI network during the flood disaster event in December 2015 at Chennai, TamilNadu, India. The interdependencies between the CI networks are modeled by using the Stochastic Colored Petri Net (SCPN) based modeling approach. SCPN is used to model a real-word process that occurs in parallel or concurrently. Furthermore, a geographic information system-based interface is integrated with the simulation model, to visualize the dynamic behavior of the interdependent HCI SCPN simulation model in a spatiotemporal environment. Such a dynamic simulation model can assist the decision-makers and emergency responders to rapidly simulate 'what if' kind of scenarios and consequently respond rapidly.

Keywords: healthcare critical infrastructure; geovisualization; geographic information system; colored petri net

1. Introduction

Understanding and rapidly responding to flood events in urban cities (cities such as Mumbai, Chennai, Hyderabad, Bangalore, etc., in India) is important for supporting its economic growth and resilience. An increase in unplanned urban settlements in metropolitan cities is resulting in the change of drainage characteristics of natural drainage areas. Hence, these natural catchments are unable to manage the increased volume of floodwater and the rate of surface runoff due to the encroachment of wetlands, floodplains, and blockage of the drainage channels due to the disposal of solid and liquid wastes [1]. Obstruction of floodways, natural water bodies causes loss of natural flood storage leading to urban floods. Urban flooding can have severe implications on the interdependent critical infrastructures. Critical Infrastructure (CI) is defined as the group of assets and technological networks or systems such as electrical supply, water supply, transport, communication, finance, healthcare, and information technology, etc., which are vital for the functioning of the economy and society [2–5].

Critical infrastructure (CI) networks are not independent functioning assets; they are interdependent. For example, the functioning of a healthcare critical infrastructure network is dependent on the electrical supply CI, water supply CI, transport CI, and communication CI, etc. The CI networks are large scale distributed systems interconnected with each other based on spatial or operational interdependencies. The interdependent CI networks form a high degree of a complex network consisting of different nodes, edges, and sets [2,3,5].

In an Interdependent CI network due to an event when a failure or disruption occurs in one of the CI network nodes, the failure propagates to the dependent CI node disrupting the subsequent second CI network such kind of domino effect type of failure is called as *"cascading failure"*. Cascading failure arises due to a failure in one of the CI network components because of spatial or logical vulnerabilities. Disruption of one of the CI services due to failure in one of the CI components (CI facilities such as hospitals, electrical substations, etc.) can initiate cascading effects within an infrastructure or, in the worst case, cause failures in other infrastructures, possibly disrupting vital services, and affecting the security and performance of the interdependent CI services or systems [4,6]. As shown in Figure 1, an interdependent CI network is a set of different types of complex CI networks consisting of different sets of nodes, edges.

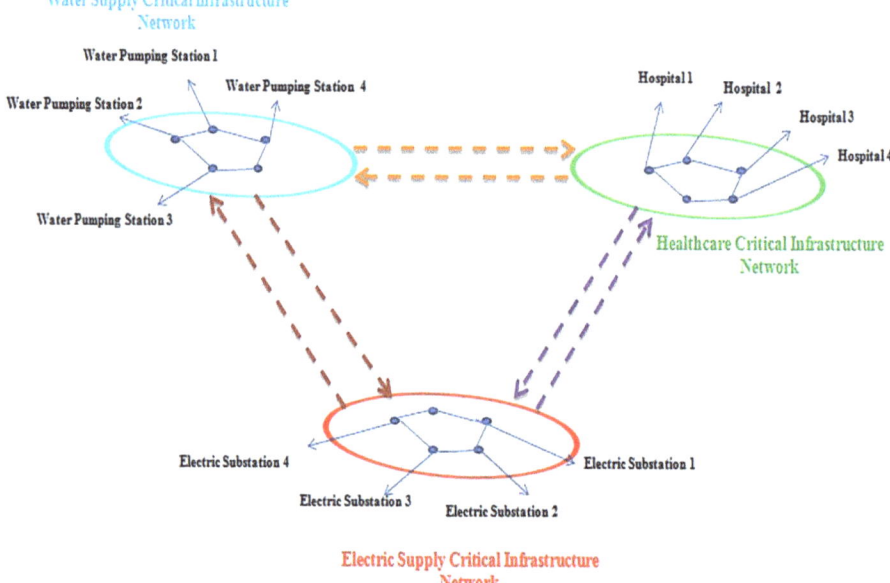

Figure 1. Interdependencies between the different Critical Infrastructure facilities nodes.

Each node in a CI network represents the CI facility. For example, in a healthcare CI network, each node represents the healthcare CI facility such as hospitals. In an electrical supply CI network, each node represents the electrical supply CI facility such as an electrical substation. The CI nodes are connected via links representing the relationship between them. In this complex interdependent network, the states of each CI node are correlated or are influenced by the state of the other CI node component. For example, the failed state of a CI facility node will disrupt the functioning of an interdependent operating CI facility node leading to a *'cascading failure'* scenario. Such an event leaves the decision-makers and emergency personnel underprepared to deal with the impact of such cascading failure disruptions.

During an urban flooding scenario, Healthcare Critical Infrastructure (HCI) represents a vital and crucial resource. As the flood levels rise and the existing HCI facilities fiercely struggle to keep up with the pace, their under-preparedness becomes evident. The healthcare operations are inevitably affected by disruptions in other critical infrastructures, and we certainly need to identify cascading scenarios and visualize the propagation of failure from one CI facility to another, which ultimately impacts the HCI facilities. In other words, the resilience of healthcare facilities cannot be treated in isolation but must be seen as part of a much bigger interdependent healthcare critical infrastructure (HCI) system [7,8].

1.1. Literature Review

Extensive research has been done on the risk assessment of a single independent critical infrastructure facility. Although such analysis has importance in risk assessment, however interdependencies among the interlinked critical infrastructures should be considered for overall vulnerability assessment. Various approaches and techniques are being used to model critical infrastructure interdependencies, often based on the purpose of the outcome of the model, such as the empirical model, agent-based model, systems dynamic model, etc. The following literature showcases the different approaches to model critical infrastructure interdependencies. Wallace et al. [9,10] modeled different infrastructure functionalities by using a uniform network flow mathematical representation. Chou and Tseng [11] proposed a knowledge discovery process, where they collected each CI facility failure history in the interdependent CI network and studied the failure patterns associated with their failure occurrence probabilities. Jha [12] developed a Bayesian Network (BN)-based model to analyze and predict the likelihood of a terrorist attack on the interdependent CI network. Barett et al. [13] Studied the interdependencies generated between the transportation CI and the communication CI due to human behavior at the time of crisis. Duenas-Osorio and Kwasinski [14] analyzed the interdependencies between the CI networks using a time series method from the post-disaster event utility restoration curves after the Chilean earthquake in 2010. Cardellini et al. [15] Used the agent-based approach to understanding the interdependencies between various interdependent CI in a single framework.

For simulation and modeling of the interdependencies between the healthcare critical infrastructure networks so far, the numbers of published studies are less. Loosemore et al. [8] analyzed the impact of an extreme event on an HCI facility and analyzed the interdependencies using rich picture diagrams. Arboleda et al. [16] developed network flow models designed to assess the impact of the loss of capability in the utility infrastructure networks on the ability of hospitals to provide adequate care for patients. Arboleda et al. [17] represented the interdependencies between different healthcare facilities and internal dependencies using a network flow model. John [18] developed an agent-based healthcare impact simulation model HCSim. The simulation model is used to assess the impact of a mass casualty event on the HCI facilities. Vugrin et al. [19] suggested that healthcare facilities need to absorb and adapt to disruptive circumstances in several ways, for example, making the structures more flood-resistant or ensuring sufficient physical capacity to absorb patients in a mass casualty event. The impact of a disaster event such as flooding on the internal and external interdependencies of a healthcare facility has been rarely addressed in the literature.

Petri Nets for Critical Infrastructure Interdependency Modeling

Petri net is a graph theory-based mathematical tool and is used to model complex network processes and analyze their performance and behavior [20,21]. Petri nets are useful to diagrammatically model concurrency and synchronization in distributed systems. Unlike the state machines, the state transitions in Petri nets are asynchronous. Various types of dynamic event-driven systems have been modeled by using Petri net, as in the real world system, events happen at the same time and the system may have many local states to form a global state.

A Petri net enables a quick and intuitive representation of the different states, events, and interdependencies between the critical infrastructure systems. The probabilistic and temporal analysis provided by the Petri net is useful in understanding the behavior of the complex system. It offers a promising approach towards the risk modeling and analysis of interdependencies of critical infrastructures. Petri net approach is modular and scalable; as it is possible to add several new CI facilities, interdependencies, activities, or events that one likes to add to an existing system. The modeling approach provides the modeler to add more details, which means that we can model a complex system at a finer level of abstraction, by implementing nets within nets (which are called as subpages in the Petri net model) [22,23]. Petri nets are explained in detail in Section 2.1. Petri net in its various extensions such as colored Petri net has been used by researchers to capture and model the interdependency among the critical infrastructures [24–28].

Gursesli et al. [25] used the Petri net to develop a model the interdependencies among various CI such as electrical supply, transportation, water supply, communication, education and, emergency services. Sultana and Chen [26] studied and analyzed the interdependencies between the elements of the infrastructure used to generate hydroelectricity such as a dam, turbine, pumping station, etc., at the onset of a flood. The interdependencies were modeled by using an extended Petri net model and the behavior was analyzed by using Markov chain analysis. Krings et al. [27] developed a generalized stochastic Petri net (GSPN) for modeling the cascading failures in an interdependent CI network. Immediate and timed transitions were used to identify a common-mode fault. The interdependencies were modeled based on a scenario where the failure of the electrical supply CI would impact the other interdependent CI. Chen et al. [28] modeled cyber-physical attacks on the smart grid using Petri Net. Laprie et al. [29] provided a Petri-net model to study the interdependencies between electric supply CI and information technology. Omidvar et al. [30] Developed a Petri net model to understand and assess the failure risk between the various CI facilities in an interdependent CI network when an earthquake occurs. Giglio et al. [31] Proposed the Petri net simulation model to be used to analyze, control, and optimize a railway traffic system. Di Febbraro et al. [32] modeled the CI interdependencies and criticality of failure events in a railway network and analyzed the vulnerabilities of the network. Szpyrka et al. [33] modeled and evaluated the risk propagation of cybersecurity with Petri nets. Petri net simulation has been widely used in the healthcare domain. Dotoli et al. [34] proposed a timed Petri net model to simulate the workflow for a hospital department. Work by Hamana et al. [35] addressed the performance evaluation and verification of a healthcare facility and its services to a specific region or territory.

The versatility of the Petri simulation means that it can be used in a wide variety of applications. Most of the work done considered the workflow of a healthcare facility or the simulation of the services provided by a healthcare facility. Our work focuses on stochastic colored Petri net-based modeling and simulating of critical interdependencies in an interdependent healthcare critical infrastructure network during a flooding disaster event.

1.2. Core Objectives

In the last five years, many urban cities in India have witnessed a stream of extreme weather patterns that have left an unmistakable path of destruction. Experiences from the Mumbai floods 2005, Kashmir floods 2014, Chennai Floods 2015, and Kerala floods 2018 in India, has shown that urban flood disasters disrupt the operations of various CI networks and services; healthcare critical infrastructure (HCI) being one of the critical and vital among them.

During an urban flooding disaster scenario, the HCI network is called upon to provide emergency services. The HCI facilities must be able to provide the flood victims and patients in the hospital with medical care, pharmaceutical supplies, pathological services, intensive care services, etc., for an extended duration and under often difficult circumstances [7]. HCI facilities are at risk of damage from internal or external sources generated by an urban flood. Due to the disruption of lifeline services such as electricity supply, water supply, etc., the patients treated at the impacted HCI facility have to be transferred to another HCI facility. Hence, there is a need to model and simulate the system dynamics of an interdependent HCI network.

Given below is a real-life What-if Scenario showcasing the criticality of interdependencies between HCI facility networks during a flooding scenario, and the need for a simulation model for the decision-makers.

"A healthcare facility is flooded. The electrical substation which provides electric supply to the hospital is inundated. Due to which the electric supply to the healthcare facility (hospital) and the water pumping facility (water pumping station) is disrupted. Due to water pumping station disruption, the hospital is cut off from water supply. At the same time, as a result of the increase in flood water level, the basement of the hospital is inundated, and the backup generators became non-operational. The loss of electrical supply, water supply, and the unpreparedness of the hospital resulted in the operational failure of the hospital. The most affected area is the intensive care unit (ICU) of the hospital, due to non-functioning medical equipment and an insufficient number of reserved oxygen cylinders for the ICU patients. The ICU patients have to be evacuated in ambulances to the nearby safer hospital. The ambulances have to transport the patients via the shortest and the safest routes".

The end-user can query the simulation model for various flooding situation-based queries such as:

- Which CI facilities are inundated?
- What is the shortest and safest route for emergency evacuation of patients from the HCI facility?
- Which roads inundated?
- How much time is left for water supply disruption?
- What would be the cascading impact on the HCI facility if there is a failure in one of its interdependent CI facilities such as disruption in an electrical CI substation?

From the above scenario, we observe that the interdependent HCI network is at its vulnerable most during a flood event, and a real-time situational simulation model will help address these vulnerabilities. There is a dire need for an interdependent HCI network dynamic simulation model during a flood event, in a spatiotemporal environment. The model should be based on real-world scenarios, which exhibit concurrency, synchronization, and randomness. Both internal and external stochastic dependencies of the HCI network have to be addressed in the simulation model.

The core objectives of this work are:

To develop a stochastic colored Petri net driven geographic information system-based simulation model, useful in understanding the status of healthcare critical infrastructures during a flooding disaster scenario. This involves understanding the impact of different flood levels on the CI facilities using probabilistic fragility curves and the complex stochastic interdependencies between the CIs. The stochastic colored Petri net model is developed with various object-oriented functions and geospatial relationships, such that the Geographic Information System (GIS) is driven by the stochastic colored Petri net model. The coupling of the Petri net and the geographic information provides the simulation model with the spatiotemporal dimension.

The entire complex dynamic simulation model is then encapsulated into a java based Geovisualization interface. The utility of the approach is evaluated and analyzed using a real-world cascading CI failure case study scenario. The case study is based on an interdependent HCI network during the flood disaster event in December 2015 at Chennai, TamilNadu, India. The ability to have a stochastic colored Petri net driven geographic information system based interdependent critical infrastructure simulation model can have an impact on real-time decision-making heuristics during a flood disaster event.

The remaining paper is organized as follows; Section 2 discusses the Methodology. Section 3 consists of the development of the Stochastic Colored Petri net (SCPN) simulation model, in a geographical environment based on the Chennai 2015 flood disaster event case study. While Section 4 presents the results, where the model predicts the propagation of cascading failure scenarios and analyzes the system dynamics of an interdependent HCI network simulation model during the Chennai 2015 flood disaster event. Conclusions are drawn in Section 5.

2. Methodology

This section describes the methodology, which consists of detailed explanation of Petri net, its variation stochastic Petri net in detail, SCPN based interdependent healthcare CI simulation model system in a spatiotemporal environment, the proposed architectural framework of the system; probabilistic assessment for interdependent healthcare critical infrastructure network and the development of an SCPN driven geographic information system based interdependent healthcare critical infrastructure simulation model.

2.1. Petri Nets

Petri net is a directed, bipartite graph as shown in Figure 2; it is a powerful mathematical tool to model a complex process, as it provides a way to disintegrate the different states of a system as mentioned earlier in Section 1.1. It is defined as a five-tuple (P, T, I, M, O). Where 'P' denotes the set of places nodes (conditions of the network). 'T' stands for transitions nodes (events in the network). 'I' stand for input functions, assigned on the directed arcs, which connect the place node to a transition node (input arc) and 'O' stands for output functions, assigned on the directed arcs which connect the transition node to a place node (output arc) in a Petri net. Furthermore, tokens are assigned in a place which is called network '*marking*' indicating the existing condition of the network. Each distinct marking in a Petri net represents a separate state of the Petri Net. An initial distribution of the tokens in the place nodes of a Petri net is called an initial marking [20,21,36].

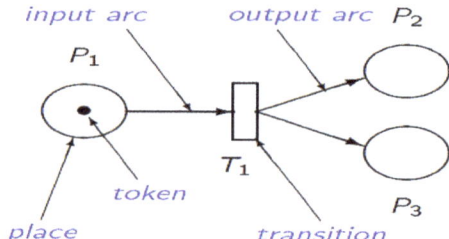

Figure 2. Basic Petri net.

- $P = \{P1, P2, P3 \ldots Pn\}$ is a set of places in the Petri Net.
- $T = \{T1, T2, T3 \ldots Tn\}$ is the limited sets of transitions, $P \cup T \neq \emptyset, P \cap T \neq \emptyset$.
- $I: P \times T \rightarrow N$ denotes the set of Input directional arcs from place to transition, where $N = \{0, 1, 2 \ldots\}$;
- $O: P \times T \rightarrow N$ denotes the set of output directional arcs from Transition to places.
- $M: P \rightarrow N$ denotes the marking of the Petri net, which defines the number of tokens present in the places, $M0$ is the initial Marking.

An initial distribution of the tokens in the place nodes of a Petri-net is called initial marking. Once the transition in the Petri net is enabled at the onset of a simulation run, the token is being fired and removed from one place node (input) to another place node (output) by the transition. There needs to be at least one enabled transition for the firing of tokens to continue or else the execution gets stopped [21,37]. In respect to critical infrastructure interdependencies modeling, the place nodes with the token markings, in the Petri net simulation model, represent the states or conditions of the CI system or their components. The transitions represent the impacts across critical infrastructure networks or their components. The CI interdependencies are stimulated by the flow of the tokens throughout the network.

Most of the studies that are present in the literature present us with Petri net simulation models that showcase the interdependencies between few CI nodes, in a small CI network. These Petri nets models cannot be used to model simulate and analyze the dynamics of the uncertainty of a large complex system. Hence, it is not possible by such Petri net models to simulate the real-life events which unfold during a flood event, which are discrete and stochastic. This limitation is addressed by developing a simulation model using Stochastic Colored Petri Net (SCPN), which increases the strength of the Petri Net and makes it possible to simulate a large real-time complex process [38,39].

The Colored Petri Nets (CPNs) [38,39] formalism is an extension of the Petri net that is particularly suited to modeling and analyzing complex interconnected systems. In Colored Petri Net, the token present in a place node is distinguished by a color, where color represents the datatype or type (such as an integer, float, string, etc.). In particular, colors can be used to model different interactions between components or transect interdependencies between them. Moreover, CPNs combines the capabilities of Petri net with those of the Standard ML programming language [39,40]. The resulting flexibility and computational power make them a suitable formalism for modeling the complex interdependencies in the critical infrastructure network. More precisely since the notion of time is essential in the problem under study, we use a timed extension of CPNs, namely, Timed Colored Petri Nets (TCPNs). Timed Colored Petri nets allow adding timing information to CPN models; this is done by associating the transitions in the CPN model with token firing times. Depending on the firing times, a Petri net simulation model can be further divided as being deterministic or stochastic [24,39,41,42]. Thus, to model the stochastic interdependencies between the Critical Infrastructures, time-critical events, and cascading effects for a real-world complex system, a timed colored Petri net is the most suitable framework

Stochastic Colored Petri Nets

Stochastic Colored Petri nets (SCPN) contain timed transitions, which are associated with a firing rate that specifies a parameter of the exponential distribution of the time period between subsequent firings of the transition. Thus, SCPN can be used to model the timing behavior of an interdependent HCI network system. The firing rates of the tokens in the SCPN are proportional to the failure probabilities of the various components of the interdependent HCI network. In Timed Stochastic Colored Petri-Net (TSCPN), a transition requires a period of delay time from occurrence-able to occurrence of an event. In this context, the duration that a transition 't' changes from the occurrence-able state to the occurrence state can be viewed as a stochastic variable 'xi'. The stochastic variable 'xi' represents the delay time consumed by a certain CI for getting affected and damaged [42,43]. A detailed explanation of a TSCPN model is given in Figure 3.

The cascading failure of the critical infrastructure nodes at various time instants forms a stochastic process. To model the stochastic interdependencies between HCI and the other CI, we need to identify the dependencies between the different variables. Such that when the process enters a particular state, it remains there for some period of (exponentially distributed) time and then moves to the next state.

To identify cascading effects and model the risk occurrence, the various parameters that need to be considered are; Probability of occurrence of the risk, the relationship between the risks and the different CI states of the interdependent HCI network and the time duration of the state of CI node when the risk will be in effect [7,39].

System analysis of Petri nets can be done using either analytical techniques such as Markov chain or simulation. Analytical techniques construct the so-called reachability graph from an SCPN, which is a labeled transition system, where each state represents a possible marking of the net. For large complex systems system analysis using analytical models such as Markov chains becomes impossible due to the state explosion problem [40].

and tools. The client interface also consists of a log window that keeps on updating the various statuses of the CI facilities. Which are if they are operating, inundation state, or a complete failure state.

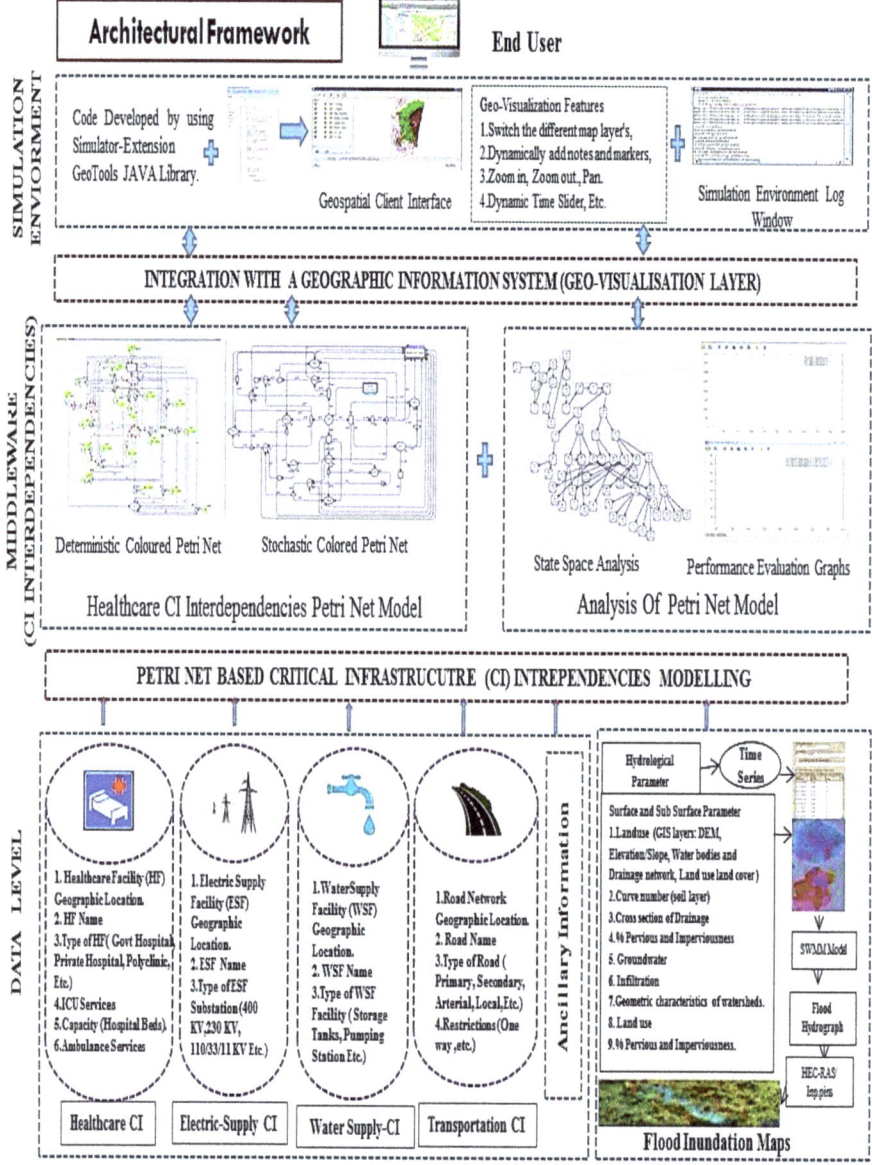

Figure 5. The proposed architectural framework for colored Petri net modeling for healthcare interdependencies during a flood event.

Temporal analysis of the HCI simulation model, as shown in Figure 6, enables us to examine and model the behavior of the interdependent healthcare CI network over time. For example, to determine whether and how the CI nodes are performing, under increasing flood levels over the time period.

For an epoch unit of time, as the states of the various nodes change in the HCI simulation model, the visualization on the interdependent HCI network for an urban flood map changes. So for each simulation run and every state change, a new map is generated. The dynamic maps help us to analyze the criticality of the situation.

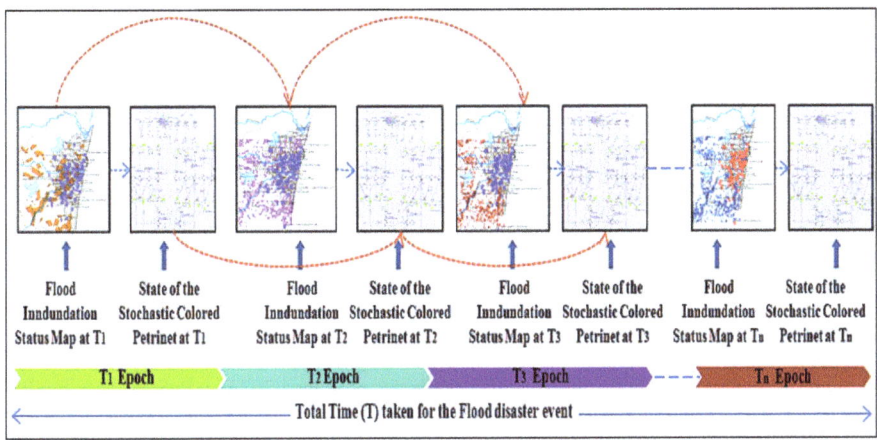

Figure 6. Temporal analysis of the SCPN interdependent HCI simulation model.

2.4. Probabilistic Assessment for Interdependent Healthcare Critical Infrastructure (HCI) Network

In a stochastic Colored Petri-net, a transition requires a period of delay time for an event to occur. That is the time duration required for a transition 't_i' to change from state 'S_1' to state 'S_2'. The time duration can be viewed as a stochastic variable 'x_i'. The stochastic variable 'x_i' represents the delay time consumed by a certain CI for getting affected and damaged. As the firing times of the transition in the Petri net are stochastic, then the probability with which the transition 't_i' will fire by time 'x_i' should be computed based on the distribution function of each transition as following:

$$f(X_i) = \int_0^{X_i} f(x)dx \qquad (1)$$

where $f(x)$ is the probability density function of the firing for transition 't_i'. For example, if the failure rate of a CI facility for a flood event corresponding to a transition 't_i' follows an exponential distribution, then the probability that transition 't_i' will fire by the time 'x' is:

$$f(X_i) = \int_0^{X_i} \lambda_i e^{-\lambda_i x} dx \qquad (2)$$

As the simulation model is based on an urban flood scenario, the CI nodes would reach a failed state due to increasing flood levels. Once the CI unit reaches a failed state, it would remain in that state until a repair action is initiated to restore the CI node to a working condition. During an urban flood scenario, the repair time of the CI node takes quite some time. As foremost, the flooding has to be controlled, so we are not considering the time taken to repair the CI node.

However, as we are simulating the domino effect of the interdependent CI network from the onset of the flood, we are interested in the time to failure component of the CI node. That is the instant at which the CI node experiences failure. These time instants are random variables, linked to the probability of an event.

Let us consider a CI node facility (electrical substation 'A') from the electrical supply critical infrastructure network. Considering the electrical substation at time t = 0 is in operating condition, the instant at a time at which it will eventually fail is a continuous random variable X ≥ 0. Where 'X' represents the time to failure of Electrical substation A. 'X' is a random variable, and its range is the set of all positive real numbers, including zero ($X \in R^+ \cup \{0\}$) [22,24,44].

The cumulative distribution function (CDF) $F_X(t)$ of the time to failure 'X' is defined as

$$F_X(t) = P\{X \leq t\} \quad (3)$$

The probability density function (PDF) of the random variable 'X' is given by

$$f_X(t) = \frac{dF_X(t)}{dt} \quad (4)$$

The hazard rate of a random variable 'X' is defined as the conditional probability that 'X' takes a value in the interval (t, t + dt), given that X > t. Where 'X 'is the time to failure of a unit, the hazard rate is called as the failure rate and is denoted by 'λ'. The failure rate of a CI facility node gives us the probability that the failure will occur in the next unit of time [31,33,35].

The time to failure is a random variable, while the Mean time to failure is the expected value, the units of which are time units (e.g., hours). The mean time to failure (MTTF) is defined as follows:

$$MTTF = H[X] = \int_0^\infty t . f_X(t) \, dt \quad (5)$$

Considering that the random variable 'X' is exponentially distributed with the failure rate 'λ',

$$f(t) = \lambda e^{-\lambda t} \quad (6)$$

$$MTTF = H[X] = \int_0^\infty t . f(t) dt = \lambda \int_0^\infty t . e^{-\lambda t} \quad (7)$$

Integrating by parts gives us

$$MTTF = \frac{1}{\lambda} \quad (8)$$

MTTF is measured as the likelihood of a system to fail and is represented as units of hours. It is used as a measure to understand the availability and reliability of the systems.

3. Development of Interdependent Healthcare Critical Infrastructure Network Simulation Model

The utility of the SCPN based interdependent HCI simulation model during a flooding disaster is shown using a comprehensive case study of a real-world situation. Using the developed system the critical infrastructure failure metric is measured, and the propagation of cascading failures in the Chennai area during the flooding event in December 2015 is evaluated, analyzed, and visualized in a spatiotemporal environment. The real-world case study showcases the dire need of the proposed simulation model system.

3.1. Healthcare Critical Infrastructure Interdependency during Chennai Flood 2015—Chennai, India

Chennai is located in the southern part of India and is the capital city of the Tamil Nadu state. It is one of the four major metropolitan cities of India. The city of Chennai and its suburb areas received heavy rainfall events during November–December 2015 that inundated the districts of Chennai, Kanchipuram, and Tiruvallur. Around midnight of 2 December 2015, land in more than 4 km radius around Adyar River, which flows through the center of Chennai was underwater.

RISAT-1 satellite data of 3 and 4 December 2015 was acquired from the National Remote Sensing Centre (NRSC), Disaster Division, Hyderabad, India. The satellite data was analyzed, and the flood inundation layer was generated. Different thematic layers of various CI facilities (example, hospitals, electrical substations, etc.) were overlaid with the flood inundation layer to generate the Chennai flood inundation map. The inundated healthcare facilities map of Chennai city during the Chennai Floods 2015 is shown in Figure 7.

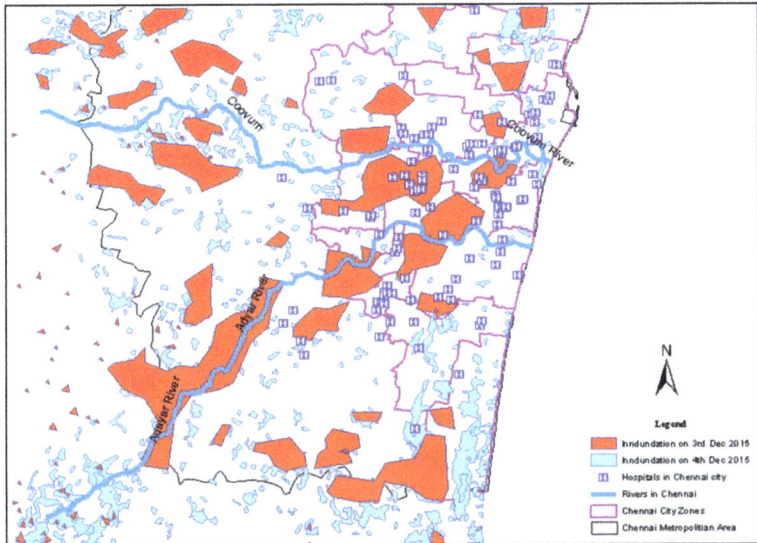

Figure 7. Inundated Healthcare facilities in Chennai during the Chennai Floods 2015. (3 December 2015 and 4 December 2015).

As floodwater levels rose in Chennai, large geographic areas got inundated; the red zones in the map show the substantial inundated regions. Critical infrastructure networks and normal life had come to a halt. Houses, hospitals, roads were flooded, communication networks went down, and there was extensive damage to the electrical power supply. The inundation and flooding of large areas of the Chennai city and suburbs of the adjoining two districts caused disruption of services from existing drinking water supply systems. On account of the inundation of large areas in the city and consequent submergence of the electrical distribution system in floodwater, most of the electrical substations were shutdown. As there was extensive damage to the electrical power infrastructure in Chennai, the electrical supply to the Chennai city was disrupted. Most of the electrical substations reported a rise of floodwater more than 4 feet.

3.2. Case Study: Interdependent HCI Network during Chennai Floods in 2015

The case study consists of a health care CI facility (hospital) in Chennai and its interdependent CI services such as electric supply CI (electric substations) and water supply CI (water pumping stations). The hospital is located in Chennai and the name of the geographical area and hospital and its interdependent CI facilities are kept confidential. During the Chennai floods 2015, the operation of the healthcare facility (*Hospital A*) and its interdependent CI also failed due to the increase in the flood level, however as the healthcare facility (*Hospital A*) was prepared for such adversities, they could evacuate the patients to a safer hospital with the help of boats and ambulances. The simulation model is been used to study another interdependent HCI network during Chennai floods, however, the example is not shown in this article. The following section describes the case study in detail.

Hospital A—Chennai floods 2015: *Hospital A* is situated in the marshlands of Chennai. The hospital is connected to the main road via a 2 km arterial road. Due to heavy rains from the 15th of

November 2015, there was significant flooding of low-lying areas. The hospital was briefly cut off from the main road. Elective procedures got stopped, but the care of the inpatients was not affected. The number of patients admitted to the hospital was under 100 because of elective admissions due to high rainfall. However, on 1 December 2015 news regarding breaching a major lake near the hospital was reported to *Hospital A*. The 2 km arterial road which connects the hospital to the main road started flooding and in few hours, the hospital was surrounded by 8 feet deep water [45].

The healthcare machinery was placed in the rooms on the ground floor of the hospital. Due to flooding, these rooms were inundated. The *Electrical Substation A* which supplies electrical supply to *Hospital A* was submerged in floodwater, due to which the electrical supply to *Hospital A* got disrupted. However, as the hospital authorities were disaster prepared, they could estimate the CI dependencies and evaluate the response time. The patients were being evacuated from Hospital *A* with the help of fishing boats and then transported to safer healthcare facilities via ambulances.

3.3. Assessing the Flood Risk at Individual Critical Infrastructure Facilities

The uncertainty around the response of critical infrastructure facilities to flood hazard makes it logical to use probabilistic fragility curves. The fragility curves are developed after analyzing the critical infrastructure facility's performance in response to the intensity of the flood hazards experienced. Fragility curves for the CI facility are developed to understand the probability of failure of the CI facility for a flood level. There are many methods to create fragility curves. However, as there are several CI facilities, it is not possible to analytically model each CI facility. Hence empirical data from past flooding events are the main source of information [46,47]. We can develop the fragility curves by analyzing the empirical data from past events, and engineering judgment is viewed as a last resort due to the subjective results it produces [46]. Hence, engineering judgment will only be used where there is no empirical data. And the relationship between the flood hazard and CI facility impact can be easily envisaged (e.g., the depth of water required to close an electrical substation).

3.3.1. Impact of Flooding on Electrical Supply Critical Infrastructure (Electrical Substation)

To analyze the impact of flooding on electrical substations, we should have the information about the location of the substation and the height of critical electrical equipment. According to Indian electricity rules the formation level (FL) of an electrical substation has to be fixed at a minimum of 600 mm higher than the surroundings based on the drainage conditions and the highest flood level in the area [48]. However, the information on failures is less and mainly in the form of the CI facility and news reports. According to the Federal Emergency Management Agency (FEMA) report [47], the functionality threshold depth for an electrical substation is 1.2 m. In a case study referring to electrical substations of a national grid [49], most of the substations had the resilience to flooding to an approximate depth of 0.3 m. By the information, from the experts working in the electrical substations; most of the substations in Chennai would shut down if the flood depth increases more than 0.5 m. The electrical supply CI facilities considered for the case study are as follows: Electrical Substations which supply electricity to Hospital A.

- Electrical Substation A [110/33/11 kV, Date of commissioning: 1 April 1992].
- Electrical Substation B [230/110 kV, Date of commissioning: 13 May 2010].

As the oldest substations commissioned is *Electrical Substation A*. The flood events, rainfall data after the year 1992, and few assumptions are considered to plot the probability of failure for *Electrical Substation A*. Table 1 below shows the probability of failure of substation for different flood levels. The fragility curve plot for *Electrical Substation A*, for various flood levels, is shown in Figure 8. The fragility curve plot shows that the flooding of the substation would start at 0.1 m and the probability of '1' indicates the complete shutdown of the substation due to flooding.

Table 1. Probability of failure of Electrical Substation A for different flood levels.

Flood Level (m)	Probability of Electrical Substation 'A' (110/11 kV) Flooding
0.1	0.333
0.2	0.475
0.3	0.67
0.4	0.84
0.5	0.968
0.6	1
0.7	1

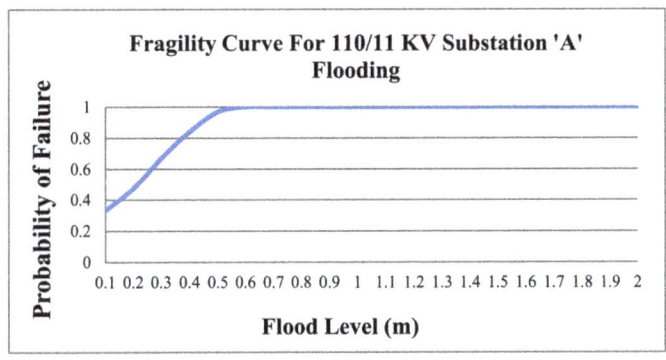

Figure 8. Fragility curve plot for Electrical Substation A (110/11 kV).

3.3.2. Impact of Flooding on Healthcare Critical Infrastructure (Hospital)

To analyze the impact of flooding on an HCI facility, data about the location of the HCI facility has to be known. The level of flood inundation level, which can affect the functioning of the healthcare facility, should also be known. As explained earlier in Section 3.2, *Hospital A* is situated in the marshlands of Chennai, close to a major lake. In 2015 floods *Hospital A* was surrounded by 8ft water. During the field visit, it was observed that the hospital is divided into two buildings having two floors each. The hospital equipment on the ground floor was affected due to 2 ft floodwater. Information collected by various sources concludes that *Hospital A* would get flooded if the flood level is around 0.6 m approximately to 2 ft. An example is given below to calculate the probability of reaching the state of flooding for *Hospital A*.

Number of Occurrence of a flood level of 0.6 m or more = 20
Number of times that Hospital 'B' has reached the flooding state = 9
Probability of reaching the state of flooding for Hospital B = 9/20 = 0.45

3.3.3. Impact of Flooding on Water Supply Critical Infrastructure (Water Pumping Station)

To analyze the impact of flooding on water pumping stations, we should know the level of floodwater level, which will cause the pumping station to stop operating. The probability of flooding of the water pumping station at *Hospital A* is calculated as follows; As the pumping station is present at the same elevation as *Hospital A*, the flood level at which the hospital will get inundated the pumping station would also reach the inundation state at the same elevation.

By analyzing the impact of flooding on each critical infrastructure, one can estimate the probability of failure of a CI facility as explained in Section 2.4. The probability of failure of a CI facility is used for providing the time delay to the transitions in the simulation model. Table 2, showcases the various timed transitions and their corresponding failure rate in our stochastic colored Petri net model.

Table 2. List of few timed transitions in the interdependent HCI stochastic colored Petri net.

Transition	Description	Transition Rate (λ)
T1	Occurrence of Flood	Deterministic
T9	The occurrence of flood affects Electrical substation A (230/110 kV)	0.96
T10	The occurrence of flood affects Electrical substation B (110/11 kV)	0.96
T11	The occurrence of flood affects Hospital A	0.45
T8	The occurrence of flood affects Water pumping station A	0.45
T10	Failure in Electrical substation A affects Electrical substation B	1
T12	Failure in Electrical substation B affects Water pumping station A	1
T13	Failure in Water pumping station A affects Hospital A	1

3.4. Stochastic Colored Petri Net (SCPN) Simulation Environment

This section describes the development of the stochastic colored Petri net model, and how the model was used to evaluate the performance of the interdependent healthcare critical infrastructure network for the Chennai Floods 2015 case study. The impacts of the risk mitigation strategies under different levels of model parameters are observed. As mentioned earlier, the interdependent healthcare CI network-based Stochastic colored Petri net is based on the case study mentioned in Section 3.2. Following are the subnets:

- Flood Simulation.
- HCI with other CI Interdependency Network.
- HCI Internal Dependencies.
- Status of the Entire Network.

(a) Flood Water Level Simulation Subnet:

As flood level in any area depends on a few variables such as rainfall, soil conditions, wind, temperatures, etc., it is considered as a random variable. It is found that there is an increase in flood levels at random intervals of time. The interdependent CI places nodes in the Petri net-based simulation model represent the states of the different CI facilities such as *Electrical substation A, Water Pumping station A, Hospital A*. In our case study, the CI facilities are located at different geographical locations with different elevations. The CI facilities are inundated at different flood water levels and at random intervals of time, considering the elevation of the CI facility. For example, *Hospital A* gets flooded for an elevation of 2 ft at time t_1. However, *Electrical substation A* might get flooded at an elevation of 3 ft at time t_9. As mentioned earlier the Petri net simulation model is been divided into four subnets. The flood simulation subnet simulates the flood levels at the various CI facilitates located at different elevations. In the flood simulation subnet, as shown in Figure 9 the flood levels vary upon the intensity of the rainfall and the geographic area, if the rainfall intensity is high then the CI facilities will get inundated at a faster rate than the rainfall at a lower intensity. Considering the *Electrical substation A* would get flooded at 3 ft, as shown in Figure 8. The token from the '*Flood simulation subnet*' arrives at '*ES1 place node*' indicating the rising flood levels at the *Electrical substation A* CI facility. The token is fired from the '*ES1 place node*' to the '*transition t_9*'.

The '*transition t_9*' is a timed transition, where the token is fired following an exponential time delay function (the rate at which the CI facility will get flooded). The transition rate is calculated based on the calculations (mentioned in Sections 2.4 and 3.3 earlier). For example, the rate at which the CI facility *Electrical substation A* will get flooded is 0.64 (the time delay for various transitions has been explained in Table 2 in Section 3.3.3). As the flood level at the *Electrical substation A* reaches 3 ft level, the '*transition t_9*' fires a token with a random timestamp to the '*flooded ES1 place node*'. The '*flooded ES1 place node*' gets enabled, as the token arrives at the place node, indicating the inundation of CI facility *Electrical substation A*.

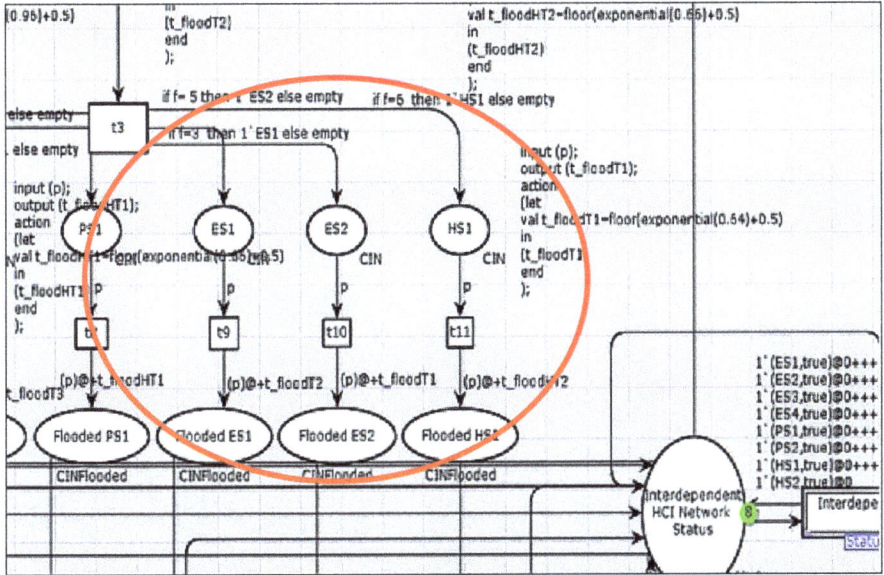

Figure 9. A snippet of the Flood Simulation Subnet.

(b) HCI with other CI Interdependency Network Subnet:

The case study from Section 3.2 is implemented by building a stochastic colored Petri net simulation model, as shown in Figure 10. The HCI with other CI interdependency network subnet is the main subnet where the cascading failure scenario from the case study has been implemented. The various CI facilities nodes in an interdependent HCI network considered for the simulation model are the following,

- Electrical Substations = 2 nodes.
- Hospitals = 2 Nodes
- Water Pumping station = 1 node
- Control Room (Command Centre) = 1 nodes
- Ambulances = 4

The flood simulation subnet provides the *"HCI with other CI interdependency network subnet"* with the flooded CI facilities place nodes. Given below is an explanation of the cascading failure simulation of *Hospital A* and its interdependent CI services form the *"HCI with other CI interdependency network subnet"* Inundation of the *Electrical substation A* results in the non-operational state of *Electrical substation A*.

The non-operational state of *Electrical substation A* enables the *'transition SF1'* to fire a token to *'P4 place node'*. The presence of a token enables the *'P4 place node'*, which represents the state of electrical service disruption to *Electrical substation B* due to failure in *Electrical substation A*. The impact of the cascading failure of *Electrical substation A* on *Electrical substation B* is simulated by firing the token from the *'P4 place node'* to *'transition SF2'*. For the *Electrical substation B* to go into a complete non-operational state, the electrical supply form *Electrical substation A* should be disrupted and the *Electrical substation B* should be inundated. The *Electrical substation B* will get inundated when the *'flooded ES2 place node'* will get enabled on receiving the token from the *'flood simulation subnet'*. As the *'transition SF2'* receives tokens from *'P4 place node'* and *'flooded ES2 place node'*, the *Electrical substation B* reaches a non-operational state.

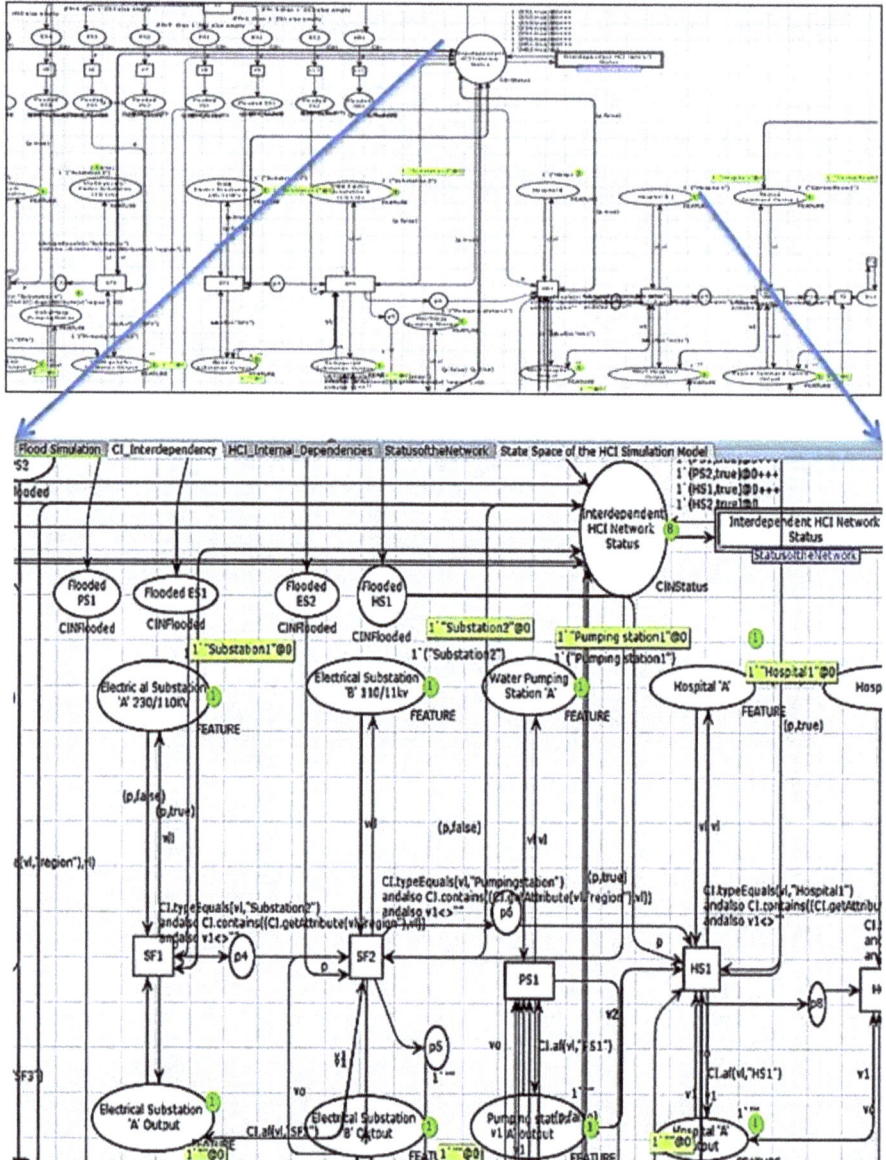

Figure 10. Interdependent healthcare critical infrastructure network colored stochastic Petri net.

The failure of *Electrical substation B* disrupts the electric supply to the *Water Pumping station A* and the *Hospital A*. This is simulated by the firing of tokens from the '*transition SF2*' to '*place node P5*' and '*place node P6*' which represent the state of electric supply disrupted to *Water Pumping station A* and *Hospital A* respectively. Another token is fired from the '*transition SF2*' to the Petri net subnet "*Status of the Interdependent HCI network*" which indicates the failure of the electrical substation 'B' CI facility node in the interdependent HCI network. Similar to the electrical substations' failure, the water pumping station arrives at a non-operational state due to a cascading failure scenario. Due to the disruption of electrical and water supply services, *Hospital A* is affected.

A healthcare CI facility such as *Hospital A* is not only dependent on external CI services such as electrical supply and water supply but also internal dependencies (explained in Section 3.4 (c)) such as oxygen supply, backup generators, battery supply, food, water, etc.). *Hospital A* checks for its internal dependencies on the *"Internal Dependencies Subnet"* of the HCI simulation model. The internal dependencies subnet (explained in Section 3.4 (c)) checks the internal dependencies in the hospital required for the operation of the hospital until the emergency services arrive.

The status results from the *"Internal Dependencies Subnet"* is been then communicated to the rescue command center requesting evacuation of patients from *Hospital A* to *Hospital C*. The command center checks in for the nearest ambulance available and sends it to the impacted hospital for the evacuation of patients. The nearest ambulance reaches the *Hospital A* for evacuation, choosing the shortest route and sends a message to the command center about reaching its destination. The *'transition HS1'* fires another token when enabled to the subnet *"Status of the Interdependent HCI network"* which indicates the failure of the *Electrical Substation A* node in the interdependent HCI. Few of the different place nodes in the subnet; the description is given in Table 3.

Table 3. Description of Few place nodes (states) in the Interdependent HCI network SCPN Subnet.

Sr.No	Name of the State (Place Node)	State (Place Node) Description
1	Flooded ES1	The place node indicates the inundation state of the *Electrical substation A* due to an increase in the flood level.
2	Flooded ES2	The place node indicates the inundation state of the *Electrical substation B* due to an increase in the flood level.
3	Flooded PS1	The place node indicates the inundation state of *Water pumping station A*, due to an increase in the flood level.
4	Flooded HS1	The place node indicates the inundation state of *Hospital A*, due to an increase in the flood level.
5	P4	The place node indicates the non-operational state of the *Electrical substation B* (Substation is inundated and electric supply is disrupted).
6	P5	The place node indicates the electric supply disruption at *Water pumping station A*, due to the non-operational state of *Electric substation B*.
7	P6	The place node indicates the electric supply disruption at *Hospital A*, due to the non-operational state of *Electric substation B*.
8	P7	The place node indicates the non-operational state of the *Water pumping station A* (water pumping station is inundated and electric supply is disrupted).
9	P8	The place node indicates the non-operational state of *Hospital A*, due to the inundation of hospital, electric supply, and water supply disruption.
10	Interdependent HCI network status	The tokens arriving at the place node indicate the non-operational state of the various CI facilities with the time stamp. The place node connects to the HCI network monitoring status subnet.

(c) HCI Internal Dependencies Subnet:

The operation of a healthcare facility depends not only on the other interconnected critical infrastructure facilities but also on a similar web of internal dependencies. The *"HCI internal dependencies subnet"* of the simulation model simulates the various internal dependencies of a healthcare facility. Figure 11 shows the subnet of the SCPN, considering the HCI internal dependencies, whereas the description of the place nodes is given in Table 4.

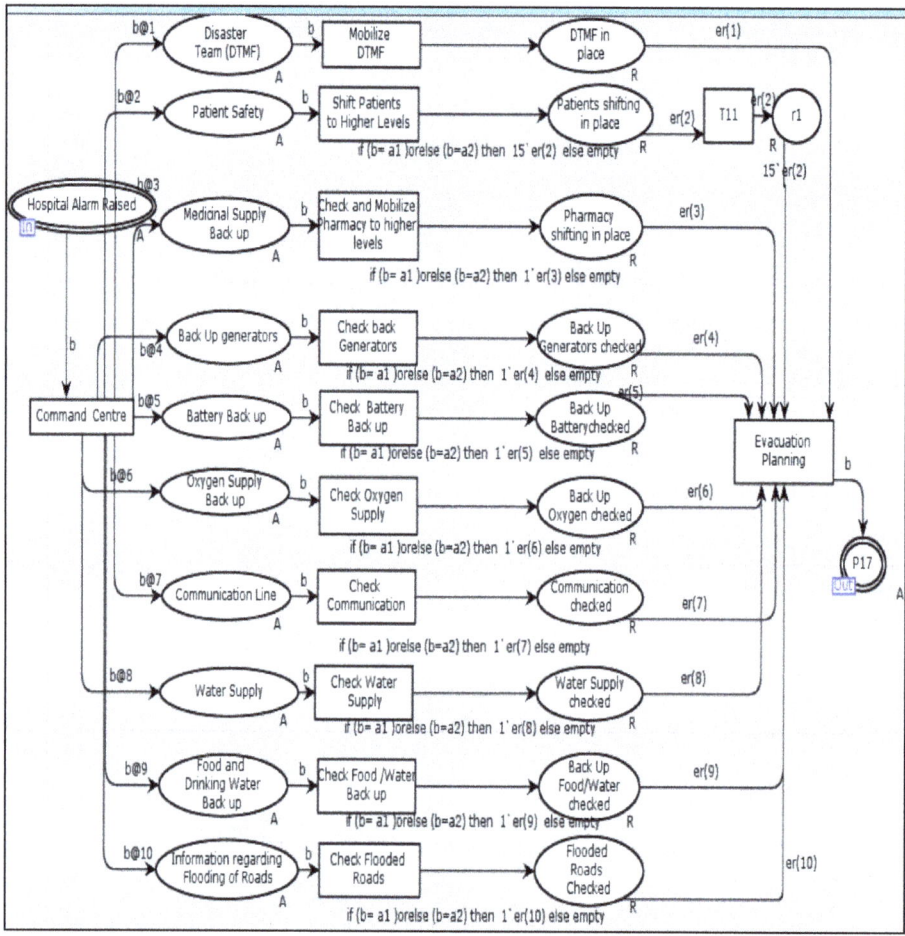

Figure 11. Healthcare critical infrastructure internal interdependencies.

Internal dependencies are related to the operational functionalities inside a healthcare facility such as back up electrical generators, food, and water supply, pharmacy supply, battery backup, oxygen supply, communication, disaster protocol, etc. For example, when an electrical CI facility node (for ex: *Electrical Substation A*) is flooded, and the electrical supply to the corresponding HCI facility node (for ex: *Hospital A*) is disrupted. The electrical backup generators have to start supplying electricity to the healthcare facility. The probability of failure and the time to failure for such generators should also be considered.

The failure of these dependencies requires immediate evacuation of patients to another safer healthcare facility. When the *'transition healthcare CI'* is enabled on the "*HCI with other CI interdependency network*" subnet is triggered, due to unavailability of electrical CI and water supply CI (for ex: *Water Pumping station A*) and inundation of the HCI facility (for ex: *Hospital A*) the "*HCI internal dependencies subnet*" is triggered. The "*HCI internal dependencies*" simulation model checks all the internal dependencies and then depending on the status of the severity of emergency at the hospital. The command center helps in evacuation of the patients to a nearby safe healthcare facility (for ex: *Hospital C*).

Table 4. Description of few place nodes in the Internal Dependencies of an HCI facility Subnet.

Sr.No	Name of the State (Place Node)	State (Place Node) Description
1	Hospital Alarm Raised	The place node indicates that the alarm state of the hospital, as the model predicts the time until the hospital might run into a non-operational state.
2	Patients shifting	The patients are shifted to secure or higher locations in the hospital, till emergency evacuation takes place.
3	Pharmacy status	The state indicates the available pharmacy status at the hospital.
4	Backup Electrical Generators status	The place node indicates the status of the backup electrical generators at the hospital.
5	Power Battery Status	The place node indicates the status of the Power Battery Status at the hospital.
6	Oxygen cylinders	The place node indicates the status of the Oxygen cylinders at the hospital.
7	Communication	The place node indicates the status of the communication lines at the hospital.
8	Food and drinking water	The place node indicates the current status of the Food and drinking water to sustain at the hospital, till evacuation.
9	Back up water supply	The place node indicates the status of the Backup water supply at the hospital
10	The status of nearby roads	The place node indicates the status of the nearby roads (Transport CI) to the hospital, if they are inundated or not.
11	Emergency Evacuation planning	After checking the internal dependencies, the hospital reports about its status to the command center for emergency evacuation

(d) Status of the Entire Network Subnet:

The status of the entire network subnet of the simulation model, as shown in Figure 12, monitors the performance of the various interdependent CI nodes. During the simulation as the CI, facility nodes reach to failure state due to the flood inundation and disruption of CI services. By analyzing the data collected from various simulation runs. We can estimate the meantime to failure of *Electrical substation A*. The interdependent CI nodes fail at different intervals of time. Every CI node will fail at a particular random time for every simulation run. Considering the mean of all the time to failure of a CI node for 'n' number of simulations will give us the meantime to failure (MTTF) of a CI node. Table 5 describes the CI facility breakdown states in the HCI interdependencies status monitoring subnet.

The place nodes "*ES1 down*" on the "*Status of the entire network*" subnet indicate the breakdown of *Electrical substation A*. Similarly when all the CI node failure transitions are triggered, it indicates that the CI nodes are disrupted and are not in operating status. This results in the collapse of the interdependent healthcare critical infrastructure network, for 'n' number of simulations, one can estimate the meantime to failure of the interdependent healthcare critical infrastructure network.

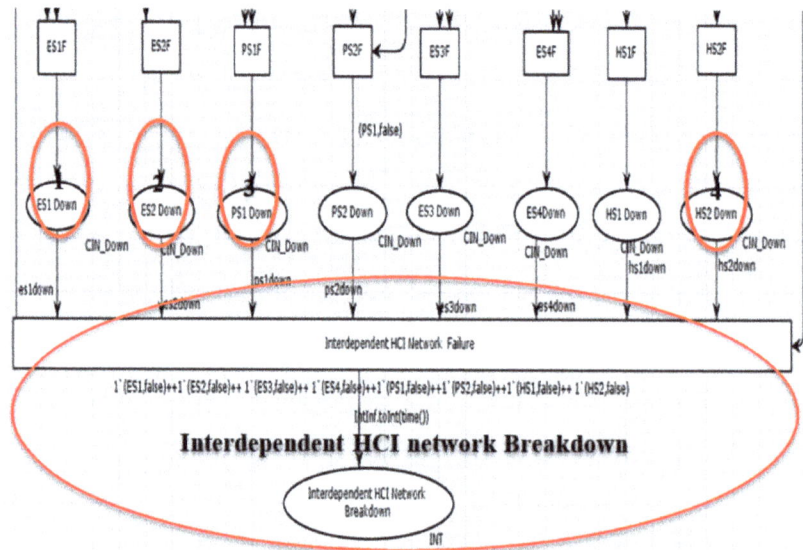

Figure 12. A snippet of HCI interdependencies status monitoring subnet.

Table 5. Description of CI facility breakdown states in the HCI interdependencies status monitoring subnet.

Sr.No	Name of the State (Place Node)	State (Place Node) Description
1	ESI Down	The place node indicates the complete failure state of the *Electrical substation A*.
2	ES2 Down	The place node indicates the complete failure state of *Electrical substation B*.
3	PSI Down	The place node indicates the complete failure state of *Water Pumping station A*.
4	HSI Down	The place node indicates the complete failure state of *Hospital A*.

4. Results

This section presents us with the results of the simulation model. System analysis of the simulation model in Section 4.1 analyzes and evaluates the temporal dimension of the SCPN based HCI simulation model based on the Chennai floods 2015 case study, whereas the spatial dimension is presented in the Section 4.2 SCPN based interdependent HCI simulation model driven geo-visualization interface.

4.1. System Analysis of the SCPN based Interdependent HCI Simulation Model

Dependability system evaluation analysis is devoted to investigating the possible manifestations of failures (when and how they can occur) and their impact on the system. The analysis is also used to prevent such failure disruptions and ways to mitigate them. Dependability system analysis provides us with solutions to evaluate the probability and the time of the first occurrence of such a catastrophic condition.

(a) Prediction of Time to Failure of a Critical Infrastructure Facility during a Flood Event

The simulated data is extracted from the states of the model and from the events that occur during the simulations. The extracted data is used to calculate the failure metric of the CI facilities and analyze the behavior of the complex model. During a simulation, the stochastic colored Petri net can contain and generate quantitative information about the performance of a system, such as the meantime to failure (MTTF) of a CI node, the number of tokens at the node place signifying the utilization of the CI node, etc. The data from the different transitions is collected by using a different data collector monitor for various CI nodes. The data collector monitor extracts numerical data from the simulation model and calculates statistics for the data, which is collected for a transition. For example, The *ES1 MTTF* data collector monitor in the HCI simulation model collects data about the time to failure of the *Electrical substation A (ES1)* place node for the '*n*' number of simulation runs.

The *Electrical substation A (ES1)* marking size monitor measures the number of tokens present in the *Electrical substation A* place node in the Petri net model. The monitor calculates the performance measure such as the average and a maximum number of tokens which are present in the *Electrical substation A (ES1)* place node during '*n*' simulation. This failure measure would help us to analyze the availability of the critical infrastructure node for service.

The results of the system analysis of the simulation model are calculated for a simulation period of 3 days of rainfall and flooding (a total of 72 h). As the simulation model is built to perform simulation indefinitely, a breakpoint monitor is required to stop the simulation. The breakpoint monitor in the Petri net model stops the simulation as per the duration required (in our case study the simulation duration was considered for 3 days (72 h).

The data from different monitors in the CPN Tools are written in different text files and a single folder for one set of simulations. Given below in Table 6 is the meantime to failures of the various CI nodes of the interdependent healthcare critical infrastructure network, for a section of the urban city Chennai during the urban flood of 2015. An example of the results shown in Table 6 is as following; Analyzing the simulation results we see that as the flood levels started increasing, the first failure occurs in *Electrical substation* A (230/110 kV) in 4.5 hours from the onset of the flood.

Table 6. Mean Time to Failure of the various CI nodes of an Interdependent HCI network, during an Urban Flood Chennai Case study.

Critical Infrastructure Node	Mean Time to Failure (MTTF) (hr)
Electrical Substation A (230/110 kV)	4.5
Electrical Substation B (110/11 kV)	7.4
Water Pumping station A	8.20
Hospital A	8.70

Due to the failure of Electrical *substation* A and increasing flood levels *Electrical substation B* (110/11 kV) is affected. The electric supply to Hospital A provided from *Electrical substation B* will get disrupted in 3 h, as it would take around 7.5 h for *Electrical substation B* to reach a complete non-operational state from the onset of the flood.

The *Water Pumping station A* is geographically located closer to *Hospital A* and due to the shutdown of *Electrical substation B*, the electric supply to the water pumping station is disrupted. The estimated time for the complete non-operational state of *Water Pumping station A* is 8.20 h from the onset of flooding. This shows that the water supply CI facility reaches a failure state an hour after the failure of the *Electrical substation B*. From the simulation results, we can infer that show that the time for *Hospital A* to reach a non-operational state is around 8.7 h from the onset of the flood. There is not much variation for the time taken to reach a non-operational state between *Hospital A* and the *Water Pumping station A*. This is because both *Hospital A* and the *Water Pumping station A* are located in the same geographic area. As the hospital gets inundated, from the simulation results we can infer that the hospital authorities can estimate that they have 3 h (approx.) for electric supply disruption, and around half an hour left for the water supply disruption. The estimation of the time frame can help the hospital authorities to arrange emergency services for the evacuation of patients and disaster prepare the hospital with the backup resources available.

The simulation model is integrated with the geographic information system, and a log window keeps on updating the status of the CI facilities if they are in an operating, inundation state, or a complete failure state. When the electric supply and water supply get disrupted to either of the hospital CI facilities, the hospital CI facilities check for the internal dependencies such as back up electrical generator, battery backup, oxygen cylinders, etc. The hospital CI facilities then request the command center for the evacuation of patients. The command center alerts the ambulance services as the hospital is reaching a failure state for the evacuation of patients. The GIS system (explained in the next Section 4.2) shows the evacuation route to a safer hospital and the same is been updated on the log window.

(b) State Space Analysis Queries for the Simulation Model

The simulation model is quite complex, as it enters into many states. The state-space for the simulation model is vast. However, we can query from the state space graph about the different states of the entire simulation model. For example, if the user wants to know the minimum path from the state where the *Electrical substation A* has inundated to the state where the entire interdependent HCI network has failed. For example, if the state where *Electrical substation A* is inundated is node 16 and the entire *HCI network failure* state node is 89 the minimum path is: [16;25; 56;76,89]. From the simulation runs we see that the failure in the electric supply CI network will increase the vulnerability of water supply CI networks. The failure of both electric supply CI and water supply CI will have a perilous impact on the HCI network. The performance simulations show that as the number of interdependencies in an interdependent HCI network increases, the more vulnerable they are.

4.2. SCPN Driven Geographic Information System

A CI facility such as a hospital, electrical substation, road, etc., in the real world, is mapped into a Geographic Information System (GIS) as a critical infrastructure geo-entity. The CI geo-entity is characterized by the type of critical infrastructure facility (such as a hospital, electric substation, water pumping station, a road segment, etc.), the geographic attributes (for example; name, represented by a polygon, point, or a line, location coordinates, etc.). The geographic attributes of a CI geo-entity are important, as the attributes help in linking the CI geo-entity to a unique spatial location and context of its environment. For example, a hospital CI geo-entity is represented as a point feature with its geographical and other attributes such as the location of the hospital, type of hospital, the capacity of beds, etc. A network of such hospital CI geo-entities would represent a thematic dataset of the hospital network.

In a stochastic colored Petri net driven geographic information system, spatial data layers related to the different CI networks such as electrical supply CI network (the geolocation of electrical substation), water supply CI network (the geolocation of water pumping station, geographic area of water bodies) and healthcare CI network (the geolocation of healthcare facilities) are combined for visual exploration of complex datasets. A JAVA (www.oracle.com/java) code is developed by using CPN tools (www.cpntools.org); Simulator Extensions Java library and Geo-Tools (www.geotools.org), which is an open-source Java, for an SCPN driven GIS simulation model. The interdependent SCPN simulation model communicates with the GIS system using the TCP/IP protocol, which is an implementation of the remote procedure call (RPC) system. Figure 13 showcases the dynamic data exchange between the SCPN simulation model and the geographic information system.

The stochastic interdependencies in the SCPN model are based on various geographical and logical based interdependency rules. Object-oriented based geospatial functions are developed such that the place nodes in the SCPN model are spatially registered, with the CI geo-entities, and the geolocation is color-coded.

The entire SCPN driven GIS model is encapsulated in a JAVA based client interface for Geovisualization as shown in Figure 14, various geospatial-based interactive components are added on the client interface such as zoom in zoom out. Dynamically add notes and markers, switching between different map layers and pan to control the display within its context, can be used by the end-users.

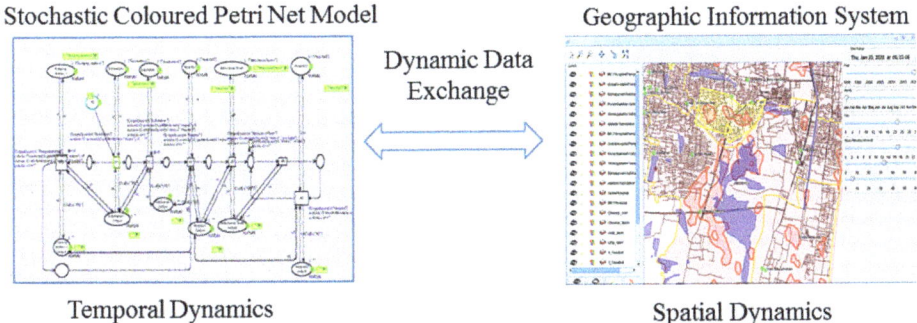

Figure 13. Stochastic Colored Petri net model-driven Geographic Information System.

The guard functions of the transition in the SCPN simulation model are based on the geospatial relation function. These guard functions act like a constraint; once the transition is enabled and the token is fired, the transition returns a Boolean result. Given below in Figure 15 is an example of a transition 'HS1' and a guard function assigned to it. The transition 'HS1' will get enabled to fire a token only when all the constraints are met. The transition first checks the CI geo entity, if it is Hospital A. When the first constraint is met, then the transition checks the region (polygon) in which the hospital A is located in. Then it would check the condition of the region if it is flooded or not. Based on the query and when the transition is fired, the geographic region on the GIS client interface is highlighted by changing the color scheme indicating the geographic region where Hospital A is situated in is "*Flooded*".

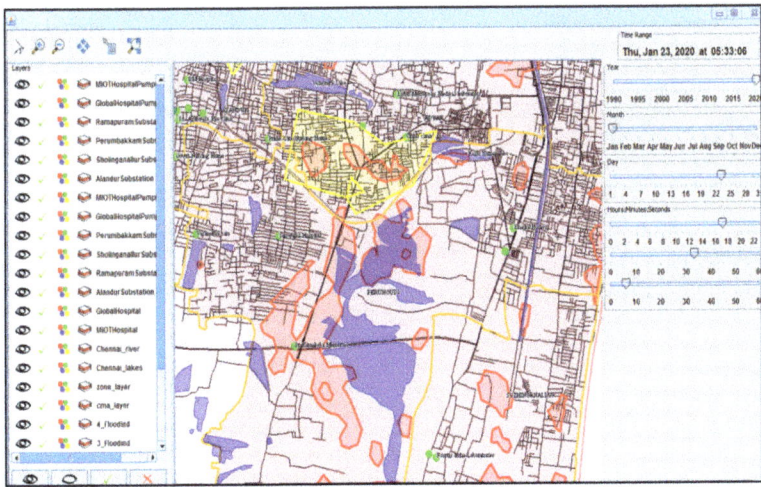

Figure 14. Geo-visualization client interface For Interdependent HCI Petri Net Simulation Model - Chennai Case Study.

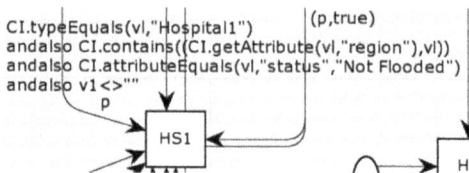

Figure 15. Transition HS1 in the SCPN model with geographical based constraints.

Various queries form the interdependent HCI SCPN simulation model can be queried with the help of different geometric, feature type, and attribute functions. The SCPN driven GIS simulation model can perform various GIS-based analyses such as attribute-based analysis, node-based analysis, spatial area-based analysis, and network-based analysis.

(a) SCPN driven GIS-based Attribute Analysis for Interdependent HCI Network

The spatial knowledge related to CI facilities in the Interdependent HCI CI network is queried from the CI spatial databases. The various place nodes in the Interdependent HCI SCPN simulation model are registered with CI spatial databases. The geospatial relationships based on the geometry of geo-entities and the geospatial based object-oriented functions in the Petri net provides the HCI simulation model with the capability of attribute analysis. The simulation model can query the CI related geographic attribute information (For ex: CI facility such as hospital location, electrical substation location, water pumping station location, etc.). A geodatabase related functions provide the end-user with attribute information about a specific CI facility in a certain geographic location.

(b) SCPN Driven GIS-based Node Analysis for Interdependent HCI Network

The geospatial functions related to the distance between two nodes provide us with information about the distance between two different CI facilities, for example; the functions display the distance between a hospital A and hospital B for the evacuation of patients. The node (point) based analysis can provide information about the attribute of the point feature, for example for node hospital A, the node base attributes provide information about the type of hospital, the capacity of the hospital, etc. As the place nodes are spatially registered, with the CI facilities, and the geolocation is color-coded. The change in the place node marking in the Petri net model would result in the change in the color scheme of the CI data objects on the GIS-based client interface. For example; The color scheme associated with the point data object registered with a hospital CI facility is blue. At this instant, there is no token present in the hospital CI place node in the Petri net model. However, when the place node is enabled with a token, the color scheme of the point data object registered with a hospital CI facility changes to red. During the simulation run, as a result of a transition being enabled, and a token is fired the SCPN simulation model state changes. As the state changes in the underlying SCPN simulation model, the behavior of the CI geo entity on the GIS-based client interface also changes.

(c) SCPN driven GIS-Based Area Analysis for Interdependent HCI Network

The Area-based analysis provides functions for polygon features. The functions are based on the geometry of the features. The functions are used to provide information about the polygon features related to critical infrastructures. GIS-based operations such as buffer can be used to identify a buffer zone of an HCI facility.

(d) SCPN Driven GIS-Based Network Analysis for Interdependent HCI Network

The transport CI geodatabase consists of nodes and links. Network operation such as proximity analysis is used to analyze the distance between the different CI nodes. Optimal route-finding operations help in determining the shortest path between two nodes (ex: healthcare facilities). This is helpful while evacuating the patients and the ambulance tries to determine the optimal path between the two healthcare facilities. Figure 16 shows the process of evacuation of patients by ambulances from Hospital A to Hospital B. When the simulation model predicts that Hospital A would reach a non-operational state in few hours from system analysis, the command center looks out for available ambulances. We see in the figure that the Ambulanceteam1 is available; the Ambulance team1 is assigned to Hospital A in the SCPN simulation model. The ambulanceteam1 looks for a safe and shortest distance to Hospital B using the optimal path functions. Once the ambulance reaches the onsite, it gives back the information to the command center. Figures 17 and 18 show us the movement of an ambulance from one hospital to another hospital evacuating patients on the GIS client interface.

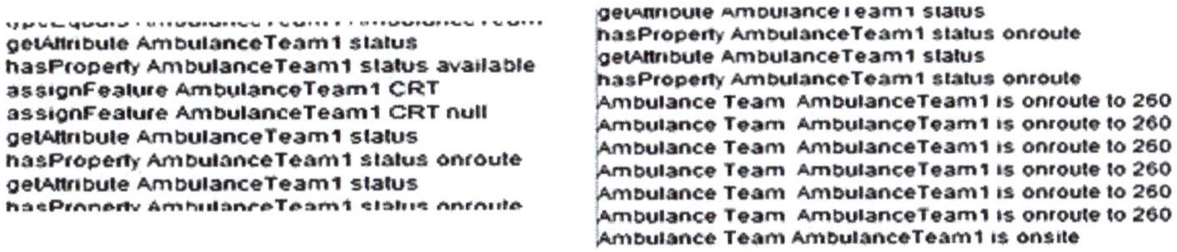

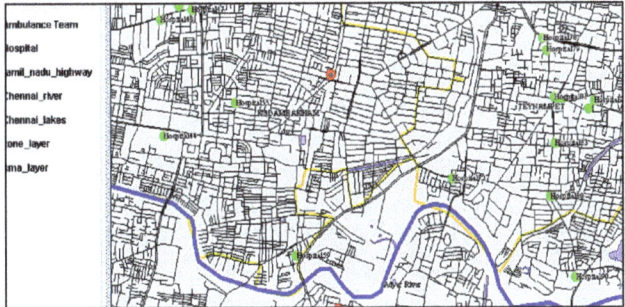

Figure 16. Ambulance using SCPN driven GIS-based Network operations.

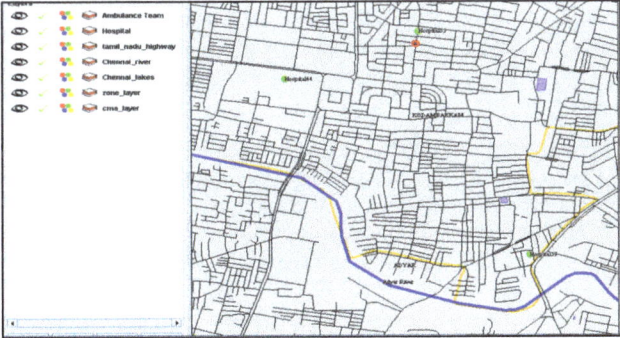

Figure 17. An ambulance (red node) starting from Hospital A.

Figure 18. Ambulance (Red node) reached to safer Hospital B.

The simulation model enables the user to analytically reason with spatial information as facilitated by interactive visual interface. The spatial data features are investigated over the period using an interactive visual interface to analyze and envisage the effect and impact of an urban flood disaster event on the interdependent healthcare CI network.

5. Conclusions

Considering the increase in extreme events today, there is an immediate need for real-time situational awareness simulation models. Critical Infrastructures and its services are the lifelines services required by society and during an extreme event the need for these services increases. The challenge of cascading failures in the interdependent HCI network is addressed in an Indian scenario. The utility of the approach is shown using a real-world case study, the dynamic performance of the interdependent healthcare critical infrastructure network and propagation of cascading failures in the Chennai area during the Chennai floods 2015 is evaluated and analyzed. The results of the system analysis of the simulation model are calculated for a simulation period of 3 days of rainfall and flooding (a total of 72 h). From the simulation runs we see that the failure in the electric supply CI network will increase the vulnerability of water supply CI networks. And the failure of both electric supply CI and water supply CI will have a perilous impact on the HCI network. From the system analysis, we can derive that the more interdependent the critical infrastructures are, the more vulnerable they are.

The simulation model will help the disaster response personnel or organizations who are managing crisis activities (e.g., Health care managers, Emergency management personnel, etc.). This work addressed this critical area to enable better preparation and management during a disaster. For instance, if the estimate from the proposed simulation model is performed, it gives insights into disruptions in electrical CI, and water supply CI and how it will impact the healthcare CI in say seven hours from now. Consequently, a hospital can plan the evacuation of critically ill patients and be better disaster prepared, thus significantly lowering the critical eventualities. The developed model can have an impact on the decision-making heuristics during a flood event. This kind of dynamic real-time understanding of the propagation of cascading failures of CI in an Interdependent CI network simulation would be a crucial component in any disaster response activities.

Author Contributions: Conceptualization, Nivedita Nukavarapu and Surya Durbha.; methodology, Nivedita Nukavarapu and Surya Durbha.; software, Nivedita Nukavarapu; validation, Nivedita Nukavarapu.; formal analysis, Nivedita Nukavarapu.; investigation, Nivedita Nukavarapu.; resources, Nivedita Nukavarapu and Surya Durbha.; data curation, Nivedita Nukavarapu.; writing—original draft preparation, Nivedita Nukavarapu.; writing—review and editing, Surya Durbha.; visualization, Nivedita Nukavarapu.; supervision, Surya Durbha.; project administration, Surya Durbha.; funding acquisition, Surya Durbha. All authors have read and agreed to the published version of the manuscript.

Funding: This research received no external funding.

Acknowledgments: The authors would like to thank the support from the Indian Institute of Technology Bombay and Disaster Division, National Remote Sensing Center (NRSC), Hyderabad, India.

Conflicts of Interest: The authors declare no conflict of interest.

References

1. Ramachandra, T.; Mujumdar, P.P. Urban Floods: Case Study of Bangalore. *J. Disaster Dev.* **2009**, *3*, 1–99.
2. Rinaldi, S.M.; Peerenboom, J.P.; Kelly, T.K. Identifying, understanding, and analyzing critical infrastructure interdependencies. *IEEE Control Syst. Mag.* **2001**, *21*, 11–25.
3. Dudenhoeffer, D.; Hartley, S.; Permann, M.; Pederson, P. *Critical Infrastructure Interdependency Modeling: A Survey of Critical Infrastructure Interdependency Modeling*; Idaho National Laboratory: Idaho Falls, ID, USA, 2006; Volume 25, p. 27.
4. Ouyang, M. Review on modeling and simulation of interdependent critical infrastructure systems. *Reliab. Eng. Syst. Saf.* **2014**, *121*, 43–60. [CrossRef]
5. Petit, F.; Verner, D.; Brannegan, D.; Buehring, W.; Dickinson, D. *Analysis of Critical Infrastructure Dependencies and Interdependencies*; Office of Scientific and Technical Information (OSTI): Oak Ridge, TN, USA, 2015.
6. Vespignani, A. Complex networks: The fragility of interdependency. *Nature* **2010**, *464*, 984–985. [CrossRef] [PubMed]
7. Nukavarapu, N.; Durbha, S. Stochastic coloured petrinet based healthcare infrastructure interdependency model. In Proceedings of the International Archives of the Photogrammetry, Remote Sensing and Spatial Information Sciences—ISPRS Archives; ISPRS Congress, Prague, Czech Republic, 12–19 July 2016.
8. Loosemore, M.; Chow, V.W.; McGeorge, D. Modelling the risks of extreme weather events for Australasian hospital infrastructure using rich picture diagrams. *Constr. Manag. Econ.* **2012**, 1–16. [CrossRef]

9. Lee, E.E.; Mitchell, J.E.; Wallace, W.A. Restoration of services in interdependent infrastructure systems: A network flows approach. *IEEE Trans. Syst. Man Cybern. Part C Appl. Rev.* **2007**, *37*, 1303–1317. [CrossRef]
10. Voeller, J.G.; Lee, E.E.; Mitchell, J.E.; Wallace, W.A. Network Flow Approaches for Analyzing and Managing Disruptions to Interdependent Infrastructure Systems. In *Wiley Handbook of Science and Technology for Homeland Security*; John Wiley & Sons: Hoboken, NJ, USA, 2009.
11. Chou, C.-C.; Tseng, S.-M. Collection and Analysis of Critical Infrastructure Interdependency Relationships. *J. Comput. Civ. Eng.* **2010**, *24*, 539–547. [CrossRef]
12. Jha, M.K. Dynamic Bayesian Network for Predicting the Likelihood of a Terrorist Attack at Critical Transportation Infrastructure Facilities. *J. Infrastruct. Syst.* **2009**, *15*, 31–39. [CrossRef]
13. Barrett, C.; Beckman, R.; Channakeshava, K.; Huang, F.; Kumar, V.A.; Marathe, A.; Marathe, M.V.; Pei, G. Cascading failures in multiple infrastructures: From transportation to communication network. In Proceedings of the 2010 5th International Conference on Critical Infrastructure, CRIS 2010, Beijing, China, 20–22 September 2010.
14. Dueñas-Osorio, L.; Kwasinski, A. Quantification of lifeline system interdependencies after the 27 February 2010 Mw 8.8 offshore Maule, Chile, earthquake. *Earthq. Spectra* **2012**, *28*, 581–603. [CrossRef]
15. Cardellini, V.; Casalicchio, E.; Galli, E. Agent-based modeling of interdependencies in critical infrastructures through UML. In Proceedings of the SpringSim '07—Proceedings of the 2007 Spring Simulation Multiconference, Norfolk, VA, USA, 25–29 March 2007.
16. Arboleda, C.A.; Abraham, D.M.; Richard, J.-P.P.; Lubitz, R. Vulnerability Assessment of Health Care Facilities during Disaster Events. *J. Infrastruct. Syst.* **2009**, *15*, 149–161. [CrossRef]
17. Arboleda, C.A.; Abraham, D.M.; Lubitz, R. Simulation As a Tool to Assess the Vulnerability of the Operation of a Health Care Facility. *J. Perform. Constr. Facil.* **2007**, *21*, 302–312. [CrossRef]
18. John, J. *Healthcare Impact Simulation Using HCSim Energy*; U.S. Department of Energy Office of Scientific and Technical Information: Oak Ridge, TN, USA, 2013.
19. Vugrin, E.D.; Verzi, S.J.; Finley, P.D.; Turnquist, M.A.; Griffin, A.R.; Ricci, K.A.; Wyte-Lake, T. Modeling Hospitals' Adaptive Capacity during a Loss of Infrastructure Services. *J. Healthc. Eng.* **2015**, *6*, 85–120. [CrossRef] [PubMed]
20. Petri, C.A. Kommunikation mit Automaten. Ph.D. Thesis, University of Bonn, Bonn, Germany, 1962.
21. Peterson, J.L. Petri Nets. *ACM Comput. Surv.* **1977**, *9*, 223–252. [CrossRef]
22. Marsan, M.A. Stochastic Petri nets: An elementary introduction. *Appl. Evol. Comput.* **1990**, *424*, 1–29.
23. Zuberek, W.M. Timed Petri nets and preliminary performance evaluation. In Proceedings of the 7th annual symposium on Computer Architecture, La Baule, France, 6–8 May 1980; pp. 88–96.
24. Marsan, M.A.; Balbo, G.; Conte, G.; Donatelli, S.; Franceschinis, G. Modelling with Generalized Stochastic Petri Nets. *ACM SIGMETRICS Perform. Eval. Rev.* **1998**, *26*, 2. [CrossRef]
25. Gursesli, O.; Desrochers, A.A. Modeling infrastructure interdependencies using Petri nets. In Proceedings of the 2003 IEEE International Conference on Systems, Man and Cybernetics. Conference Theme—System Security and Assurance (Cat. No.03CH37483), Washington, DC, USA, 8 October 2004.
26. Sultana, S.; Chen, Z. Modeling flood induced interdependencies among hydroelectricity generating infrastructures. *J. Environ. Manage.* **2009**, *90*, 3272–3282. [CrossRef] [PubMed]
27. Krings, A.; Oman, P. A simple GSPN for modelling common mode failures in critical infrastructures. In Proceedings of the 36th Annual Hawaii International Conference on System Sciences, HICSS 2003, Big Island, HI, USA, 6–9 January 2003.
28. Chen, T.M.; Sanchez-Aarnoutse, J.C.; Buford, J. Petri net modeling of cyber-physical attacks on smart grid. *IEEE Trans. Smart Grid* **2011**, *2*, 741–749. [CrossRef]
29. Laprie, J.-C.; Kanoun, K.; Kaâniche, M. Modelling Interdependencies Between the Electricity and Information Infrastructures. *Appl. Evol. Comput.* **2007**, *4680*, 54–67.
30. Omidvar, B.; Malekshah, M.H.; Omidvar, H. Failure risk assessment of interdependent infrastructures against earthquake, a Petri net approach: Case study-power and water distribution networks. *Nat. Hazards* **2013**, *71*, 1971–1993. [CrossRef]
31. Giglio, D.; Sacco, N. A Petri net model for analysis, optimisation, and control of railway networks and train schedules. In Proceedings of the 2016 IEEE 19th International Conference on Intelligent Transportation Systems (ITSC), Rio de Janeiro, Brazil, 1–4 November 2016.

32. Di Febbraro, A.; Giglio, D.; Sacco, N. On analyzing the vulnerabilities of a railway network with Petri nets. *Transp. Res. Procedia* **2017**, *27*, 553–560. [CrossRef]
33. Szpyrka, M.; Jasiul, B. Evaluation of cyber security and modelling of risk propagation with Petri nets. *Symmetry* **2017**, *9*, 32. [CrossRef]
34. Dotoli, M.; Fanti, M.P.; Iacobellis, G.; Martino, L.; Moretti, A.M.; Ukovich, W. Modeling and management of a hospital department via petri nets. In Proceedings of the 2010 IEEE Workshop on Health Care Management, WHCM, Venice, Italy, 18–20 February 2010.
35. Hamana, S.; Augusto, V.; Xie, X.; Ieee, F. A Timed Petri Net Approach for Verification of Territorial Healthcare Information Systems. In Proceedings of the 2016 IEEE International Conference on Automation Science and Engineering (CASE), Fort Worth, TX, USA, 21–25 August 2016.
36. Murata, T. Petri Nets: Properties, Analysis and Applications. *Proc. IEEE* **1989**, *77*, 541–580. [CrossRef]
37. Peterson, J.L. A note on colored Petri nets. *Inf. Process. Lett.* **1980**, *11*, 40–43. [CrossRef]
38. Jensen, K.; Kristensen, L.M. *Coloured Petri Nets: Modelling and Validation of Concurrent Systems*; Springer: Berlin/Heidelberg, Germany, 2009.
39. Wells, L. Performance analysis using CPN tools. In Proceedings of the 1st International Conference on Performance Evaluation Methodolgies Tools—Valuetools '06, Pisa, Italy, 11–13 October 2006; p. 59.
40. Jensen, K. In Proceedings of the Sixth Workshop and Tutorial on Practical Use of Coloured Petri Nets and the CPN Tools, Aarhus, Denmark, 24–26 October 2005; p. 300.
41. Jensen, K. Coloured petri nets. In *Lecture Notes in Computer Science (Including Subseries Lecture Notes in Artificial Intelligence and Lecture Notes in Bioinformatics*; Springer: Berlin/Heidelberg, Germany, 1987.
42. Jensen, K. *Coloured Petri Nets: Basic Concepts, Analysis Methods and Practical Use*; Springer: Berlin/Heidelberg, Germany, 1996.
43. Van der Aalst, W.M.P.; Stahl, C.; Westergaard, M. Strategies for modeling complex processes using colored Petri nets. In *Lecture Notes in Computer Science (Including Subseries Lecture Notes in Artificial Intelligence and Lecture Notes in Bioinformatics*; Springer: Berlin/Heidelberg, Germany, 2013.
44. Malhotra, M.; Trivedi, K.S. Dependability Modeling Using Petri-Nets. *IEEE Trans. Reliab.* **1995**, *44*, 428–440. [CrossRef]
45. Pandey, S.; Kaliamoorthy, I.; Reddy, M.S.; Rajakumar, A.; Pillai, B.; Micheal, J.C.J.; Kancherla, R.; Rela, M.; Varghese, J. Safe emergency evacuation of a Tertiary Care Hospital during the 'once in a century' floods in Chennai, India. *Indian J. Crit. Care Med.* **2016**, *20*, 104–108. [CrossRef]
46. Sill, B.B.L.; Kozlowskf, R.T. Analysis of Storm-Damage Factors for Low-Rise Structures. *J. Perform. Constr. Facil.* **1997**, *11*, 168–177. [CrossRef]
47. Federal Emergency Management Agency. *Seismic Performance Assessment of Buildings*; FEMA P-58. vol. 1, no. September; Federal Emergency Management Agency: Washington, DC, USA, 2012; p. 278.
48. Precautions, G.S. *Indian Electricity Rules, 1956*; Government of India, Ministry of Power, Central Electricity Board: New Delhi, India, 1956.
49. Peace, J.; Seidel, S.; Peace, J. *Business Weathering The Storm: Building Business Resilience Building Business Resilience*; Center for Climate and Energy Solutions: Arlington, VA, USA, 2013.

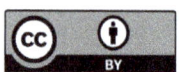

© 2020 by the authors. Licensee MDPI, Basel, Switzerland. This article is an open access article distributed under the terms and conditions of the Creative Commons Attribution (CC BY) license (http://creativecommons.org/licenses/by/4.0/).

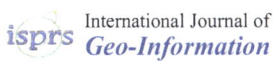

Article

A Multi-factor Spatial Optimization Approach for Emergency Medical Facilities in Beijing

Liang Zhou [1,2], Shaohua Wang [2,*] and Zhibang Xu [1,3]

1   Faculty of Geomatics, Lanzhou Jiaotong University, Lanzhou 730070, China; zhouliang@lzjtu.edu.cn (L.Z.); xzbang@whu.edu.cn (Z.X.)
2   Institute of Geographic Sciences and Natural Resources Research, CAS, Beijing 100101, China
3   School of Resource and Environment Science, Wuhan University, Wuhan 430079, China
*   Correspondence: wangshaohua@lreis.ac.cn

Received: 13 April 2020; Accepted: 30 May 2020; Published: 1 June 2020

Abstract: The outcomes for emergency medical services (EMS) are highly dependent on space-time accessibility. Prior research describes the location of EMS needs with low accuracy and has not integrated a temporal analysis of the road network, which accounts for varying mobility in a dynamic transportation network. In this study, we formulated a network-based location-allocation model (NLAM) and analyzed the spatial characteristics of emergency medical facilities within the fifth ring road in Beijing by considering time, traffic, and population characteristics. The conclusions are as follows: (1) The high demand area for EMS is concentrated in the areas in middle, north, and east during the daytime (8:00–20:00) and in the middle and north during the nighttime (20:00–8:00). From day to night, the centroid of the potential demand distribution shifts in the Western and Southern areas. (2) The road traffic data is sampled 20 times throughout the week, and variations in the average driving speed affect a higher mean driving speed on the weekend. This primarily impacts the main roads, due to these roads experiencing the greatest fluctuation in speed throughout the week of any roadway in the study area. (3) Finally, the 15-min coverage of emergency medical facilities are sampled 20 times in one week and analyzed. Fortunately, there is 100% coverage at night; however, due to traffic congestion, there were a few blind coverage areas in the daytime. The blind area is prevalent in Shijingshan South Station and the Jingxian Bridge in the South fifth ring.

Keywords: emergency medical facilities; traffic jam; megacity; network-based location-allocation model; Beijing

1. Introduction

High-quality educational and medical resources are the primary purpose pursued by urban residents. However, the spatial distribution of educational and medical facilities is uneven. In particular, the regional imbalance of medical services is more prominent, and medical treatment becomes a prominent factor affecting people's livelihood [1]. The proportion of medical technology is the highest factor among influencing aspects, followed by charges, medical ethics, and traffic convenience [2]. The attractive radiation range of high-level hospitals is far beyond the scope of space accessibility in general, which has caused a certain degree of the shortage of medical resources. Although China was promoting the medical classification system in 2015, it has not been enforced. It remains uncertain, for the impact of accessibility on medical services has changed. Compared with other medical services, emergency medical services are more dependent on the accessibility of time and space. Medical personnel rush to the scene in the quickest possible time, and the corresponding rescue measures can significantly improve the survival rate of patients [3]. Therefore, it is essential to improve the regional equilibrium allocation of emergency medical facilities with high accessibility. For the megacities with more than 10 million people, the improvement and optimization of the spatial distribution of emergency medical facilities has become a critical part of the healthy development of the city.

The existing research is executed with all medical service facilities (including comprehensive hospital, specialist hospital, hospital, emergency medical facilities, clinic, and so on), mainly from three aspects, including the analytics and evaluation of medical service facilities [1,4], study on the spatial and temporal accessibility of medical facilities services and its influencing factors [5–7], and the location selection and spatial optimization of medical service facilities [8–10]. There is relatively little research on emergency medical facilities for megacities. Chen et al. (2016) used the floating car global positioning system (GPS) to analyze the impact of traffic congestion on the space-time accessibility of emergency medical facilities in downtown Guangzhou [11]. Guo Zengxun et al. (2012) analyzed the temporal and spatial distribution of 120 emergency needs in urban areas using the Beijing emergency center dispatch information database [12]. The research of all medical service facilities consider multifactors such as the hospital's grade, capacity, and facilities level. However, only the space-time accessibility will be considered for emergency medical facilities when responding to emergency needs (this will not be considered in the extreme case of the nearest emergency ambulance). Therefore, the research on the spatial layout of emergency medical facilities needs to consider factors such as population, time, and traffic. First of all, quantitatively simulate potential first aid needs; then, carefully consider time and traffic factors to analyze the spatial accessibility and coverage of emergency medical facilities, and, finally, optimize for the shortcomings. Some scholars consider the availability and efficiency of facilities, such as the gravity model [13] and its derived mobile search method [14], and the location-allocation model (also called the LA model). Since the 1970s, the location-distribution model has been widely used in site selection studies in education [15,16], firefighting [17], medical [18], and emergency facilities [19]. The existing spatial optimization of medical service facilities using the location-allocation model [8,9] has deficiencies in these two issues. First, the shape of the residential area or the neighborhood committee or village committee is the request point. The second is using the road speed without the time and area difference as the impedance parameter of the road network. In actual situations, the demand for emergency medical services is generated at work, life, or place of residence and needs to be expressed more meticulously. In the same way, the traffic conditions of roads also change with time and location. There are differences in traffic speeds between the peak traffic period and the peak period and the main road sections and suburban road sections. Studies have shown that there is a definite spatial and temporal difference in the accessibility of emergency medical facilities under the influence of transportation factors [6]. Therefore, a more detailed simulation of traffic factors is also required when performing coverage analysis.

Multisource location data such as the floating-car data, mobile terminal location-based service (LBS) positioning data, network data, map, and point of interest (POI) data have provided solutions to the deficiencies mentioned above. The POI data using the electronic map platform can be used to obtain the location of work, life, or place of residence as a request point for emergency medical services. The traffic situation data calculated based on the floating car global positioning system (GPS), mobile terminal location-based service (LBS) positioning, and mobile internet user volunteered geographic information (VGI) collection [20] can help obtain traffic speed information for different road sections at different times. The POI data has been proved to be of great significance in facility planning, urban space, and rescue analysis [21,22], and it has been applied in urban research [23–25]. The GPS and VGI data of floating cars are also widely used in urban traffic and spatial analysis research [25,26].

There are three classes of location models for emergency medical services (EMS), including covering models, p-median models, and p-center models [27]. The objective of covering models for EMS is to provide covering the demand point within a distance limit and budget constraints. The covering models contain the location set covering problem (LSCP) [28] and the maximal covering location problem (MCLP) [29]. The LSCP aims to locate the smallest number of EMS facilities that are required to cover all EMS demand points [30]. The MCLP model for EMS seeks the maximal coverage with a given number of facilities [31]. The objective function for the p-median model for EMS is to minimize the total distance between the demand points and the facilities [32–34]. The p-center model for EMS tends to find the center of a circle that has the smallest radius to cover the destinations [35,36]. It is essential to optimize the EMS for considering multifactors using location models [37].

This study aims to improve the problems in the study of the space layout of existing emergency medical facilities and consider time, traffic, population, and other factors to study the spatial layout of urban emergency medical facilities. First, by using POI facility data combined with population distribution grid data to more closely simulate the potential demand distribution of emergency medical services, then using the collected traffic data of different time and road sections to simulate the road traffic conditions at different times. Finally, the location-distribution model was used to quantitatively measure the coverage of urban emergency medical facilities, combined with the lack of optimization and improvement. The study aims to enhance the scientific and practical research of the spatial layout of urban emergency medical facilities.

2. Study Area and Method

2.1. Study Area

The study selected Beijing within the fifth ring road (area of approximately 668.40 km^2) as the study area, mainly based on the following considerations. First, the city of Beijing is large in scale and densely populated, and the spatial layout and optimization of emergency medical facilities are more urgent and typical. Second, Beijing's urban functional areas are staggered and complicated, and the traffic situation is complex and dynamic. The significance and value of emergency medical facility coverage in functional urban areas and traffic conditions in complex cities are significant. The permanent population of Beijing was approximately 21.7 million by the end of 2015. There were 10,425 institutions related to health, including 701 hospitals, 30 disease prevention and control centers (epidemic stations), 19 maternal and child health clinics, and 1979 community health centers, with 111,555 beds in total, including 104,644 hospital beds, as shown in Figure 1. During the year of 2015, a total of 163.4797 million visits were made to Beijing hospitals. Beijing is home to the highest quality of medical resources in China, and its scope of influence is, to some extent, covered by the whole country, because high-quality hospitals also have a strong appeal to patients in that specific field. In contrast, emergency medical facilities serve more local populations. This study focuses on emergency medical facilities to address the challenges for the distribution, coverage, and optimization of medical emergency medical facilities in the context of traffic congestion.

2.2. Data Preprocessing

The dataset in this research mainly included real-time traffic data, emergency location data, population data, POI facility data, road network data, and administrative divisions and other data. Emergency site data, POI facility data, and real-time traffic data are all available via Python Reptiles from the Open Maps Open Platform (http://lbs.amap.com/). The first-aid site and POI data were obtained in August 2016. The first-aid site was the emergency center in the Gaode POI three-level classification. After data deduplication, 80 first-aid sites in the study area were obtained. After data preprocessing, the POIs have been obtained a total of 187,700 of the nine major categories. The population grid data was produced by Worldpop (http://www.worldpop.org.uk/), with a spatial resolution of 100 meters [38]; real-time traffic data was mainly used to obtain the road traffic speed information under the Gaode traffic situation interface. The acquisition time was 8/15-8/21/2017. A continuous week of data was collected to distinguish road traffic conditions at different times on weekends and weekdays. The collection time points were 0, 6, 7, 8, 9, 10, 12, 15, 17, 18, 19, 20, and 21 o'clock. After removing the inaccurate and incomplete information, a total of 634,200 pieces of data on road speed were obtained. It should be pointed out that the road traffic data provided by Golder did not cover some low-level roads. The road network data came from OpenStreetMap (http://www.openstreetmap.org/). Other data, such as the regional administrative data, came from the national basic geographic information database, and the statistical data came from the Beijing Statistical Yearbook 2016.

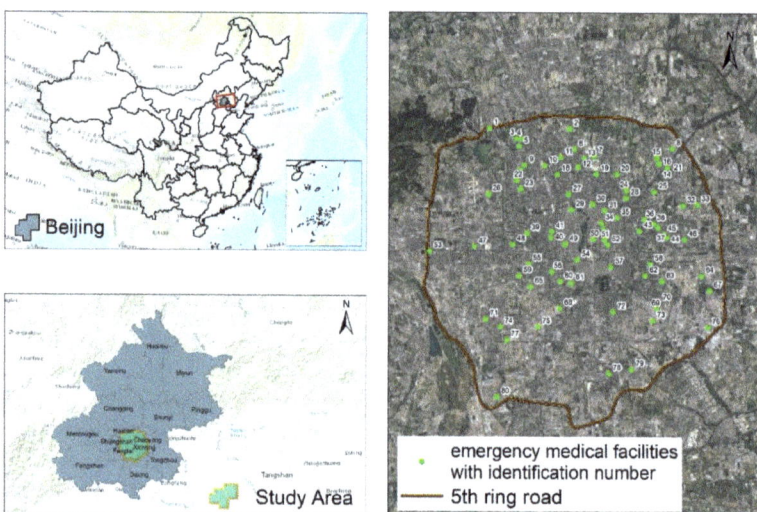

Figure 1. Study area and locations of the emergency medical facilities in Beijing.

2.3. Method

The methodology of this study was mainly divided into three parts, including the spatial identification of the potential needs of emergency medical services, the construction of multitemporal traffic network, and the coverage analysis of multitemporal emergency medical facilities.

2.3.1. Spatial Identification of Potential Demands for Emergency Medical Services

The potential demands of emergency medical services involve three elements, including time, place, and person, which can be summarized as which people have the potential for emergency medical services at which sites. At the present stage, subject to technical and data reasons, it is unrealistic to obtain full-time spatial locations for all people. This paper adopted a compromise strategy. It considered human work and living activities and divided them into two-time intervals. Then, found out where the person may be located in the two times frames and used the population data to simulate the spatial distribution of people at different places. Specifically, the time was first divided into two periods of daytime (8:00–20:00) and night (20:00–8:00 on the following day). Most people mainly stayed in workplaces during the daytime and stayed in residential and accommodation areas. In this situation, we could find and classify the corresponding POI categories. The population grid raster data was used to extract and obtain the estimates of personnel for each POI site by a geographic information system (GIS). Finally, the POI data was used to estimate the population of each POI site as the population field value. Using 100*100 m as the minimum grid unit for the kernel density analysis, the results of kernel density analysis were used to characterize the spatial distribution of the potential emergency demands. The higher the density, the more the population, the higher the demand for potential emergency medical services, and vice versa, the lower the demand for emergency medical services.

Table 1 shows the main activities of urban residents at different temporal periods. The analysis method mainly involved in this section is the kernel density analysis. The kernel density analysis was used to calculate the density of an element in its surrounding neighborhood. It utilized a kernel function to get the value per unit area based on a point or polyline feature to fit each point or polyline to a smooth conical surface. Only points or line segments that fell within the neighborhood were considered for computing the density. If there was no point or line segment within the neighborhood of a particular cell, the cell was assigned a null value. We used the default search radius (bandwidth) based on the space configuration and the number of input points. This method corrected spatial outliers without causing a large search radius. Using the population field gave some elements more weight than other elements, depending on how important they were. The kernel functions of the study were based on the quadratic kernel function described in Silverman's book [39].

Table 1. The main places of activities for urban residents in different periods. POI: point of interest.

Time	Major categories	Detailed Category of POI
8:00–20:00	Residential, Corporate company, Science and Technology Culture, Food and Beverage Services, Leisure Services, Transportation Station Type, Financial Venues, Government Agencies	Villas, dormitories, residential areas, residential quarters, and dual-use commercial and residential buildings; company companies; museums, archives, art galleries, planetariums, libraries, cultural palaces, science and technology museums, exhibition halls, convention centers, schools, scientific research institutions, training institutions, media organizations, cultural and art groups, driving schools, and scientific and educational cultural venues; tea houses, pastry shops, cafes, fast food restaurants, cold drinks shops, dessert shops, foreign restaurants, Chinese restaurants, casual dining establishments, and catering-related venues; sports venues, entertainment venues, leisure venues, theaters, and resorts and convalescent places; subway stations, port terminals, railway stations, airport-related, and coach stations; securities companies, insurance companies, banks, and financial service agencies; and industrial and commercial tax agencies, public security agencies, transportation vehicle management, society-relevant groups, foreign institutions, government agencies, and social organizations.
20:00–8:00	Residential and Accommodation services	Villa, dormitory, residential area, residential area, commercial and residential dual-use buildings, hotels, guest houses, and hotel accommodation services.

2.3.2. Multitemporal Traffic Network Construction

Traffic congestion is an important factor influencing the temporal and spatial differences in the accessibility of emergency medical services [6]. Therefore, it is essential to consider the road network modeling for traffic conditions at different times. First, we collated traffic situation data that was crawled to obtain the traffic speed at each time of each road segment and then used the road network data to create a network dataset and, according to the driving speed and the road length, the driving time of each road was calculated and the driving time was taken as the cost impedance of the road. Thus, a plurality of road network datasets were obtained, including traveling time at different times. The key to the research was the crawling, processing accuracy, and real-time performance of traffic situation data. Since the traffic situation data collected through the Gaode API was segmented data—that is, the speeds of different sections of a road were different—after the time dimension was superimposed, the speed of each section of each road was different at different times of the day. While in a network analysis, if a road is broken into small sections at different speeds at different times, the computational complexity will increase exponentially, and the number of small sections after an interruption will increase dramatically. Therefore, this study adopted the following preprocessing method. Road data with traffic speed in each period was converted into a 10*10 meter raster grid. The average speed of each raster grid at the same time in different days reflected the average speed of the road. The gaode traffic congestion data itself also had coverage blind areas; all speed-free road sections used the average speed of all other roads at the same time as their driving speed. In addition, in the construction of road network datasets, considering that ambulances have road priority, they can be free from road turning, traffic lights, and road direction. Therefore, appropriate settings were selected when the corresponding road network parameters were set. When the road impedance was set, the impedance field of the road was set to use the travel time. This travel time field can be defined as the value the road length dividing the corresponding road speed.

2.3.3. Multitime Status Analysis of Emergency Medical Facility Coverage

The analysis of the coverage of emergency medical facilities at multiple times is mainly to measure and analyze the arrival coverage of existing emergency medical facilities at different time points for all potential emergency medical service demand sites. This process involves three factors, including emergency medical facility sites, potential emergency medical service demand locations, and road traffic conditions. The emergency medical sites are fixed, and most of them are open 24 h. The spatial distribution of potential emergency medical services at different times has been identified, and road network data at different points in time have been established. Therefore, the research purpose in this section was to calculate the coverage of the existing emergency medical facilities using the public service coverage model according to the corresponding road traffic conditions for the needs of potential emergency medical services at different times. Specifically, the POI site for the potential emergency medical service in the corresponding time period was set as a request point, the POI site for the emergency medical place was set as a facility point, and a plurality of times were established based on the time. The demand POI sites for the potential emergency medical service in the corresponding period were set as the demand points. The emergency medical site POI was set as a facility, and based on the established road network dataset for multiple times, the "maximum coverage" algorithm in the "location-allocation" model was used to calculate the coverage of the emergency vehicle within 15 min ("Emergency Center Construction Standards" (BAN 117-2016). The minimization impedance algorithm was used to simulate the site selection optimization for the possible coverage blind spots.

The study used the L-A model, which suitably locates facilities to ensure that the requirements of the demand point are met most efficiently. The L-A model has a variety of algorithms that assign demand points to facilities while locating facilities. For an emergency medical facility, on the one hand, the emergency medical services of the hospital must arrive at as many places as necessary for emergency treatment within the specified response time. On the other hand, the first-aid site should make it easier for the ambulance to reach the demand place within the minimum travel cost. We propose a Network-based Location-Allocation Model (NLAM), including the maximum coverage (also called the maximal coverage location problem, MCLP) and the minimum impedance problem (also called p-median algorithm), along road networks.

(i) For possible coverage blindness, the p-median model can be used to perform a simulated siting of emergency medical facilities, which refers to setting facilities at appropriate locations so that the sum of all weighted costs between the demand point and solution at the facility can be minimized. The p-median model selects the facility that minimizes the sum of the weighted impedance (response point assigned to a facility multiplied by the impedance to that facility). We proposed a p-median model along the road network based on the formulation of the ReVelle–Swain model (1970) [11].

The notion is shown:

- P = total number of population
- M = total number of demand points
- i = index of demand points ($i = 1, 2, \ldots, M$)
- W_i = the weighted value of the population associated at the demand point ($P = \sum_{i=1}^{M} w_i$)
- N = total number of potential candidates for the EMS location

- j = index of potential EMS facility sites (j = 1, 2, ..., N)
- d_{ij} = the shortest-path distance between demand node i and potential EMS facility j along the road network
- p = the number of optimal locations

The mathematical description of this model is described as follows:

$$\text{Minimize } f = \sum_{i=1}^{M} \sum_{j=1}^{N} w_i * d_{ij} * x_{ij} \tag{1}$$

subject to:

$$\sum_{j=1}^{N} x_{ij} = 1, \quad i = 1, 2, 3, \ldots, M \tag{2}$$

$$x_{ij} \leq y_j, \quad i = 1, 2, 3, \ldots, M, \quad j = 1, 2, 3, \ldots, N \tag{3}$$

$$\sum_{j=1}^{N} y_j = p \tag{4}$$

$$x_{ij} = \{0, 1\}, \quad i = 1, 2, 3, \ldots, M, \quad j = 1, 2, 3, \ldots, N \tag{5}$$

$$y_j = \{0, 1\}, \quad j = 1, 2, 3, \ldots, N \tag{6}$$

The objective function (1) is to minimize the sum for all demand points of the network distance to their closest EMS facility. Constraint (2) requires that all demand points are to be assigned to only one EMS facility point. Constraint (3) allows demand point i to assign to a point j only if there is an open EMS facility at this location. Constraint (4) ensures that exact p EMS facility locations are to be chosen among the N potential ones. In Formulation (5), x_{ij} equals 1 if the demand at node i is allocated to the facility at site j and equals 0, otherwise. In Formulation (6), y_j equals 1 if an EMS facility is located at site j and equals 0, otherwise.

(ii) For the current coverage of emergency medical facilities, the maximum coverage location problem model is mainly used for the location facilities, so that as many request points as possible are allocated to the impedance interruptions of the facility points being solved. The algorithm handles the request as follows. Request points outside the impedance cutoff at all facilities will not be allocated. If a demand point is only within the impedance interruption of one facility, the request point will assign all of its request weights to the facility. If a demand point is within an impedance interruption at two or more facilities, the demand point will assign all of its request weights to the nearest facility only. The mathematical description of this model is as follows:

$$\text{Maximize } \sum_{i} w_i * y_i \tag{7}$$

subject to:

$$\sum_{j \notin N_i} x_j \geq y_i \quad \forall\, i \tag{8}$$

$$\sum_{j} x_j = p \tag{9}$$

$$x_j = \{0, 1\} \quad \forall\, j \tag{10}$$

$$y_i = \{0, 1\} \quad \forall\, i \tag{11}$$

The objective of Function (7) was to maximize the amount of the covered EMS demand. Constraint (8) defined whether the EMS coverage had been provided to a given EMS demand i based on the location decisions. Constraint (9) specified that the p EMS facility locations were to be chosen among the N potential ones. Constraints (10) and (11) defined the integer siting and coverage variables. If a facility location j was providing coverage, then x_j equaled 1; otherwise, x_j equaled 0. If the demand i was covered, the decision variable y_i was equal to 1; otherwise, y_i was equal to 0.

3. Results

3.1. Spatial Distribution of Potential Needs for Emergency Medical Services

According to the characteristics of the population and functional space, using the 187,700 points of POI data obtained, the spatial distribution of potential demand for emergency medical services at different times in the study area is shown in Figure 2. The darker color denotes the higher POI density after the weight of the population in the area and the higher demand for potential emergency medical services. The shallower color indicates the lower POI density of the weight of the superimposed population in the area and the lower demand for potential emergency medical services. Figure 1 identifies potential high-demand areas during the daytime (08:00–20:00) in Zhongguancun, Wudaokou, Xidan North Street, Chaoyangmen, Sanlitun, Guomao, Dawang Road, Wangfujing, Chongwenmen, and Century City. The high-demand areas are mostly concentrated in the Central, Northern, and Eastern parts of the study area, and the areas between the East Third Ring Road and the Northwest three-fourth ring are most prominent. The potential high-demand areas at night (20:00- 08:00 on the following day) are distributed in the front gates of Dashilan, Yong'anli, Jinsong, Dongzhimen, Lianchichi Road, Chongwenmen Ciqikou, Suzhou Bridge, Chegongzhuang—Guanganmen, and Wukesong. The high-demand areas are mostly concentrated in the Central and Northern parts of the study area, and the "Haidian Huangzhuang-Beijing West Railway Station" is more widely distributed along the line. Based on the analysis of daytime and nighttime, the potential demand for emergency medical services in the study area is mostly distributed within the Fourth Ring Road, and the area outside the area between the South third ring and the fourth ring is even more pronounced. From day to night, the direction of distribution of the potential demand for emergency medical services shifted westward and southward. The use of statistical zoning tools to analyze the demand for potential medical emergency services in the major administrative districts of the Fifth Ring Road found that the total number of daytime and nighttime demand was, in descending order: Chaoyang District, Haidian District, Xicheng District, Dongcheng District, and Fengtai District.

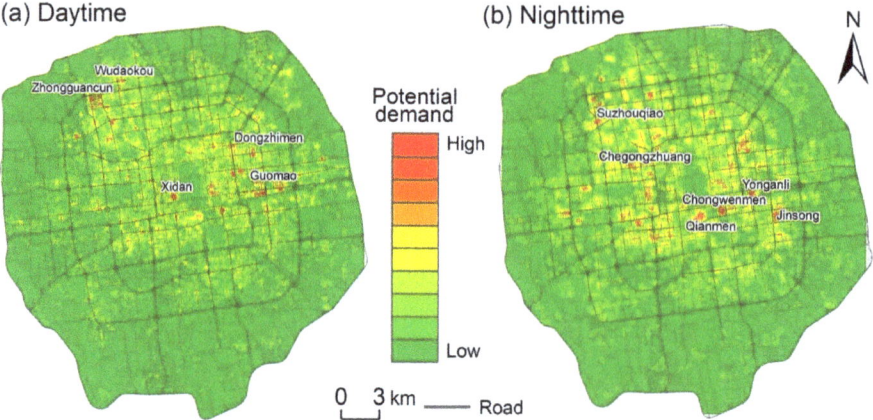

Figure 2. Spatial distribution of the potential demand for emergency services at different times: (**a**) daytime and (**b**) nighttime.

3.2. Spatial Distribution of Multitemporal Traffic Conditions

Using the collected 644,200 traffic data, according to the method described in the previous section, the traffic speeds of the roads in the study area at different times were first obtained through data preprocessing. Extensive computations were performed on average road speeds at 20 time points on all weekdays and weekends in the study area, as shown in Figure 3a. From the analysis of the period, during the morning peak (07:00–09:00) and the evening peak (17:00–19:00), the average driving speed decreased significantly, and the average driving speed had a slight rebound at noon. Comparing working days and weekends, the average speed of the weekends at the same time was mostly slightly higher than the working day. The average speed at 06:00 in the morning on weekends was slightly higher than at midnight, since people have more nightlife activities in the early morning on weekends The average driving speed at noon on the weekend compared with at noon on the working day was slightly higher, because the residents' trips during weekends have a certain time delay compared with on working days. Further, using the highest value of the speed of each road at different times minus the lowest value, the difference in speed was obtained as in Figure 3b. It can be found that the road segments with relatively large differences were mostly along the ring roads, among which, the ten road segments with the most extreme differences were concentrated in the Wufangqiao section of the East fifth ring of the Jingha Expressway and the Majialou Bridge section of the South Fourth Ring Road of the Jingkai Expressway. In order to accurately measure the coverage of emergency medical facilities, the road network was modeled at 20 time points on weekdays and weekends using the speed data of each road at the time. The obtained road speed distribution is shown in Figure 4.

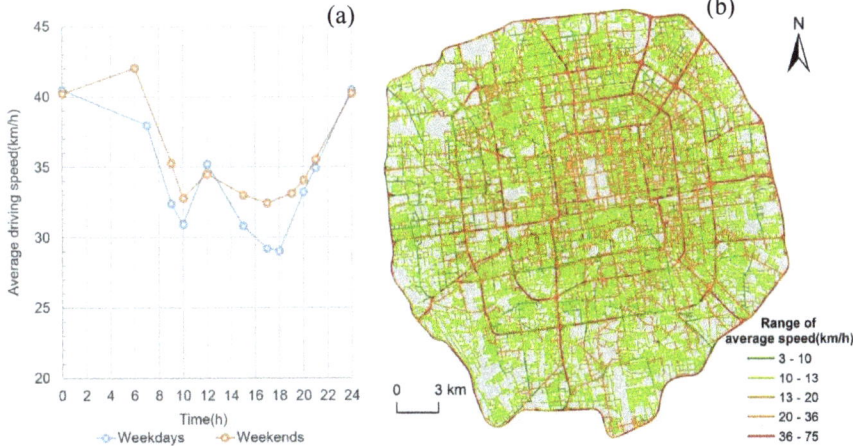

Figure 3. The average vehicle speed: (**a**) at different times; (**b**) on each road segments.

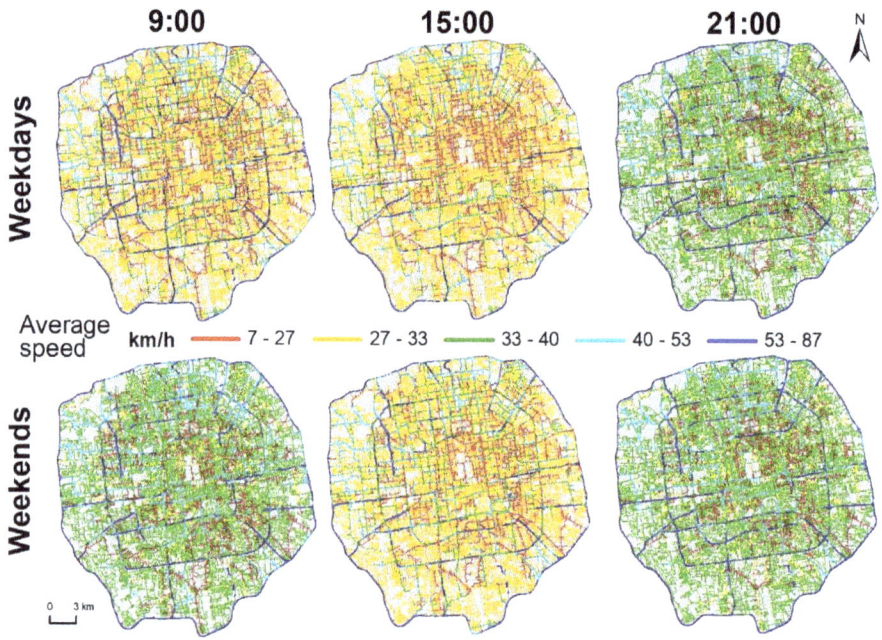

Figure 4. Speed at different times of each road in the study area.

3.3. Coverage Analysis of Multitime Status Emergency Medical Facilities

Based on the road network modeled for 20 time points on the working day and weekend, the "location-distribution" model was further analyzed, and it was found that the overall coverage of emergency medical facilities in the study area was relative high (Table 2 and Figure 5). From the perspective of spatial coverage, full coverage can be achieved within 15 min in the night period (20:00–8:00), divided by whether it was a working day or a weekend. There were very few coverage blind spots in emergency medical facilities during the daytime (08:00–20:00). In the spatiotemporal view, different traffic conditions at different time points made the space of the same emergency center cover in 15 min to make a difference. At the same time, due to the influence of time and traffic, the coverage of emergency medical facilities fluctuated, and the time at which coverage fell was basically in line with the traffic peak hours. In order to find the blindness area from spatial coverage due to traffic factors, POI facilities that cannot be covered at different points in time need to be further extracted to explore their spatial characteristics and get the optimal solution of the model.

Table 2. The coverage of emergency medical facilities at different times.

Working day (time)	9:00	10:00	12:00	15:00	17:00	18:00	20:00	21:00	0:00	7:00
Coverage (%)	99.99	99.94	99.99	99.95	99.81	99.84	100	100	100	100
Weekend (time)	9:00	10:00	12:00	15:00	17:00	19:00	20:00	21:00	0:00	6:00
Coverage (%)	99.99	99.99	99.99	99.99	99.99	99.97	100	100	100	100

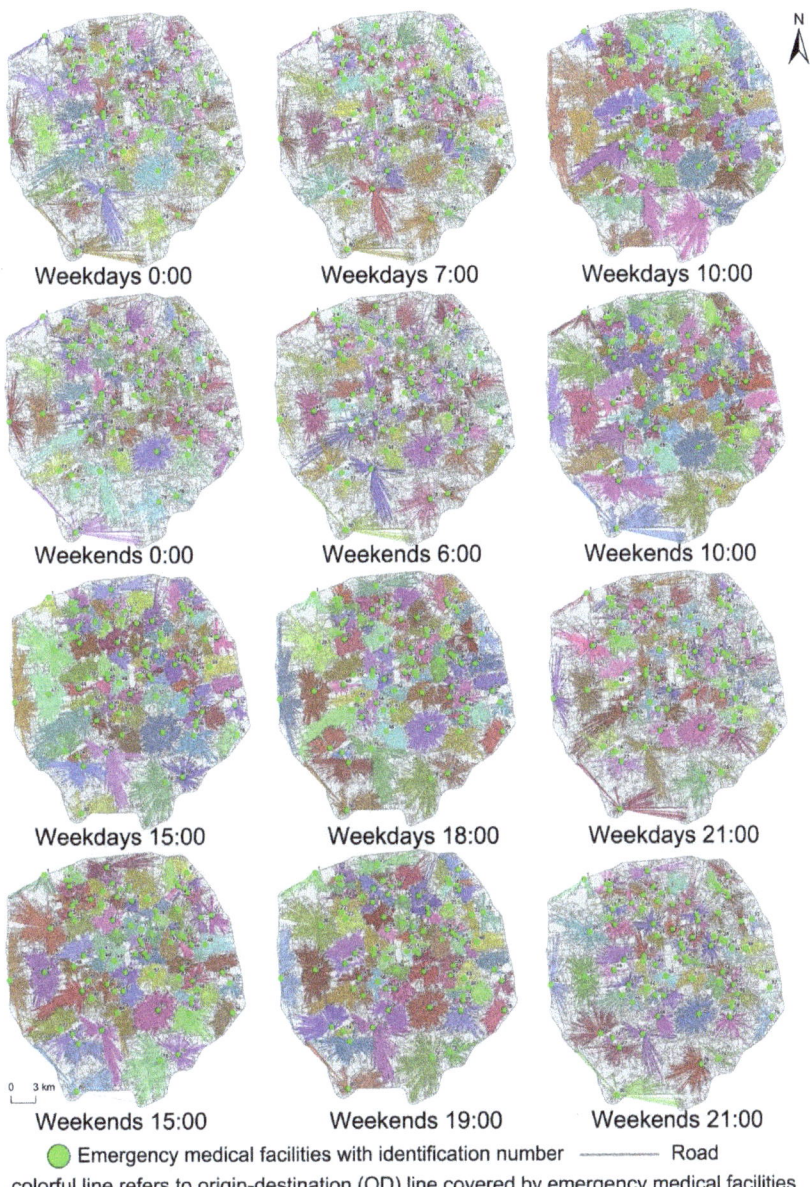

Figure 5. The coverage distribution of emergency medical facilities at different times.

The POI facilities were extracted that failed to be covered at different time points, and the results were merged. The results are shown in Figure 6a. There were two main areas that could not be covered during part of the day, including parts of the Shijingshan South Station and the Southern Fifth Ring Road Jingxian Bridge. The Shijingshan South Station did not cover POIs on a small area (six sites). The scale of uncovered sites along the South Fifth Ring Road Jingxian Bridge varied from 1-36 in different times. Considering that the Shijingshan South Railway Station has a small scope of uncovered sites on the one hand, on the other hand, there is a first-aid center (The first-aid center was not involved in the analysis, because it was not in the study area) in the Jingxi District of Chaoyang Hospital, which is close to the Northwest of Ximenkou Bridge on the West Fifth Ring Road. Therefore, the main coverage blindness area and optimized area are in the Southern Fifth Ring Road Jingxian Bridge (Figure 6b).

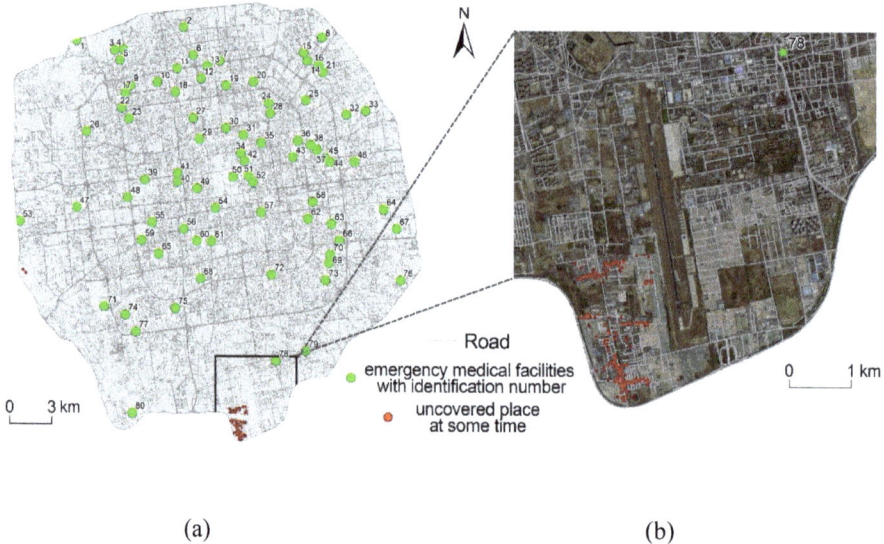

(a)   (b)

Figure 6. The blind coverage area of emergency medical facilities at some times: (**a**) the whole study area; (**b**) the Southern Fifth Ring Road Jingxian Bridge area.

Since the number of facilities within the Jingxianqiao area is not large enough, the construction of a new emergency center will make waste. If the method of reconstructing the road from the perspective of improving the road traffic conditions will also have a higher cost, a simple and effective solution is to find an existing medical facility in the area and transform it to have the function of an emergency center. This step can be performed by the following method. First, all medical facilities in the area are selected as candidates for the "location-allocation" model. Then, use the "minimum impedance" model to calculate and find the medical facilities that can cover the area with the least time-cost and upgrade it as an emergency medical service solution covering this area. The computational process was based on the road network at 17:00 on the most stressful working day. The final candidate was Beijing Wanbo Brain Health Traditional Chinese Medicine Hospital. It should be noted that the possibility of being an emergency medical facility is only discussed here from the perspective of spatial accessibility, subject to the lack of our medical professional knowledge.

4. Conclusions and Discussion

This study takes the urban emergency medical facilities in the Wuhan District in Beijing as the research object and comprehensively considers time, traffic impedance, and population factors to study the spatial distribution characteristics. First, using the POI facility data and population distribution grid data, the spatial distribution of potential medical emergency service needs during the day (8:00–20:00) and night (20:00–8:00) were identified. Then, using the collected traffic situation data, the road network was modeled according to the traffic conditions at different times. Finally, the emergency medical coverage at different time points in the study area was quantified using the algorithm in the "location-allocation" model, further combining the inadequacies of the proposed improvement direction. The main conclusions obtained in this paper are as follows:

(1) The distribution of potential emergency medical service needs during the two periods in the study area was identified based on the characteristics of the population and the space of residence and residence. During the day (8:00–20:00), high-demand areas for potential emergency medical services are mainly distributed in Zhongguancun, Wudaokou, Xidan North Street, Sanlitun, Guomao, Dawang Road, and other places, gathering in the Central, Northern, and Eastern parts of the study area. The high demand areas for potential emergency medical services during the night (20:00–8:00) were mainly distributed in Dashilan, Yong'anli, Chegongzhuang-Guang'anmen, Lianhuachi East Road, and other places, mostly in the Middle and North of the study area. From daytime to nighttime, the direction distribution center of potential demand shifted to the west and south. The total demand for potential emergency medical services in the major administrative regions of the study area are, in descending order: Chaoyang District, Haidian District, Xicheng District, Dongcheng District, and Fengtai District.

(2) Statistical analysis of the road traffic situation data were obtained, modeling the road network at 20 temporal ranges on the working days and weekend. Statistical analysis found that the average speed of all roads in the study area at the same time last weekend was mostly slightly higher than the working day. However, the average speed at midnight on weekends was slightly higher than the midnight on weekdays; the probable reason is that there is a certain delay in the travel of weekend residents compared to working days. The average driving speed at 6:00 in the morning on weekends is slightly higher than that at midnight, because people have more nightlife activities and less morning activities on the weekends. The roads at very different speeds at different time points are mostly ring roads. The ten road sections with the most extreme differences are concentrated in the Wufangqiao section of the East fifth ring of the Jingha Expressway and the Majialou Bridge section of the South Fourth Ring Road of the Jingkai Expressway.

(3) Based on the road network model at 20 time points on weekdays and weekends, the 15-min coverage of emergency medical facilities under the 20 time points in the study area was quantitatively measured, and optimization suggestions were given for coverage blind spots. The overall coverage of emergency medical facilities was relatively high. In the nighttime (20:00- 8:00), including working days and weekends, full coverage of the ambulances were achieved for 15 min. At some time points during the daytime (8:00–20:00) on the weekdays and weekends, there were very few coverage areas for emergency medical facilities, which were mainly distributed in parts of the Shijingshan South Railway Station and the Southern Fifth Ring Road Jingxian Bridge. Affected by time and traffic factors, the coverage of emergency medical facilities fluctuates, and the time at which coverage falls is basically in-line with traffic peak times. Further, the blind spot for the coverage of the Yinxianqiao area in the South Fifth Ring Road was considered. Considering the characteristics of the location and the scope of the uncovered point, the corresponding simulation site selection was given.

In this study, we did not consider the parallel method to solve the multifactor spatial optimization problem. We will integrate a high-performance spatial analysis method and spatial cloud computing algorithm [40–42] into the spatial optimization for a large-scale dataset to improve the efficiency in a future work. The multifactor spatial optimization approach is essential to understand the current worldwide emergency regarding the pandemic of COVID-19. In the next step, we will use a multifactor spatial optimization model for the testing site selection of COVID-19 with spatial coverage and the space-time traffic network.

Author Contributions: Conceptualization, Shaohua Wang and Liang Zhou; investigation, Zhibang Xu; methodology, Shaohua Wang, Zhibang Xu, and Liang Zhou; resources, Zhibang Xu; software, Shaohua Wang; and writing—original draft, Shaohua Wang and Liang Zhou. All authors have read and agreed to the published version of the manuscript.

Funding: This study was funded by the National Natural Science Foundation of China (Grant No. 41701173 and No. 41961027), National Key Research and Development Project (2016YFC0803106), China Postdoctoral Science Foundation (No. 2016M600121).

Conflicts of Interest: The authors declare no conflicts of interest.

References

1. Zheng, W.; Jiang, H.; Ai, H. Analysis of regional inequalities of basic medical resources supply in China. *Geogr. Res.* **2015**, *34*, 2049–2060.
2. Chen, Y.; Yunqing, M.; Shuzhang, L. Research and Analysis of Influencing Factors on the Patient's Medical Treatment Selection. *Chin. J. Soc. Med.* **2012**, *29*, 110–111.
3. Pons, P.T.; Haukoos, J.S.; Bludworth, W.; Cribley, T.; Pons, K.A.; Markovchick, V.J. Paramedic response time: Does it affect patient survival? *Acad. Emerg. Med.* **2005**, *12*, 594–600. [CrossRef]
4. Guagliardo, M.F. Spatial accessibility of primary care: Concepts, methods and challenges. *Int. J. Health Geogr.* **2004**, *3*, 3. [CrossRef]
5. Oppong, J.R.; Hodgson, M.J. Spatial accessibility to health care facilities in Suhum District, Ghana. *Prof. Geogr.* **1994**, *46*, 199–209. [CrossRef]
6. Xia, T.; Song, X.; Zhang, H.; Song, X.; Kanasugi, H.; Shibasaki, R. Measuring spatio-temporal accessibility to emergency medical services through big GPS data. *Health Place* **2019**, *56*, 53–62. [CrossRef] [PubMed]
7. Zhong, S.Y.; Yang, X.; Chen, R. The accessibility measurement of hierarchy public service facilities based on multi-mode network dataset and the two-step 2SFCA: A case study of Beijing's medical facilities. *Geogr. Res.* **2016**, *35*, 731–744.
8. Pulver, A.; Wei, R. Optimizing the spatial location of medical drones. *Appl. Geogr.* **2018**, *90*, 9–16. [CrossRef]
9. Delen, D.; Erraguntla, M.; Mayer, R.J.; Wu, C.N. Better management of blood supply-chain with GIS-based analytics. *Ann. Oper. Res.* **2011**, *185*, 181–193. [CrossRef]
10. Nasrabadi, A.M.; Najafi, M.; Zolfagharinia, H. Considering short-term and long-term uncertainties in location and capacity planning of public healthcare facilities. *Eur. J. Oper. Res.* **2019**, *281*, 152–173. [CrossRef]
11. ReVelle, C.S.; Swain, R.W. Central facilities location. *Geogr. Anal.* **1970**, *2*, 30–42. [CrossRef]
12. Guo, Z.; Yu, H.; Lu, Q. Region and Time Distribution of 120 EMSS Demand in Main Districts of Beijing. *Chin. Gen. Pract.* **2012**, *26*, 29.
13. Hansen, W.G. How accessibility shapes land use. *J. Am. Inst. Plan.* **1959**, *25*, 73–76. [CrossRef]
14. Yang, D.H.; Goerge, R.; Mullner, R. Comparing GIS-based methods of measuring spatial accessibility to health services. *J. Med. Syst.* **2006**, *30*, 23–32. [CrossRef] [PubMed]
15. Cooper, L. Location-allocation problems. *Oper. Res.* **1963**, *11*, 331–343. [CrossRef]
16. Menezes, R.C.; Pizzolato, N.D. Locating public schools in fast expanding areas: Application of the capacitated p-median and maximal covering location models. *Pesqui. Oper.* **2014**, *34*, 301–317. [CrossRef]
17. Murray, A.T. Optimising the spatial location of urban fire stations. *Fire Saf. J.* **2013**, *62*, 64–71. [CrossRef]
18. Harper, P.R.; Shahani, A.K.; Gallagher, J.E.; Bowie, C. Planning health services with explicit geographical considerations: A stochastic location–allocation approach. *Omega* **2005**, *33*, 141–152. [CrossRef]
19. Li, X.; Zhao, Z.; Zhu, X.; Wyatt, T. Covering models and optimization techniques for emergency response facility location and planning: A review. *Math. Meth. Oper. Res.* **2011**, *74*, 281–310. [CrossRef]
20. Goodchild, M.F. Citizens as sensors: The world of volunteered geography. *GeoJournal* **2007**, *69*, 211–221. [CrossRef]
21. Niyomubyeyi, O.; Pilesjö, P.; Mansourian, A. Evacuation Planning Optimization Based on a Multi-Objective Artificial Bee Colony Algorithm. *ISPRS Int. J. Geo Inf.* **2019**, *8*, 110. [CrossRef]
22. Li, X.; Xu, G.; Chen, E.; Zong, Y. Learning recency based comparative choice towards point-of-interest recommendation. *Expert Syst. Appl.* **2015**, *42*, 4274–4283. [CrossRef]
23. McKenzie, G.; Janowicz, K.; Gao, S.; Yang, J.A.; Hu, Y. POI pulse: A multi-granular, semantic signature–based information observatory for the interactive visualization of big geosocial data. *Cartogr. Int. J. Geogr. Inf. Geovis.* **2015**, *50*, 71–85. [CrossRef]
24. Santos, F.; Almeida, A.; Martins, C.; Gonçalves, R.; Martins, J. Using POI functionality and accessibility levels for delivering personalized tourism recommendations. *Comput. Environ. Urban* **2019**, *77*, 101173. [CrossRef]
25. Zhang, S.; Tang, J.; Wang, H.; Wang, Y.; An, S. Revealing intra-urban travel patterns and service ranges from taxi trajectories. *J. Transp. Geogr.* **2017**, *61*, 72–86. [CrossRef]
26. Zhu, D.; Wang, N.; Wu, L.; Liu, Y. Street as a big geo-data assembly and analysis unit in urban studies: A case study using Beijing taxi data. *Appl. Geogr.* **2017**, *86*, 152–164. [CrossRef]
27. Jia, H.; Ordóñez, F.; Dessouky, M. A modeling framework for facility location of medical services for large-scale emergencies. *IIE Trans.* **2007**, *39*, 41–55. [CrossRef]

28. Toregas, C.; Swain, R.; ReVelle, C.; Bergman, L. The location of emergency service facilities. *Oper. Res.* **1971**, *19*, 1363–1373. [CrossRef]
29. Church, R.; ReVelle, C. The maximal covering location problem. *Pap. Reg. Sci.* **1974**, *32*, 101–118. [CrossRef]
30. Daskin, M.S.; Stern, E.H. A hierarchical objective set covering model for emergency medical service vehicle deployment. *Transp. Sci.* **1981**, *15*, 137–152. [CrossRef]
31. Eaton, D.J.; Daskin, M.S.; Simmons, D.; Bulloch, B.; Jansma, G. Determining emergency medical service vehicle deployment in Austin, Texas. *Interfaces* **1985**, *15*, 96–108. [CrossRef]
32. Dzator, M.; Dzator, J. An effective heuristic for the P-median problem with application to ambulance location. *Opsearch* **2013**, *50*, 60–74. [CrossRef]
33. Ahmadi-Javid, A.; Seyedi, P.; Syam, S.S. A survey of healthcare facility location. *Comput. Oper. Res.* **2017**, *79*, 223–263. [CrossRef]
34. Grekousis, G.; Liu, Y. Where will the next emergency event occur? Predicting ambulance demand in emergency medical services using artificial intelligence. *Comput. Environ. Urban* **2019**, *76*, 110–122. [CrossRef]
35. Chanta, S.; Mayorga, M.E.; McLay, L.A. Improving emergency service in rural areas: A bi-objective covering location model for EMS systems. *Ann. Oper. Res.* **2014**, *221*, 133–159. [CrossRef]
36. Daskin, M.S.; Owen, S.H. Two New Location Covering Problems: The Partial P-Center Problem and the Partial Set Covering Problem. *Geogr. Anal.* **1999**, *31*, 217–235. [CrossRef]
37. Afshari, H.; Peng, Q. Challenges and solutions for location of healthcare facilities. *Ind. Eng. Manag.* **2014**, *3*, 12.
38. Lloyd, C.T.; Sorichetta, A.; Tatem, A.J. High resolution global gridded data for use in population studies. *Sci. Data* **2017**, *4*, 1–17. [CrossRef]
39. Silverman, B.W. *Density Estimation for Statistics and Data Analysis*; CRC Press: Boca Raton, FL, USA, 1986.
40. Zhou, L.; Dang, X.W.; Sun, Q.K.; Wang, S.H. Multi-scenario simulation of urban land change in Shanghai by random forest and CA-Markov model. *Sustain. Cities Soc.* **2020**, *55*, 1–10. [CrossRef]
41. Heitzler, M.; Lam, J.C.; Hackl, J.; Adey, B.T.; Hurni, L. GPU-accelerated rendering methods to visually analyze large-scale disaster simulation data. *J. Geovis. Spat. Anal.* **2017**, *1*, 3. [CrossRef]
42. Wang, S.; Zhong, Y.; Wang, E. An integrated GIS platform architecture for spatiotemporal big data. *Future Gener. Comput. Syst.* **2019**, *94*, 160–172. [CrossRef]

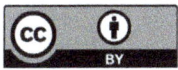

© 2020 by the authors. Licensee MDPI, Basel, Switzerland. This article is an open access article distributed under the terms and conditions of the Creative Commons Attribution (CC BY) license (http://creativecommons.org/licenses/by/4.0/).

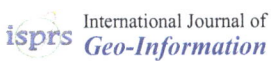

Article

Using GIS for Disease Mapping and Clustering in Jeddah, Saudi Arabia

Abdulkader Murad * and Bandar Fuad Khashoggi

Department of Urban and Regional Planning, Faculty of Architecture and Planning, King Abdulaziz University, Jeddah 21589, Saudi Arabia; bkasoghie@stu.kau.edu.sa
* Correspondence: amurad@kau.edu.sa

Received: 15 April 2020; Accepted: 15 May 2020; Published: 18 May 2020

Abstract: Geographic information systems (GIS) can be used to map the geographical distribution of the prevalence of disease, trends in disease transmission, and to spatially model environmental aspects of disease occurrence. The aim of this study is to discuss a GIS application created to produce mapping and cluster modeling of three diseases in Jeddah, Saudi Arabia: diabetes, asthma, and hypertension. Data about these diseases were obtained from health centers' registered patient records. These data were spatially evaluated using several spatial–statistical analytical models, including kernel and hotspot models. These models were created to explore and display the disparate patterns of the selected diseases and to illustrate areas of high concentration, and may be invaluable in understanding local patterns of diseases and their geographical associations.

Keywords: GIS; urban health; health clusters; kernel density; hotspot analysis

1. Introduction

Disease mapping has been historically considered as one of the most important public health issues, derived from an understanding of the relationship between health and location. Understanding this relationship has attracted the attention of scientists and researchers for decades [1,2]. The actual start of using the disease mapping method was in 1854, when Dr. Snow mapped a cholera outbreak that hit the city of London, England [1,3,4]. However, one of the most useful functions of GIS in public health is its mapping outputs [5]. Disease mapping technology, has been evolving remarkably, is one of the most important GIS technologies [6]. Nowadays, this technology is increasingly being used as an effective tool in disease surveillance by GIS [7].

Studies on the geographical distribution of diseases can be categorized into three main classes: disease mapping, disease clustering and ecological analysis. GIS-based disease mapping depends on identifying a number of aspects, the most important of which are locations of disease occurrence, patterns of disease spread, environmental risk factors that lead to disease spread and socio-economic data, in order to analyze spatial relationships within the affected area [8,9]. GIS-based disease clustering studies aim to evaluate whether a disease is clustered geographically, and, if so, the locations of the clusters. Moreover, these types of studies are based on an examination of potential environmental risk factors that may appear at a specific location and represent a potential hazard, such as the risk of pollution [10]. Ecological analysis studies are relevant within epidemiological research, as they focus on analyzing the geographical distribution of disease in relation to explanatory covariates, usually at an aggregated spatial level [11].

Healthcare studies rely heavily on GIS-based mapping and clustering technologies to draw a general visualization that aims to control a spread of diseases and identify disadvantaged populations at a geographical level [12,13]. Several studies have shown that GIS is a useful tool for the mapping and clustering of disease. For example, Gould and Wallace [14] used GIS to map cases of HIV/AIDS in the United States in the 1980s. They mapped the locations of disease occurrence and patterns of potential spread. They also tried to control the disease using the clustering method. In another example, Braga et al. [15] mapped lung cancer disease in two Italian cities to determine disease rates at the level of urban clusters using Kernel and Bayesian methods. Eisen and Eisen [16] discussed how to use GIS to prevent and control diseases such as malaria and West Nile virus. In addition, Rasam et al. [17] used GIS-based cholera disease mapping to identify patterns of disease spread in the Sabah area of Malaysia. The disease mapping relied on the use of the cohort technique to determine the pattern of disease spread. As a result, it became clear that the disease was spreading from person to person through contaminated water. Photis [18] investigated GISs that can deal with healthcare issues by using disease mapping technology that can improve planning policies and assess possible intervention scenarios. Furthermore, in the United States, a GIS-based measles disease mapping method was used to detect the locations of disease occurrence and determine the spread patterns. As a result, it became clear that disease rates were high in areas with children who had not received vaccination against the disease. The disease mapping method contributed to identifying areas lacking health services and finding the best locations for these services, especially after the maps showed the locations and number of disease cases, as well as the time period related to the disease spread [19].

At the analysis level, to obtain the precise outputs for disease mapping, the quality of the spatial data used in the analysis should be evaluated based on a number of elements, i.e., (1) positional accuracy, (2) thematic accuracy, (3) temporal accuracy, (4) completeness, (5) logical consistency, and (6) usability [20]. Disease incidence data may be represented differently when mapping disease cases or counts within tracts, compared to mapping disease structures based mainly on estimates of complex models [11]. The geographical incidence of disease uses, as its fundamental unit of observation, the locations of cases of the disease being studied. Important data and information about environmental risks and potential exposure can be identified through residential addresses [21]. The simplest possible mapping form is the depiction of disease rates at specific sets of locations. For events, the locations of case events should be mapped. To count within tracts, there should be a representation of the number of events within the tracts of arbitrary areas with the locations and numbers of cases events [22].

A set of analytical and statistical methods may be performed by GIS software for disease mapping and clustering. These methods can support research investigations of the spatial distribution of diseases and its spread by integrating and modeling spatial data in a way that helps pinpoint cases and exposures, characterize spatial trends, identify disease clusters, correlate different sets of spatial data, and test statistical hypotheses [23]. The most important analytical and statistical methods of disease mapping and clustering within the GIS software are: (1) a kernel density estimation method that is used to produce spatial distribution maps of epidemic diseases by modeling disease risk prediction [24], (2) a weighted standard deviational ellipses method that can compare the spatial distributions of the diseases and identify their possible spatial directions, and (3) a hotspot analysis method that is used to calculate the Getis–Ord Gi* statistic to identify where the selected health conditions will be more concentrated [25,26].

Some analytical and statistical methods have been applied to analyses of health services using GIS in Jeddah, Saudi Arabia. For example, Murad [27] discussed the application of GIS for the catchment area of health centers in Jeddah using the straight-line allocation (SLA) technique, which defines health center catchment areas based on a closest proximity approach. Murad [28] measured the accessibility to public health centers in Jeddah by using the Euclidean distance and drive-time methods. A cumulative model was created to determine the level of accessibility in each district of the city depending on estimating distance from a road and from health centers. Furthermore, Murad [9] used GIS mapping for hospital planning in Jeddah and produced several thematic maps related to hospital location and analysis, including classifications of health supply and accessibility to hospitals locations. All previous GIS applications for health in Jeddah only covered the supply side of health services. No study has mapped health disparities based on the location of diseases in Jeddah. To fill this gap, we outline new research focusing on patient distribution and disease disparities in Jeddah. The paper seeks to answer the questions of how GIS can be used to map disease locations in Jeddah city, and how this technology can be applied to analyze spatial clustering and determine whether any unusual clusters of health conditions exist in Jeddah, and to identify which places have unusually high or low prevalences of diseases.

2. Materials and Methods

2.1. Study Area

Jeddah is located on the west shore of Saudi Arabia, 12 m above sea level. It is approximately 949 km from the capital city Riyadh and 79 km from the holy city of Makkah. The area of Jeddah is approximately 1765 km^2. Over time, the city has expanded its services, including transportation, communication, and health projects, as well as public utilities like water, electricity, and other infrastructure projects. Demographically, Jeddah is populated by approximately 4.1 million people (2015), which makes it the second largest city after the capital city, Riyadh. The average household size is 5.2, and 41% of the population are aged 23 and below, while 3% are aged 65 or older. Health services in Jeddah city are provided through three main sectors: the Ministry Of Health network of hospitals and primary healthcare centers that are distributed throughout the city, other governmental institutions, and the private sector. This paper covers only primary healthcare centers that are operated by the Ministry of Health.

2.2. Methods for Disease Mapping and Clustering in Jeddah City

This study seeks to create a GIS application to produce mapping and cluster modeling of three diseases in Jeddah, Saudi Arabia: diabetes, asthma, and hypertension. To build this application, we firstly captured three GIS coverages: the road network, health center locations, and population districts. The nonspatial data linked to those coverages included the health capacity, number of patients (diabetes, asthma, and blood-pressure), number of people living in each district of the city, and the population density of the district. Data concerning the three diseases were collected from the records of registered patients at the health centers in Jeddah. Secondly, several analytical and statistical models were used to map and cluster the three diseases in order to detect their various spatial patterns and identify the trend of their prevalence in Jeddah. An initial spatial analysis of the data was based on the use of classification tools provided by ESRI (Redlands, CA, USA), within the ArcGIS Software. These analytical tools clarified the spatial distribution patterns of diseases at the level of Jeddah districts. Several data classification methods can be used for GIS applications. These include defined interval, manual interval, equal interval, geometrical interval, Quantile, natural breaks, and standard deviation. The created data was classified using the natural breaks method, which is based on the Jenks Natural Breaks algorithm. The natural break method produces Class breaks that identify the best group similar values and maximize the differences between classes. Based on this classification method, the features are divided into classes whose boundaries are set where there are relatively big differences in the data values.

Moreover, we used an analytical function called standard deviational ellipses. This function can compare the spatial distributions of the three diseases and identify their possible spatial directions in a location such as Jeddah. A weighted standard deviational ellipse was selected based on the number of patients in each health center location. This tool provides a way of measuring the trend for a set of points or areas by calculating the standard distance separately in the x-, y- and z-directions. These measurements define the axes of an ellipse (or ellipsoid) encompassing the distribution of features. The ellipse is referred to as the standard deviational ellipse, since the method calculates the standard deviation of the x- and y-coordinates from the mean center to define the axes of the ellipse. This tool is useful for various GIS applications and studies including, for example, the mapping of distributional trends for a set of crimes, groundwater well samples for a particular contaminant, comparing the size, shape, and overlap of ellipses for various racial or ethnic groups, plotting ellipses for a disease outbreak over time, and examining the distribution of elevations for storms of a certain category.

For further investigation, this study used the Kernel model in the ArcGIS Software to determine clusters of health conditions at the level of Jeddah districts. The Kernel estimation can identify the spatial disparities of the three diseases. Finally, we used a statistical model called Getis–Ord Gi* to model the spatial diffusion of the selected diseases. The application of this model was based on the datasets available for each disease within each health center in Jeddah. The hotspot analysis tool in ArcGIS was used to calculate the Getis–Ord Gi* statistic for each feature in a dataset. The resulting z-scores and p-values defined where features with either high or low values clustered spatially. For statistically significant positive z-scores, the larger the z-score, the more intense the clustering of the high values (hot spots). For statistically significant negative z-scores, the lower the z-score, the more intense the clustering of the low values (cold spots). The hotspot analysis results are useful for determining where the selected health conditions will be more concentrated, and, eventually, which and where health services should be available.

3. Results

3.1. Spatial Distribution of Diseases

GIS can assist with updating and mapping health event prevalence, and is used as a supporting tool for surveillance and as a decision-making tool by which to control health conditions and disease. GIS can be used to map the geographical distribution of the prevalence of a disease, the trends of disease transmission, and spatially model the environmental aspects of disease occurrence. The created geo-database of health in Jeddah incorporates three types of health conditions: diabetes, asthma, and blood-pressure. For the first type of spatial analysis of these data, ArcGIS (produced by ESRI) data classification tools were used. These tools can help researchers understand the spatial distribution and classification of health conditions. Looking at the output of health event classification in Figures 1–3, asthma patients are highly concentrated in the north east of the city. These parts of the city are considered highly urban developed locations, producing large number of asthma patients, as confirmed in studies that have suggested that there is more asthma in urban than in rural areas in many parts of the world. Early studies from Africa (South Africa, Ethiopia, Kenya, and Ghana) reported that populations living in rural areas (i.e., those not exposed to the effects of an urban or western lifestyle) experienced a very low burden of allergic disease, with a traditional, rural way of living providing a possible protective cover. Similar studies from Asia (China, Japan, Korea, India, and Saudi Arabia) confirmed the urban–rural gradient due to exposure to different allergens, air pollution, affluence, and diet in the development of asthma and allergy [29]. Meanwhile, hypertension and diabetes patients are located more in the central and northern city districts. These city districts are considered as high-density locations, confirming that patterns of diabetes and hypertension patients follow the population density pattern in Jeddah. These are the results of the initial analysis for defining the spatial distribution of health conditions.

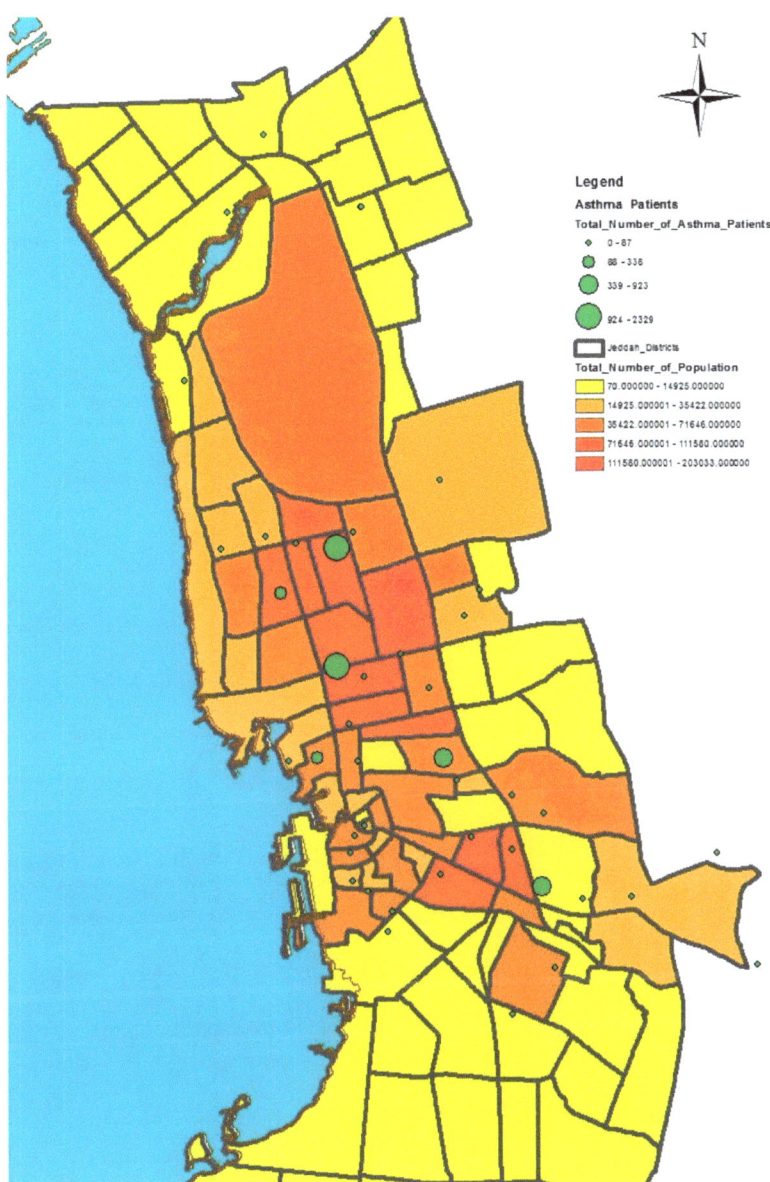

Figure 1. Spatial distribution of asthma patients.

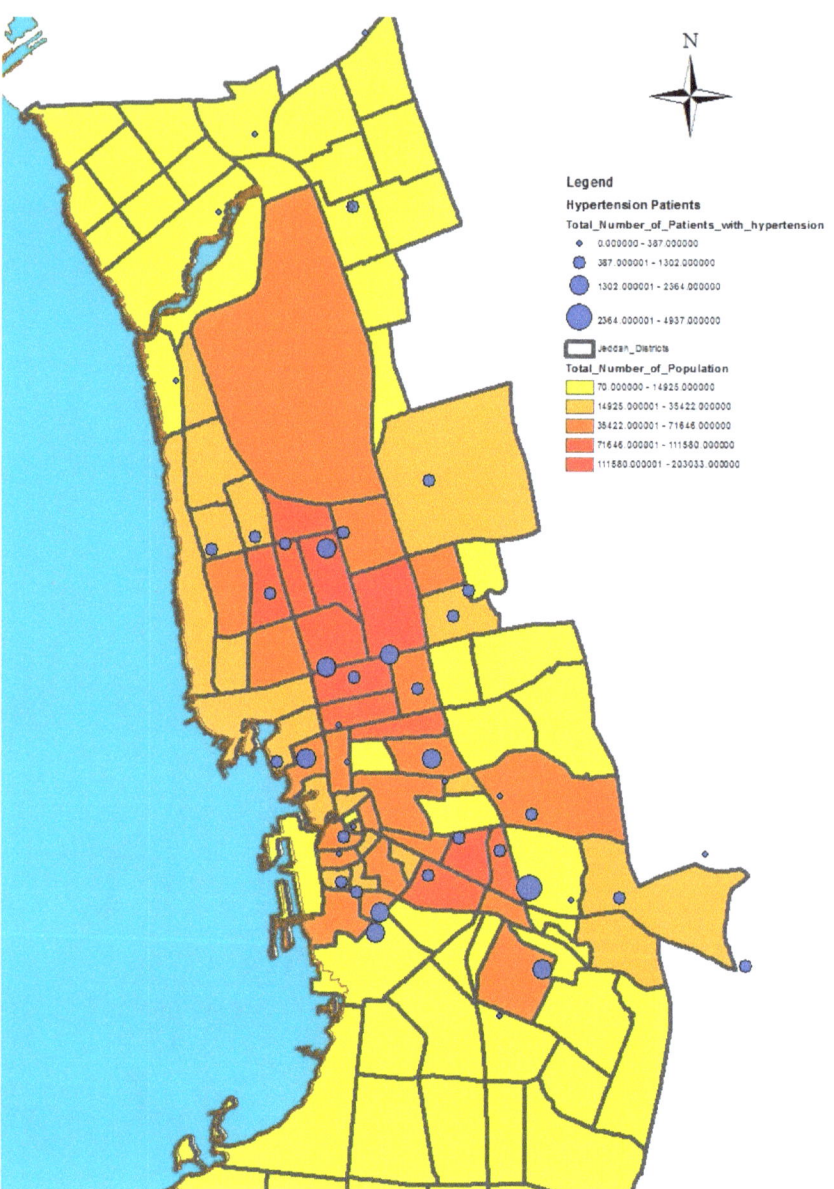

Figure 2. Spatial distribution of hypertension patients.

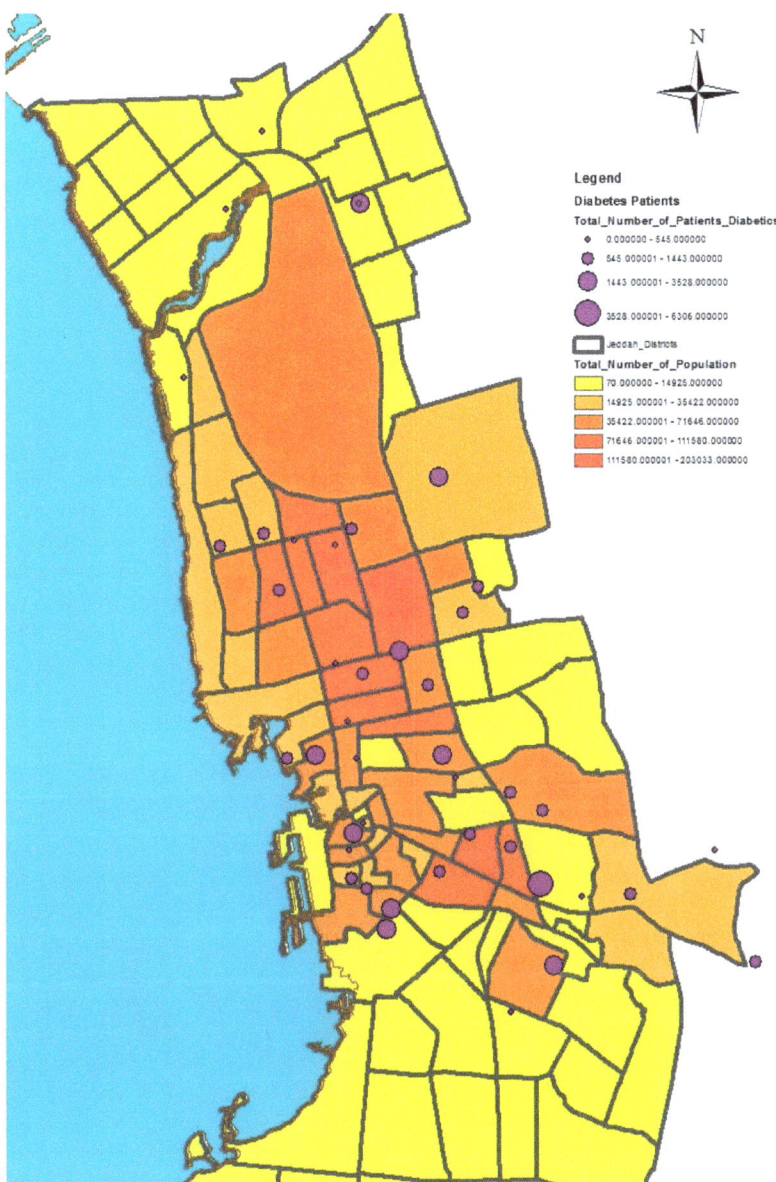

Figure 3. Spatial distribution of diabetes patients.

A further analysis was applied to these data using a spatial statistic function called the standard deviational ellipses, which measures the orientation and direction of features, providing a tool for abstracting spatial trends. This type of analysis is useful for comparing the distributions of categories of health conditions. Although GIS analysis can provide a sense of orientation by drawing features on a map, calculating the standard deviational ellipse clarifies the trend. This tool can be used to calculate the standard deviational ellipse using either the locations of the features or the locations influenced by an attribute value associated with the features. The latter is termed a "weighted standard deviational ellipse" [25]. Much research has emphasized the importance of using the function of standard deviational ellipses in analyzing the spatial distribution of health conditions categories. For example, Eryando et al. [30] used the standard deviational ellipse function, statistical analysis, overlap analysis, and environment variables to map the spatial distribution of malaria in the district of Sukabumi, Indonesia, where a malaria outbreak occurred from 2004 to 2012. The study relied on data collection through Global Positioning System (GPS) plotting and field surveys based on data of positive malaria cases (2011–2012) derived from healthcare centers in the district of Sukabumi. The axis of standard deviation ellipses showed a skewed distribution towards the northwest southeast. Environmental factors such as an anomaly of rainfall and temperatures led to the outbreak of malaria, particularly in warm and high areas. The development and metabolism of vectors were supported by the physical environment in the Sukabumi District. Mapping the spatial distribution of malaria provides an initial visualization that can help in formulating possible intervention priorities. As a result, the use of the standard deviational ellipse function contributed to understanding the geographical factors that led to the occurrence of malaria, and determining prevalence trends based on specific geographical patterns. In another example, Dong et al. [31] used the standard deviational ellipse function to investigate the directional trend and determine the presence of spatial-temporal clustering of influenza A(H7N9) in China from March 2013 to December 2014. The study relied on identifying three phases characterized by a high epidemic infection. The standard deviational ellipse was used at each phase to investigate the directional trend of epidemic spread using statistical scans to identify patterns of spatial-temporal clusters of the epidemic spread. It appeared that the directional trend of the epidemic was from the eastern coast to the southeast, with a future directional trend of transmitting the epidemic to the central and western areas of China. As a result, defining the spatial-temporal patterns of the epidemic A(H7N9) provided general insights into understanding the dynamics of the epidemic's spread in China.

In this study, we selected a weighted standard deviational ellipse based on the number of patients with diabetes, asthma, and blood pressure at each health center in Jeddah city. This tool creates a new feature class containing an elliptical polygon centered on the mean center for all features. The attribute values for these output ellipse polygons include two standard distances (long and short axes), the orientation of the ellipse, and the case field. The orientation represents the rotation of the long axis measured clockwise from noon.

Figures 4–6 show the output of the standard deviational ellipses for the three health conditions in Jeddah. The directional orientation for asthma patients is less than that for hypertension and diabetes patients. In other words, asthma patients are more concentrated in the northeast of the city, while hypertension and diabetes patients are spread most widely over the north, south, and southeast.

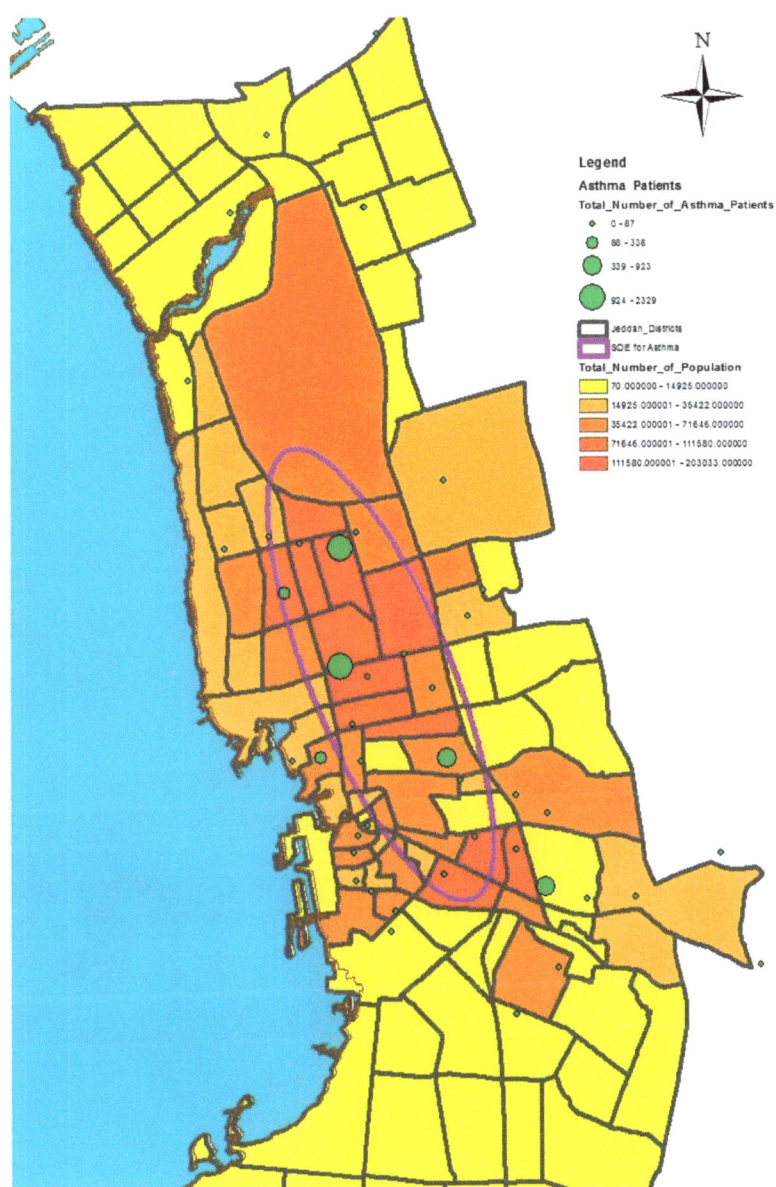

Figure 4. Standard deviational ellipses for asthma patients.

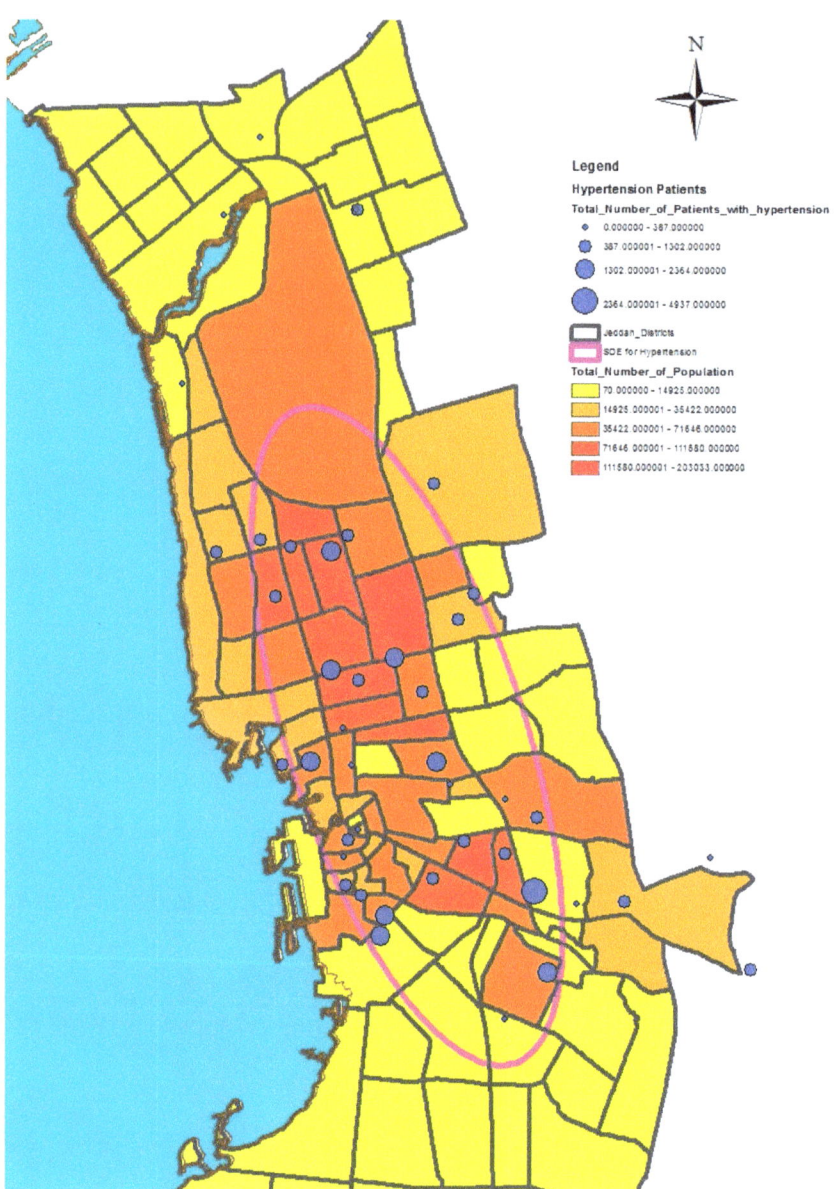

Figure 5. Standard deviational ellipses for hypertension patients.

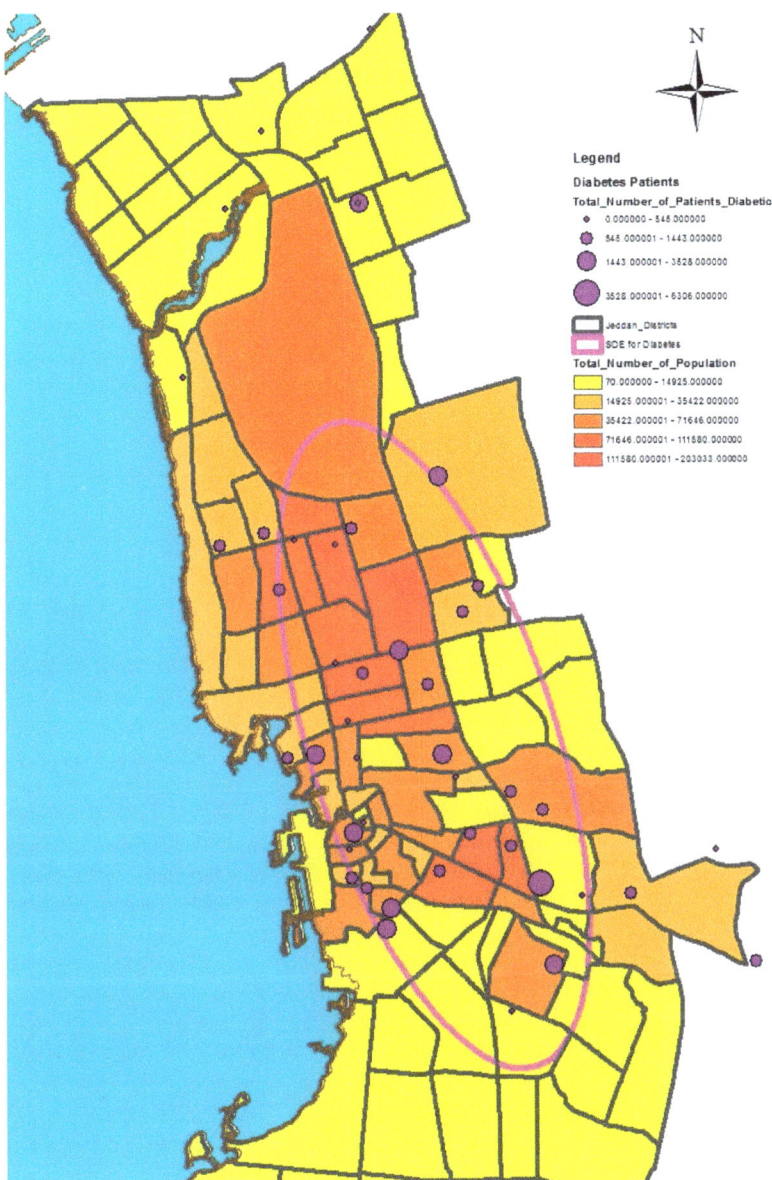

Figure 6. Standard deviational ellipses for diabetes patients.

3.2. Identifying the Spatial Disparities of Diseases

This paper has used kernel density estimation in the ArcGIS software (produced by ESRI) to identify clusters based on the spatial disparities of the aforementioned health conditions in Jeddah. This tool is also useful in identifying high-risk areas and visualizing transmission directions of diseases; thus, it contributes to formulating possible intervention priorities related to the provision of health service resources. The kernel density estimation was used to depict the density of service providers (number per unit area) as a continuous spatial variable, with peaks representing areas of with good access and valleys indicating areas with poor access. The kernel density estimation calculates the magnitude per unit area from the point or polyline features using a kernel function to fit a smoothly tapered surface to each point or polyline. Possible uses of Kernel density include analyzing the density of houses or crimes for community planning, or exploring how roads or utility lines influence wildlife habitat. The population field could be used to weight some features more heavily than others, or to allow one point to represent several observations. For the presented application, point features (health centers location) were used as the input data of this model. The population field is the number of patients with asthma, diabetes, or hypertension. The search radius value was selected as 10,000 square kilometers.

The algorithm used to determine the default search radius of the kernel model, also known as the bandwidth, is as follows:

(1) Calculate the mean center of the input points. If a population field other than 0 was selected, this and all following calculations will be weighted by the values in that field.
(2) Calculate the distance from the (weighted) mean center for all points.
(3) Calculate the (weighted) median of these distances (D_m).
(4) Calculate the (weighted) standard distance (SD).
(5) Apply the following formula to calculate the bandwidth:

$$Search\ Radius = 0.9 \times \min\left(SD, \sqrt{1\frac{1}{\ln(2)}} \times D_m\right) \times n^{-0.2}$$

where n is the number of points if no population field is used or if a population field is supplied, and n is the sum of the population field values.

Many studies have emphasized the importance of using kernel density estimation to identify spatial disparities and risk areas of diseases. For example, Z. A. Latif [32] used Kernel density estimation to map a dengue outbreak in order to produce a risk map in Selangor, Malaysia. The aim of this method was to locate hotspots. The results showed that eight areas could be classified as high-risk. In addition, Chaikaew, Tripathi, and Souris [33] used GIS-based spatial analyses to identify patterns of diarrhea disease prevalence in Chiang Mai province, Northern Thailand. The analysis relied on using a set of analytical and statistical methods such as quadrant analysis (QA), nearest neighbor analysis (NNA), and spatial autocorrelation analysis (SAA) to visualize the spatial patterns of the disease in the province. Moreover, kernel density estimation was used to determine hotspots of diarrhea based on the collection of patient data at the village level and population censuses from 2001 to 2006. Hotspot maps based on kernel density estimation revealed cluster patterns and the spatial direction of the prevalence of the disease. As a result, the method can contribute to developing a system to monitor and prevent disease outbreak.

Figures 6–9 show the results of the kernel density services for the selected types of patients in Jeddah. The density for asthma patients shows a high concentration in the northeast city districts, while hypertension and diabetes patients were concentrated in the central and northern city districts. These results therefore identify the spatial clusters of the selected health conditions in Jeddah.

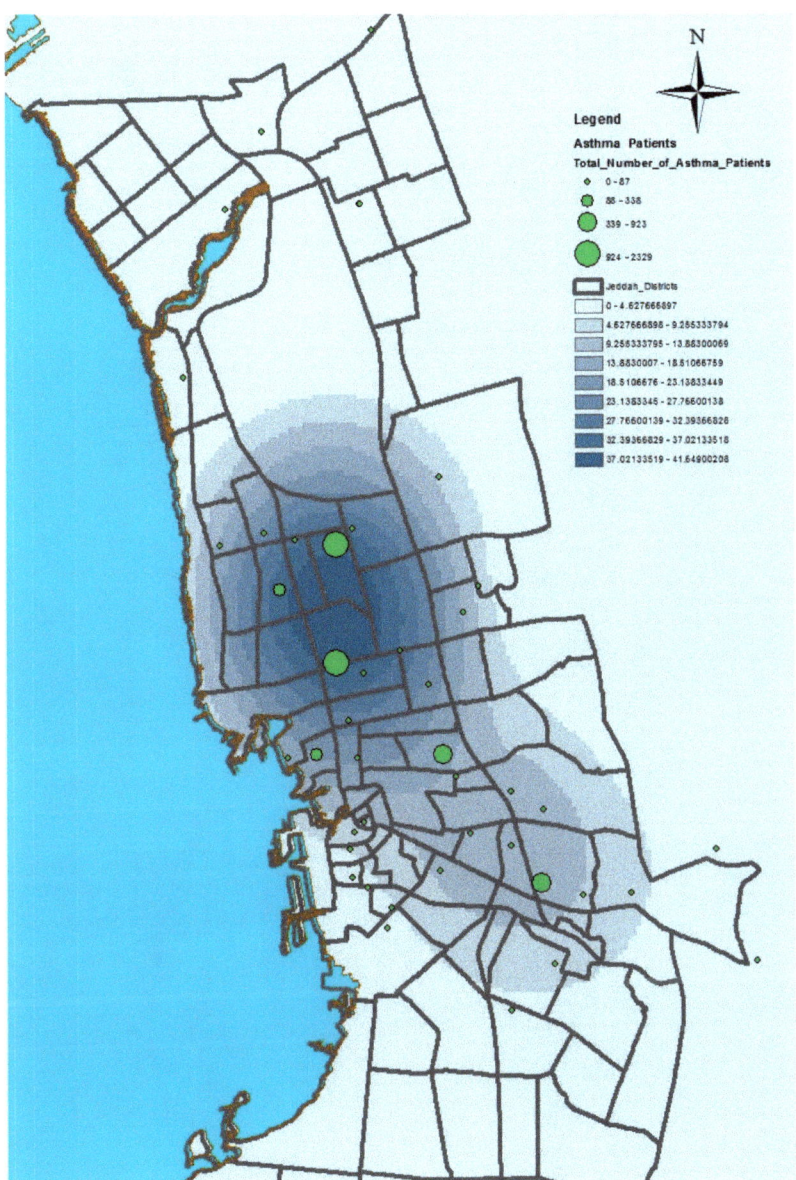

Figure 7. Kernel density for asthma patients.

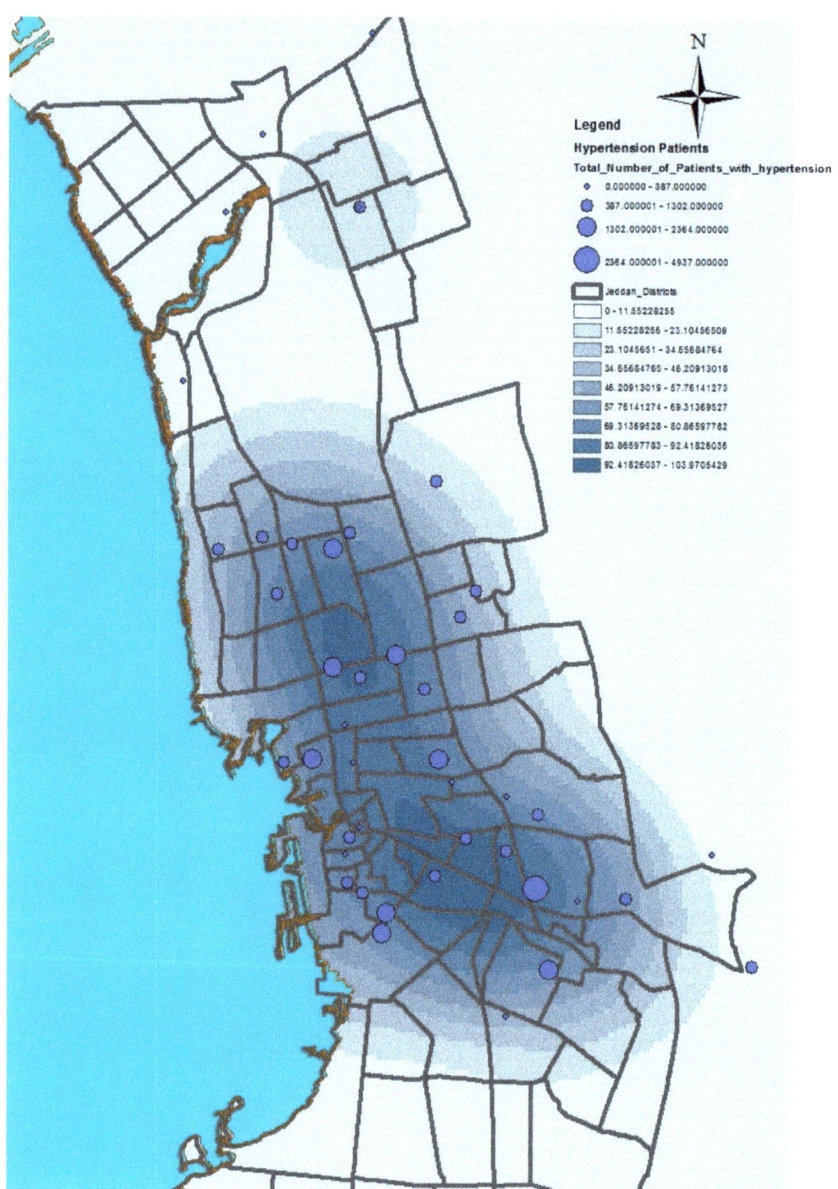

Figure 8. Kernel density for hypertension patients.

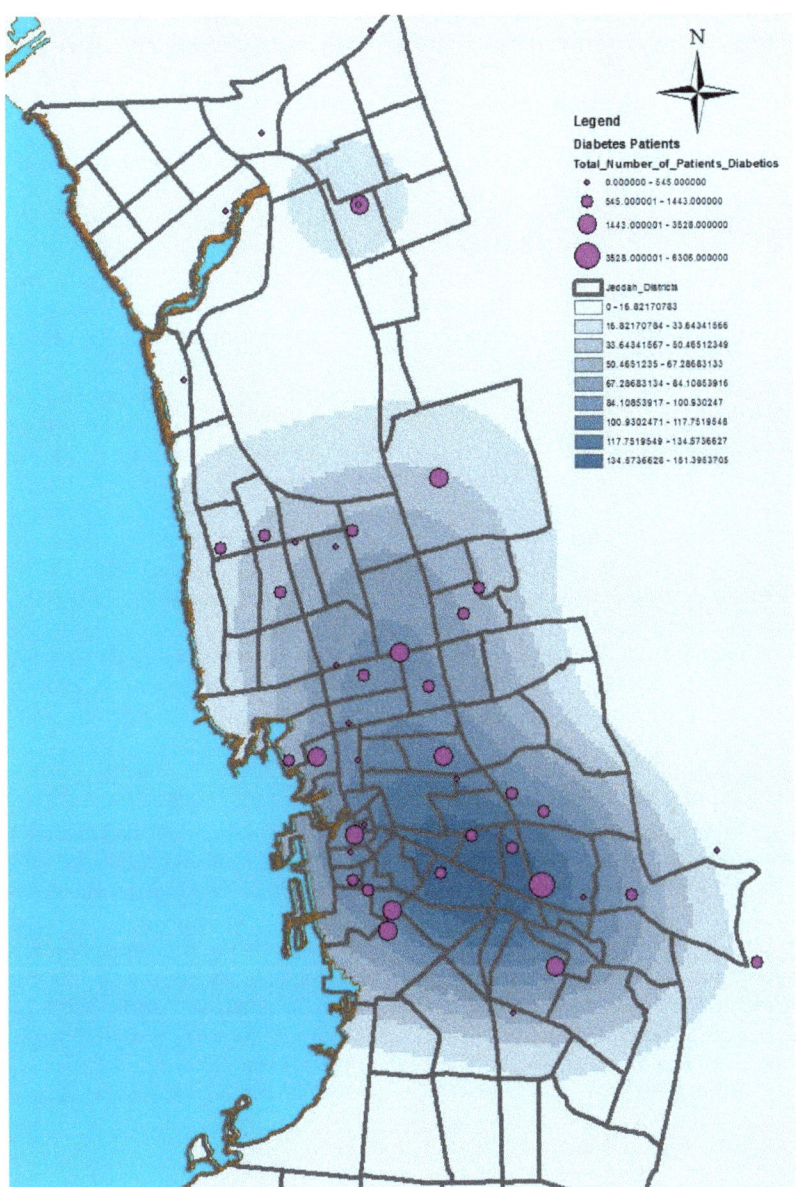

Figure 9. Kernel density for diabetes patients.

3.3. Modeling the Spatial Diffusion of Diseases

GIS software can be used by health professionals to predict the spatial location and diffusion of health conditions. The geographical patterns of interactions between infected and susceptible individuals are crucial for understanding how and where infectious diseases spread. Spatial diffusion describes the movement of phenomena, people, goods, ideas, innovations, and diseases through space and time. Sometimes, diseases follow a pattern of contagious diffusion, spreading gradually outward from a point of origin to nearby locations. In hierarchical diffusion, diseases spread via the urban hierarchy, starting in large cities and spreading over time to medium-sized cities, before arriving in smaller cities and towns. Network diffusion refers to the spread of disease through transportation or networks. As with the other types of diffusion, network diffusion reflects the geographical and social structuring of human interactions. Today, the emerging trend in epidemic modeling is to focus on individuals rather than larger populations or nodes through the use of agent-based modeling. Agent-based models simulate the behavior and interactions of individuals to generate insights about populations and communities.

One of the analytical tools used to identify the spatial diffusion of diseases is the Getis-Ord Gi* statistic based on hotspot analyses. For example, Saxena et al. [34] used the methods of Getis-Ord Gi* and Standard Deviational Ellipse to define a spatial distribution pattern, identify hotspots, and map a directional distribution trend of Plasmodium vivax (Pv) and Plasmodium falciparum (Pf) occurrences in Ranchi, India. The study relied on malaria epidemiological data from 2007–2009, derived from 328 subcenters of the 14 primary health centers (PHCs) in the district. The results showed that there was randomness in the pattern of spatial distribution (Pv); in contrast, the spatial distribution of occurrence (Pf) was significantly clustered. During the period of 2007–2009, there was a downward trend in the number of subcenters associated with the (Pv) hotspot category; in contrast, there was an upward trend in the high (Pf) risk subcenters. Moreover, from 2008 onwards, a shifting trend in (Pf) diffusion was noted from the north-west to western direction. In another example, Carnes and Ogneva-Himmelberger [35] used a set of analytical and statistical tools, including the Getis-Ord-Gi* statistic (hot spot analysis), to analyze the distributional trends of West Nile Virus in the United States from 2000 to 2008. The maps revealed that the directional trend of the virus cases was from east to west. Moreover, the analysis of hotspots revealed that metro areas in large cities and rural areas had high rates of virus cases. As a result, the outputs of this study assisted in formulating strategies to overcome West Nile Virus diffusion. The application of hotspot analysis can be found in crime analysis, epidemiology, voting pattern analysis, economic geography, retail analysis, traffic incident analysis, and demographics.

In this study, a GIS was used to model the prevalence of the three selected diseases based on data that were available from health centers in Jeddah. The Getis–Ord Gi* statistic model was applied to the collected data to model the spatial diffusion of the health conditions in Jeddah. The hotspot analysis tool in ArcGIS was used to calculate the Getis–Ord Gi* statistic for each feature in each dataset. The results of a hotspot analysis are shown in Figures 10–12. The asthma analysis showed hotspot locations in the central city districts and coldspot locations in the north and south. This means that asthma patients are more concentrated in the central city districts. The modeling of hypertension patients shows that coldspot locations are only located in the north of the city, whereas the remaining city districts have a high number of hotspots. In other words, hypertension patients are spread over several city districts, except for the northern parts of the city, where few suffer from hypertension. The results of the diabetes modeling showed that hotspot locations are grouped in the central and southern city districts, and coldspots are grouped in the northern city districts. The hotspot analysis results are useful for determining where the selected health conditions are more concentrated, and, eventually, which and where health services should be made available.

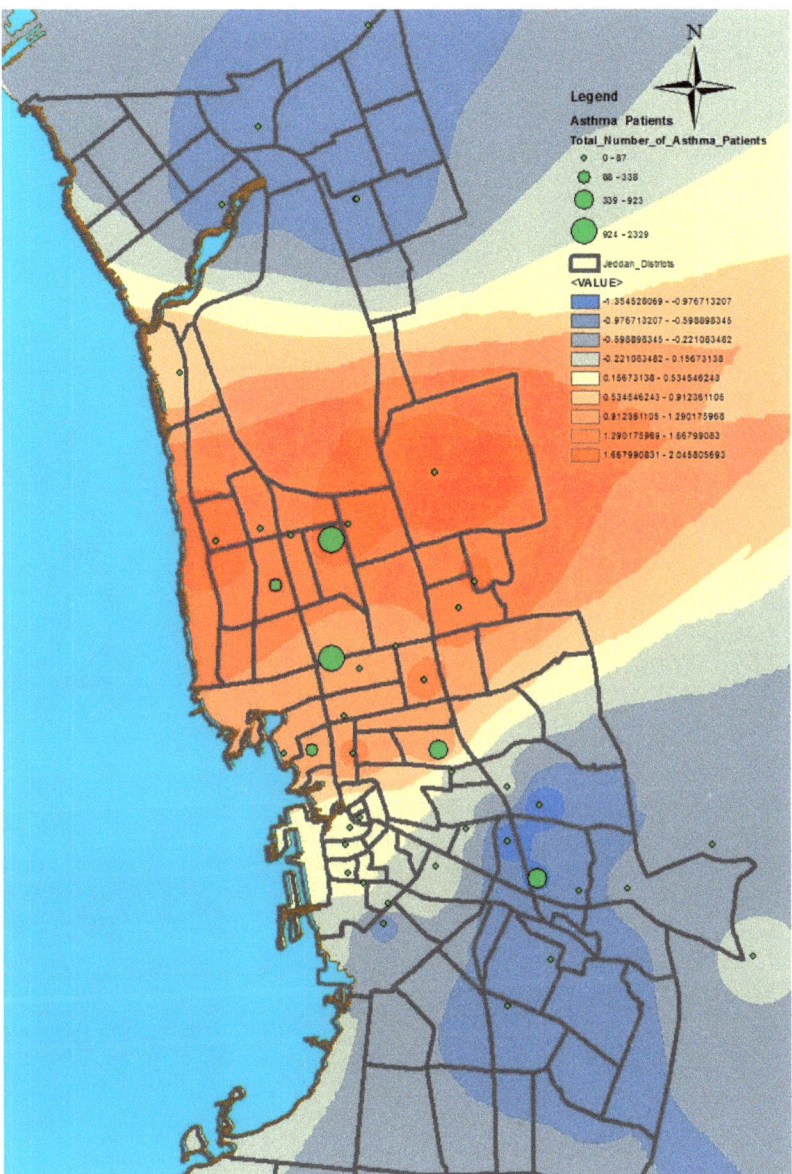

Figure 10. Hotspot analysis for asthma patients.

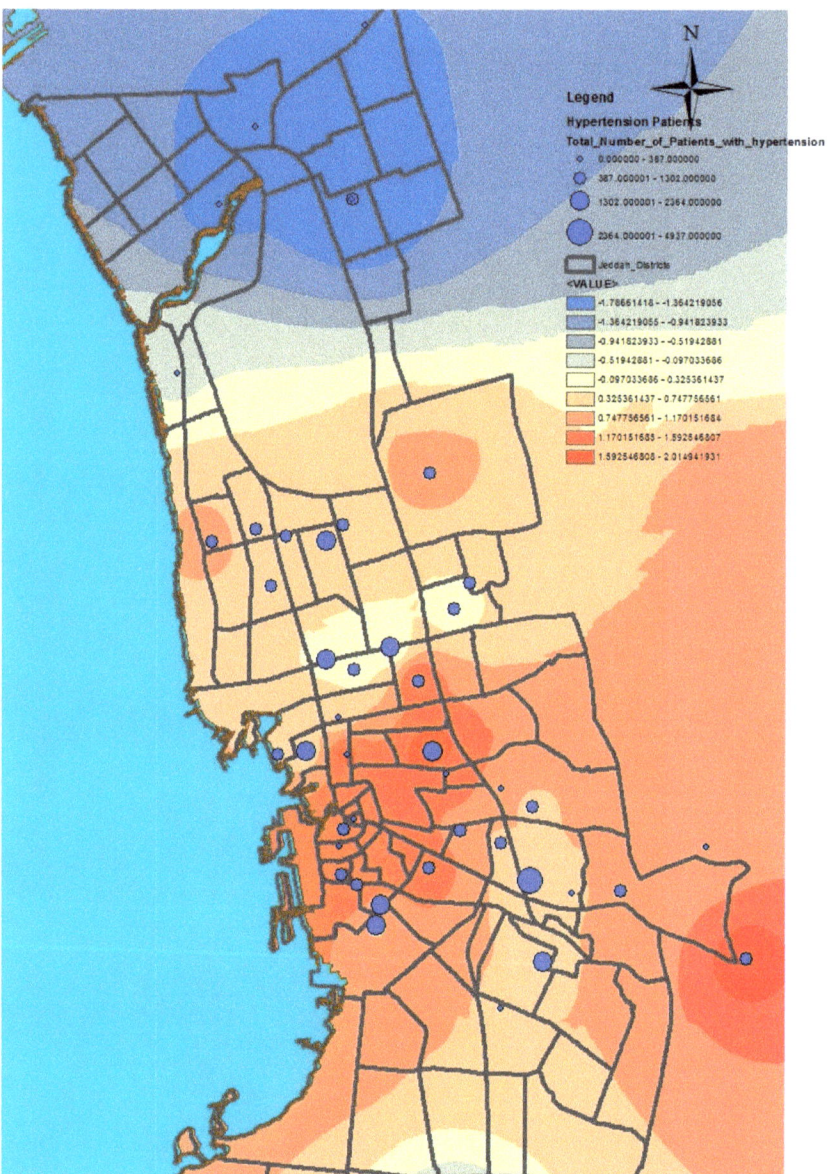

Figure 11. Hotspot analysis for hypertension patients.

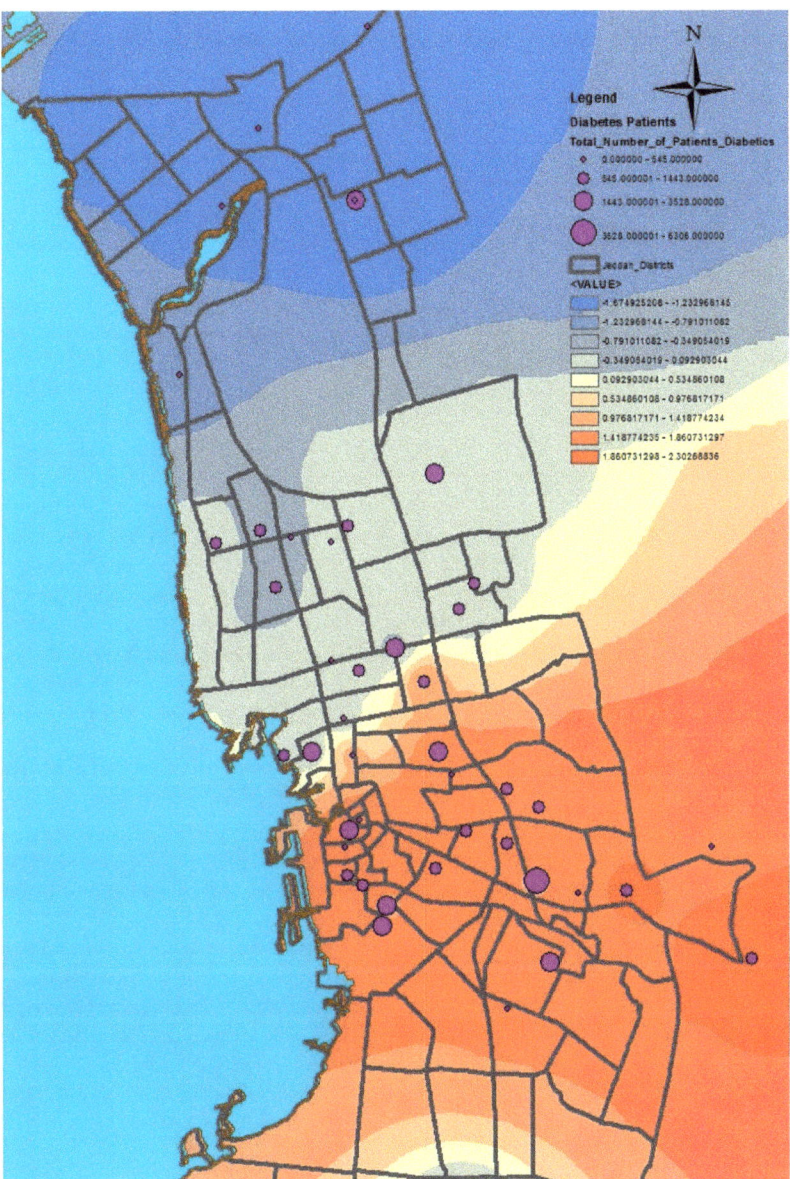

Figure 12. Hotspot analysis for diabetes patients.

4. Discussion

The use of GIS in health care studies has increased, and its applications have become more sophisticated. For example, GIS can be used for exposure modeling as a tool to study cancer incidence in a population exposed to airborne dioxins. An assessment of the relationship between the environment and health needs to develop statistical methods and epidemiological techniques capable of broad analyses and visualization. Nevertheless, recent GIS technologies have contributed to disease control and related decision-making through the effective updating, mapping, and monitoring of disease.

In addition, GIS can map trends of disease spread and provide a visualization of how the diseases occur by modeling the environmental risk factors causing the disease.

The traditional method of disease control, based on empirical observations, is laborious, expensive, and time-consuming. However, by applying GIS techniques to map disease presence, density, and spatial diffusion, the root causes of diseases and sources of infection can be determined. For example, Srinath et al. [36] analyzed and mapped the spread of disease in the US state of Texas using GIS, and also investigated the environmental factors that contribute to promoting the spread of diseases. In their study, they emphasized that there is a strong relationship between disease spread and environmental factors which requires the development of new spatial methods to enhance epidemiological research. According to Geanuracos [37], public health researchers are increasingly shifting their attention from models of disease etiology, which focus exclusively on individual risk factors, to models that also consider the complex and powerful effects of the socio-physical environment. It has been observed that many diseases are spread excessively within endemic areas or cores, for example, sexually transmitted infections (STIs) and (HIV/AIDS). These areas are often characterized by high levels of racial/ethnic segregation, low socioeconomic status, and high rates of homicide and other criminal activities. One of the most important foundations for epidemiology is the investigation of the possible clustering of diseases in order to consider whether such clusters need further investigation, whether they are likely to be chance occurrences, or whether they reflect a rational interpretation of the spatial distribution of the at risk population. Spatial clustering methods are exploratory tools that help researchers and policymakers to understand complex geographic patterns. Knowing whether clusters exist and where they are located provides an important foundation for health research and policy formulation. Responding to community concerns, however, only addresses a fraction of potential clusters and is likely to miss clusters in communities that lack political and economic strength. Spatial clustering analysis is an effective tool in the surveillance of public health, especially when spatial clustering methods are integrated; this will inevitably contribute to discovering the factors and causes of health issues through conducting more exploratory and investigative analyses. We used a GIS to define and model the spatial clusters of three diseases in Jeddah (diabetes, hypertension, and asthma). This was achieved using the kernel model and the Getis–Ord Gi* statistic model.

5. Conclusions

GIS technology has been applied in the public health sector to map various diseases. The development of GIS technology has contributed to improving healthcare through disease mapping and clustering, the detection of disease spread trends, the identification of the spatial and temporal distribution of infection vectors, as well as the control and surveillance of infectious diseases. In this study, we selected three diseases in Jeddah, Saudi Arabia for analysis: diabetes, hypertension, and asthma. Data about these diseases were collected from health center records. GIS-based clustering models, including kernel and Getis-Ord Gi* statistic models, were used to define the locations of clusters of the selected diseases. The results show different clusters for each disease, and will be useful for health planners in Jeddah to improve the supply health services in the resulting cluster locations.

Author Contributions: Conceptualization, Abdulkader Murad and Bandar Fuad Khashoggi; Methodology, Abdulkader Murad; Software, Abdulkader Murad; Formal Analysis, Abdulkader Murad; Data Curation, Abdulkader Murad; Writing-Original Draft Preparation, Abdulkader Murad and Bandar Fuad Khashoggi; Writing-Review & Editing, Abdulkader Murad and Bandar Fuad Khashoggi; Visualization, Abdulkader Murad; Supervision, Abdulkader Murad. All authors have read and agreed to the published version of the manuscript.

Funding: This research received no external funding.

Conflicts of Interest: The authors declare no conflict of interest.

References

1. Geraghty, E. Why Health is so Spatial. 2016. Available online: https://www.youtube.com/watch?v=3p7OFICg9Ak (accessed on 30 January 2020).
2. Krieger, N. Place, space, and health: GIS and epidemiology. *Epidemiology* **2003**, *14*, 384. [CrossRef] [PubMed]
3. GISGeography. The Remarkable History of GIS. 2015. Available online: https://gisgeography.com/history-of-gis/ (accessed on 3 February 2020).
4. ESRI. GIS for Public Health Today and Tomorrow. 2020. Available online: https://www.esri.com/news/arcuser/0499/umbrella.html (accessed on 3 February 2020).
5. Wilkinson, P.; Grundy, C.; Landon, M.; Stevenson, S. GIS in public health. In *GIS and Health*; Gatrell, A., Loytonen, M., Eds.; Tylor and Francis: Abingdon, UK, 1998; pp. 179–189.
6. Kirby, R.; Delmelle, E.; Eberth, J. Advances in spatial epidemiology and geographic information systems. *Ann. Epidemiol.* **2016**, *27*, 1–9. [CrossRef] [PubMed]
7. Fletcher-Lartey, S.M.; Caprarelli, G. Application of GIS technology in public health: Successes and challenges. *Parasitology* **2016**, *143*, 1–15. [CrossRef] [PubMed]
8. Nicol, J. Geographic information system within the national healths, the scope for implementations. *Plan. Outlook* **1991**, *34*, 37–42. [CrossRef]
9. Murad, A. Using GIS for planning public general hospitals at Jeddah city. *Environ. Des. Sci.* **2005**, *3*, 3–22. [CrossRef]
10. Lawson, A.; Browne, W.; Vidal-Rodeiro, C. *Disease Mapping with Winbugs and Mlwin*; John Wiley & Sons: Chichester, UK, 2003.
11. Maheswaran, R.; Craglia, M. *GIS in Public Health Practice*; CRC Press: New York, NY, USA, 2004; pp. 32–34.
12. Koch, T. *Cartographies of Disease: Maps, Mapping, and Medicine*; ESRI Press: Redlands, CA, USA, 2005.
13. American Hospital Association. Mapping Medicare Disparities. 2018. Available online: https://www.aha.org/system/files/2018-12/mapping-medicare-disparities-issue-brief.pdf (accessed on 7 April 2020).
14. Gould, P.; Wallace, R. Spatial structures and scientific paradoxes in the AIDS pandemic. *Geogr. Ann.* **1994**, *76*, 105–116. [CrossRef]
15. Braga, M.; Cislaghi, C.; Luppi, G.; Tasco, C. A Multipurpose, interactive mortality atlas of Italy. In *GIS and Health*; Gatrell, A.C., Löytönen, M., Eds.; Taylor and Francis: London, UK, 1998; pp. 125–138.
16. Eisen, L.; Eisen, R. Using geographic information systems and decision support systems for the prediction, prevention, and control of vector-borne diseases. *Annu. Rev. Entomol.* **2011**, *56*, 41–61. [CrossRef]
17. Rasam, A.; Ghazali, R.; Noor, A.; Mohd, W.; Hamid, J.; Bazlan, M.; Ahmad, N. Spatial epidemiological techniques in cholera mapping and analysis towards a local scale predictive modelling. *IOP Conf. Ser. Earth Environ. Sci.* **2014**. [CrossRef]
18. Photis, Y.N. Disease and health care geographies: Mapping trends and patterns in a GIS. *Health Sci. J.* **2016**, *10*, 1–8.
19. Sones, M. Reveal: Mapping and Tracking the Spread of Deadly Diseases. 2019. Available online: https://www.esri.com/about/newsroom/blog/reveal-mapping-and-tracking-the-spread-of-deadly-diseases/ (accessed on 18 December 2019).
20. Santos, A.S.; Medeiros, N.G.; dos Santos, G.R.; Filho, J.L. Use of geostatistics on absolute positional accuracy assesment of geospatial data. *Bull. Geod. Sci.* **2017**, *23*, 405–413. [CrossRef]
21. Lawson, A.; Kleinman, K. *Spatial and Syndromic Surveillance for Public Health*; John Wiley & Sons: New York, NY, USA, 2005; p. 57.
22. Lawson, A.; Cressie, N. Spatial statistical methods for environmental epidemiology. *Handb. Stat.* **2000**, *18*, 357–396.
23. Carroll, L.N.; Au, A.P.; Detwiler, L.T.; Fu, T.; Painter, I.S.; Abernethy, N.F. Visualization and analytics tools for infectious disease epidemiology: A systematic review. *J. Biomed. Inform.* **2014**, *51*, 287–298. [CrossRef]
24. Gatrell, A.; Senior, M. Health and health care application. In *Geographical Information System Principles and Application*; Longley, P., Goodchild, M., Maguire, D., Rhind, D., Eds.; John Wiley & Sons: Chichester, UK, 1999; pp. 925–938.
25. Esri. How Directional Distribution Standard Deviational Ellipse Works. 2020. Available online: https://pro.arcgis.com/en/pro-app/tool-reference/spatial-statistics/h-how-directional-distribution-standard-deviationa.htm (accessed on 2 May 2020).

26. Esri. How Hot Spot Analysis (Getis-Ord Gi*) Works. 2020. Available online: https://pro.arcgis.com/en/pro-app/tool-reference/spatial-statistics/h-how-hot-spot-analysis-getis-ord-gi-spatial-stati.htm (accessed on 2 May 2020).
27. Murad, A. Defining health catchment areas in Jeddah city, Saudi Arabia: An example demonstrating the utility of geographical information systems. *Geospat. Health* **2008**, *2*, 151–160. [CrossRef]
28. Murad, A. Using geographical information systems for defining the accessibility to health care facilities in Jeddah City, Saudi. *Geospat. Health* **2014**, *8*, 661–669. [CrossRef]
29. Hussain, S.; Farhan, S.; Alnasser, S. Time trends and regional variation in prevalence of asthma and associated factors in Saudi Arabia: A systematic review and meta-analysis. *Biomed Res. Int.* **2018**, *2018*, 9. [CrossRef]
30. Eryando, T.; Susanna, D.; Pratiwi, D.; Nugraha, F. Standard deviational ellipse (SDE) models for malaria surveillance, case study: Sukabumi district-Indonesia, in 2012. *Malar. J.* **2012**, *11*, P130. [CrossRef]
31. Dong, W.; Yang, K.; Xu, Q.; Liu, L.; Chen, J. Spatio-temporal pattern analysis for evaluation of the spread of human infections with avian influenza A(H7N9) virus in China, 2013–2014. *BMC Infect. Dis.* **2017**, *17*, 704. [CrossRef]
32. Latif, Z.A.; Mohamad, M.H. Mapping of dengue outbreak distribution using spatial statistics and geographical information system. In Proceedings of the 2nd International Conference on Information Science and Security (ICISS), Seoul, Korea, 14–16 December 2015; pp. 1–6.
33. Chaikaew, N.; Tripathi, N.; Souris, M. Exploring spatial patterns and hotspots of diarrhea in Chiang Mai, Thailand. *Int. J. Health Geogr.* **2009**, *8*, 36. [CrossRef]
34. Saxena, R.; Nagpal, B.; Das, M.; Srivastava, A.; Gupta, S.; Kumar, A.; Jeyaseelan, A.; Baraik, V. A spatial statistical approach to analyze malaria situation at micro level for priority control in Ranchi district, Jharkhand. *Indian J. Med Res.* **2012**, *136*, 776–782.
35. Carnes, A.; Ogneva-Himmelberger, Y. Temporal variations in the distribution of west Nile virus within the United States, 2000–2008. *Appl. Spat. Anal. Policy* **2011**, *5*, 211–229. [CrossRef]
36. Srinath, I.; Szonyi, B.; Esteve-Gassent, M.; Lupiani, B.; Gautam, R. Geographical information systems: A tool to map and analyze disease spread. *Online J. Public Health Inform.* **2013**, *5*. [CrossRef]
37. Geanuracos, C. Use of geographic information systems for planning HIV prevention interventions for high-risk youths. *Am. J. Public Health* **2011**, *97*, 1974–1981. [CrossRef]

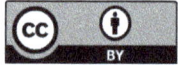

© 2020 by the authors. Licensee MDPI, Basel, Switzerland. This article is an open access article distributed under the terms and conditions of the Creative Commons Attribution (CC BY) license (http://creativecommons.org/licenses/by/4.0/).

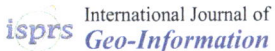

Review

Issues of Healthcare Planning and GIS: A Review

Bandar Fuad Khashoggi and Abdulkader Murad *

Department of Urban and Regional Planning, Faculty of Architecture and Planning, King Abdulaziz University, Jeddah 80210, Saudi Arabia; bkasoghie@stu.kau.edu.sa
* Correspondence: amurad@kau.edu.sa; Tel.: +966-541009024

Received: 3 March 2020; Accepted: 25 May 2020; Published: 27 May 2020

Abstract: *Introduction:* For the past 2400 years, the spatial relationship between health and location has been a concern for researchers. Studies have been conducted for decades to understand such a relationship, which has led to the identification of a number of healthcare planning issues. Geographic Information Systems (GIS) technology has contributed to addressing such issues by applying analytical approaches at the level of epidemiological surveillance and evaluating the spatial inequality of access to healthcare. Consequently, the importance of reviewing healthcare planning issues and recognition of the role of GIS are integral to relevant studies. Such research will contribute to increasing the understanding of how to apply analytical approaches for dealing with healthcare planning issues using GIS. *Methods:* This paper aims to provide an examination of healthcare planning issues and focuses on reviewing the potential of GIS in dealing with such issues by applying analytical approaches. The method of a typical literature review was used through collecting data from various studies selected based on temporal and descriptive considerations. *Results:* Researchers have focused on developing and applying analytical approaches using GIS to support two important aspects of healthcare planning: first, epidemic surveillance and modeling, despite a lack of health information and its management, and, second, evaluating the spatial inequality of access to healthcare in order to determine the optimum distribution of health resources. *Conclusion:* GIS is an effective tool to support spatial decision-making in public health through applying the evolving analytical approaches to dealing with healthcare planning issues. This requires a literature review before preparing relevant studies, particularly because of the continuous development of GIS technologies.

Keywords: GIS; healthcare planning; health geomatics; public health

1. Introduction

The relationship between health and place has long been acknowledged [1] and a concern of scientists and researchers. The Hippocratic treatise was written 2400 years ago, to describe "Airs, Waters, and Places" [2]. Intensive research continued to examine the relationship between health and place by producing maps of disease over 200 years ago [3], which led to the founding of epidemiology in the early 19th century by geographers [2].

However, there are many major issues affecting public health, which have led to geographical studies with an important and effective role in understanding a spatial relationship between the place and health, and enhancing aspects of community health, in addition to planning healthcare services [4]. In addition, understanding the relationship between health and place has led to the emergence of a number of healthcare planning issues that affect the public health of people. In general, the incompatibility between supply and demand is the basis for issues of healthcare service planning, where the disparity between supply and demand creates an imperfect healthcare system. In other words, spatial planners should represent the healthcare services in geographical areas in line with the size of demand in such areas. Truthfully, it cannot be said that there is an ideal healthcare system globally; for example, there is no ideal healthcare system in the southern-world countries. Furthermore, when looking at the northern-world countries that are more developed than the southern-world countries, we find that there is similar inequality, where many urban areas are disadvantaged in terms of utilizing healthcare services [5]. Hence, the interest of researchers and spatial planners has focused on how to deliver healthcare services equitably and effectively to all individuals of society. Fortunately, the recent emergence of GIS has enhanced the understanding of the spatial relationship between health and place, thus, it is considered as an effective tool for dealing with healthcare planning issues [6].

From this standpoint, before starting work on any study of healthcare planning, a review should be undertaken of the most important issues that have attracted the interest of researchers and spatial planners during the past three decades, and that remain a focus today. In addition, what is the role of GIS, as a helpful tool, in dealing with these issues? A literature review will be a useful contribution in providing a a broad understanding of how analytical approaches related to GIS are applied to dealing with healthcare planning issues.

This paper seeks to provide a useful contribution in addition to what has been presented within previous studies and research, where it demonstrates in a different way a number of healthcare planning issues, and highlights analytical approaches using GIS in dealing with these issues. The paper will contribute to reaching the most important issues that need further investigation, analysis and visualization to be considered as future trends that health organizations and officials should deal with using GIS technology. Moreover, the paper will discuss the most important challenges and obstacles that health organizations and officials face in applying GIS. The focus of the presented paper will be on a number of issues that have not been extensively discussed in most of the previous studies and research as the authors have believed. Accordingly, the objectives of this paper are as follows:

1. Identifying the most important historical gaps related to health geomatics based on understanding the spatial relationship between health and place. This will contribute to defining the most important healthcare planning issues that health organizations, institutions and researchers have been dealing with using GIS technology.
2. Discussing five independent issues related to healthcare planning, unlike most previous studies and research that focused on reviewing one or two major issues (e.g., epidemiological planning or health resources allocation).
3. Presenting a largest possible number of useful GIS analytical approaches related to each discussed issue of healthcare planning. This will contribute to defining the gaps that need further investigation, analysis and visualization under each issue.

2. Methods

This paper aims to provide a literature and critical review to examine healthcare planning issues, and the potential of GIS in dealing with those issues. The method of a typical literature review was used in this paper to recognize how to use GIS in applying analytical approaches for decision-making associated with healthcare planning. In addition, this method will help in identifying recent trends, the written research regarding the use of GIS in dealing with healthcare planning issues, and the issues that require further investigation. The literature review included a set of studies, articles, and papers about public health, healthcare planning, and GIS modeling that were published between 1978 and 2020. The literary review was undertaken between October 2019 and mid-March 2020, when the authors of the present paper reviewed 132 titles. After review, this paper focussed on 73 titles, while 59 titles were excluded because they lacked at least one of these attributes: (1) focus on the healthcare aspect; (2) focus on the GIS aspect; (3) available full text or (4) a detailed description supporting results and recommendations. However, the reader is first introduced to a brief history of health geomatics and the emergence of GIS. This will contribute to understanding the relationship between health and place, and the developments of this relationship over history. This follows a review of the health concept, in addition to a review of the spatial planning concept, and its role in providing an effective healthcare system. Finally, we discuss healthcare planning issues, and present the role of GIS in

3. Results

3.1. Brief History of Health Geomatics and GIS

The relationship between health and place was discovered in the distant past. The identifcation and study of this relationship began with the father of medicine, Hippocrates. In his treatise, which is about airs, waters, and places, he mentions that people who live in rough, mountainous country at high elevation, which is characterized by well water and great differences of climate associated with the various seasons, will have large physiques and display hardiness and bravery, with no small degree of wildness in their character. On the other hand, he mentioned that people who live in low, stifling lands that have cold winds and warm water, will be neither large nor slight but rather broad, and bravery and hardiness are not an integral part of their natural characters. Consequently, he deduced that people who live on lowlands near waterways were more likely to develop malaria. In addition, Hippocrates (Figure 1) also wrote about topics such as the different characteristics of cities and how they influence the public health of people [1].

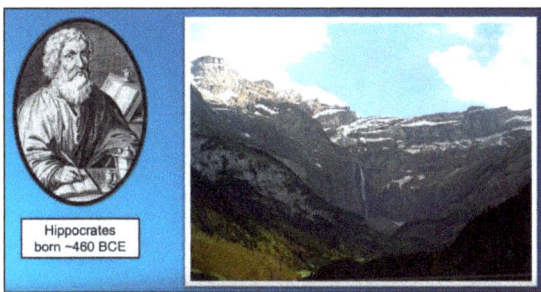

Figure 1. Hippocrates and relationship between health and place. (Source: [1]).

Another example dates to almost 1500 years ago, specifically to the Persian physician and spatial thinker, Al-Razi (Figure 2), who found the best location to build a hospital in Baghdad City. Al-Razi made his spatial decision by placing pieces of meat in wooden columns in different places in Baghdad City. He checked the pieces to determine where the last piece became spoiled. He then decided to build the hospital in the location of that piece because it was free from smoke and dirt, and thus was the cleanest and healthiest of the options, providing a space for patients in need of air that was fresh and free from contaminants [1].

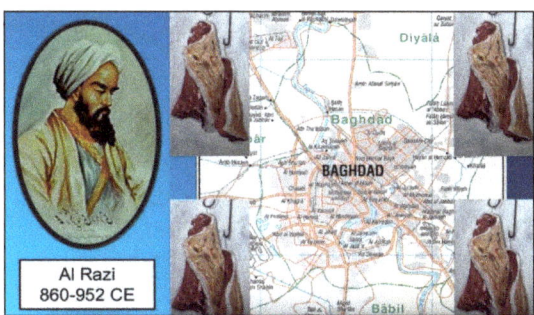

Figure 2. Al-Razi and the best location for building a hospital in Baghdad City (Source: [1]).

However, according to Koch and Tom [7] and Geraghty [1], the first spatial health map of plague disease spread was produced in Bari, Italy, 1694 (Figure 3). The plague is considered one of the most fearful diseases of all. At that time, nothing was known of what caused the plague disease or its spread. The plague was contained through three spatial decisions. These decisions were designed within the health map produced by the royal auditor Philip Arrieta. First, there was a coastal patrol to contain the active disease. Second, a wall separated the active area of the disease from healthy areas, with tents placed to symbolize troops to enforce the quarantine. Third, there was a general cordon to protect the full province, and this cordon was also monitored by troops. As shown in the figure below, cities were represented using simple drawings of either a church (with a cross) or a hospital (without a cross), and trees were used to show uninhabited areas.

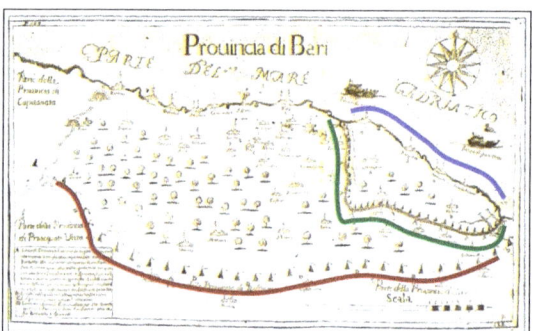

Figure 3. The first spatial health map of the plague disease in Bari, Italy, 1694. (Source: [1]).

The history of GIS in the field of spatial health actually began in 1854 when the cholera epidemic hit the city of London, England. Indeed, this epidemic killed at a rate of 500 people per week. The hero of this issue was Dr. Snow, who is known as the father of modern epidemiology. Dr. Snow took a different approach in dealing with this epidemic through drawing spatial maps that included a number of represented features relevant to the disease (e.g., outbreak locations, roads, property boundaries, and water lines). As shown in Figure 4, when he added these features to the map, he discovered that cholera cases existed along water lines, with a significant number of deaths (black color on the map) centered around the water pump. Hence, spatial maps proved that cholera cases were spreading through water, while many believed that the disease was spreading through air [1,8]. According to GisGeography [8], Dr. Snow's cholera epidemic map was an effective bridge linking geography and public health; in other words, he emphasized that there was a relationship between the place and health. This map is considered to be the beginning of the spatial analysis that later supported the field of epidemiology, specifically in studying the spread of diseases. Dr. Snow's work proved that GIS is an effective tool for solving problems and making spatial decisions.

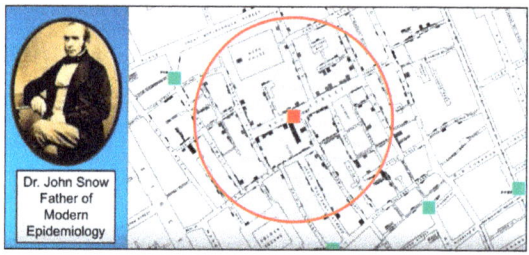

Figure 4. Spatial distribution of cholera cases in London, England, produced by Dr. Snow, 1854.(Source: [1]).

The work of Dr. Snow enhanced a continuation of the GIS concept to support public health, especially in epidemiology [9]. Historically, one of the leading works in the history of GIS and health was published in 1875 when Alfred Haviland produced the first atlas of color maps for cancer disease in the Divisions and Counties of England and Wales to locate areas with a high cancer rate. He used the maps to prepare an argument based on environmental risk factors of the disease, of which the most important was mineral production [10,11]. Later, the work of Haviland (Figure 5), reflected the importance of GIS in studying cancer, where it contributed to enhancing the analytical capabilities of epidemiologists and health officials. Thus, his work has enabled officials to detect environmental risk factors and their relationship to cancer, especially in the 1970s. In the present day, GIS can be used to produce cancer maps with a set of statistical and spatial analyses [12].

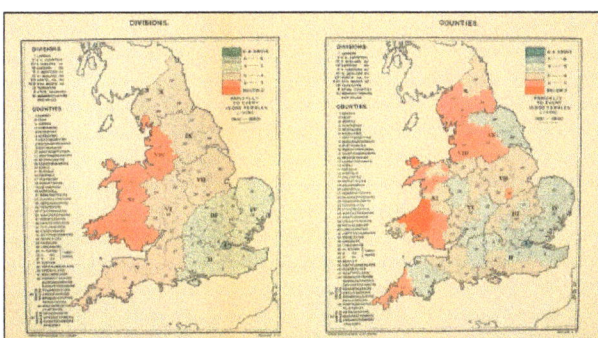

Figure 5. One of the atlas maps of geographical distribution of cancer disease in the Divisions and Counties of England and Wales, produced by Haviland, 1875 (Source: [13]).

The spatial maps produced by the preceding works were printed on paper. The transition from paper maps to digital maps ocurred after the emergence of computer systems, specifically in the period between 1960 and 1990, during which the leading GIS systems were developed and marketed, including the software of Esri [8]. According to Clarke et al. [14], computer systems were applied to geographical sciences during the 1960s, while GIS was applied to scientific fields during the 1970s. That contributed to producing maps easily, and facilitated the overlap of urban and health planning maps for selecting suitable areas and locations for expansion based on several criteria. Moreover, the process of managing spatial (geographic) databases was also facilitated.

However, one of the leading global organizations that has used GIS software in healthcare planning and disease control is the Center for Disease Control and Prevention (CDC), which began using GIS in the 1990s [15]. The CDC was established on July 1, 1946, in Atlanta, Georgia, USA. Initially, the primary mission of this center was to prevent malaria from spreading across the nation. The center faced major challenges to overcome mosquitoes with a budget of USD 10 million and only 400 employees, while the healthcare services provided were few. In addition, there was a scarcity of medical epidemiologists in the USA during that period. However, despite these challenges, disease control was the primary goal of the CDC, and gradually the center overcame its difficulties to contribute to improving people's public health [16].

During the 1990s, GIS technology became a major tool at the CDC. The center used this technology for improving people's public health by surveillance of diseases, allocation of health resources, assessment of environmental risks, and management, analysis and modeling of spatial data [15]. However, according to the WHO [17], nearly 17 million people die from heart disease and stroke annually, with smoking and an unhealthy diet among the most important factors leading to these diseases. Consequently, at the beginning of the millennium, the CDC, in cooperation with the WHO, launched the "Atlas of Heart Disease and Stroke" based on ArcGIS technology (Figure 6). This project is considered one of the leading and most successful models in improving public health globally.

The purpose of designing this atlas was to provide an accessible reference for decision-makers in public health, ultimately leading to the reduction of heart disease and stroke-related deaths in the US by allocating health resources according to needs within specific geographic areas.

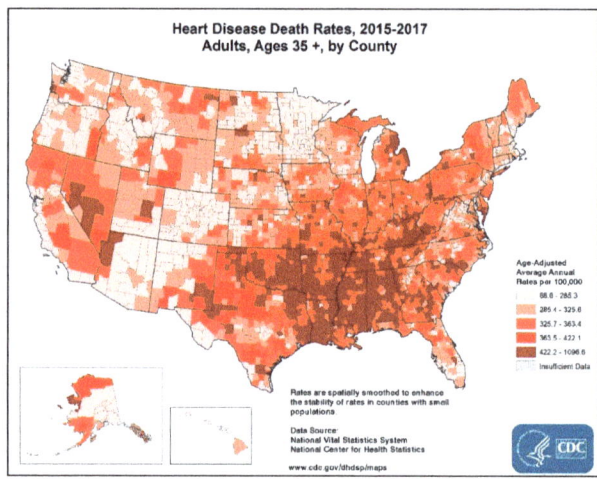

Figure 6. Example of atlas maps of heart disease and stroke produced by the Center for Disease Control and Prevention (CDC). (Source: [18]).

GIS technology and software have evolved since 2000, especially in methods of spatial analysis and modeling of public health [19]. For example, according to Aghajani [20], the International Health Organization in Europe proposed the use of GIS to detect diseases in contaminated water areas in 2003. GIS contributed to caring for patients and managing their movements to ensure that they avoid disease areas. In addition, in 2006, the Environmental Protection Agency proposed a strategic plan for GIS to investigate a West Nile virus outbreak in Pennsylvania, USA. By studying and analyzing a number of factors that contributed to spreading the virus easily, such as mosquitoes, blood transfusion, breastfeeding, and hospital infection, the agency succeeded in determining the original location and extent of transmission of the virus through healthcare centers using GIS. However, development of GIS technology and software in the period since 2000 has also contributed to emerging new trends that enhance using GIS as a tool for improving public health. These trends are considered as issues in health planning, the most important of which are the monitoring of epidemic diseases, accessibility and utilization of healthcare, disease mapping and its spread patterns, health information management, and allocation of health resources [21]. Although the examples covered in this section may not cover the entire history of GIS development, they identify individuals and institutions that have played a major role in the development of GIS and its relationship with public health.

3.2. Overview of Healthcare Planning

Health is a basic human right that every individual should be able to enjoy at the highest possible level [22]. However, it is an elusive term and can be defined in different ways; according to the WHO, health is the foundation upon which physical and mental strength and social well-being is based [23]. In light of this definition, it is clear that a healthy society can contribute to supporting social and economic development, where its individuals will be more productive and effective due to their good mental and physical ability and high social well-being. However, there is a strong correlation between economic growth and healthcare; whenever rate of economic growth increases, governments will provide equitable and balanced healthcare that meets all the needs of society's individuals. On the other hand, economic growth may not support the provision of equitable healthcare due to several reasons, the most important of which are the lack of available health resources and the weak preparation and implementation of short- and long-term plans for distributing healthcare services across geographic areas that have different population densities [24].

During the 1970s, the WHO and UNICEF adopted the "Health for All" strategy globally due to weakening health levels of people caused by a number of factors, the most important being poverty, and poor living conditions and nutrition. This strategy sought to achieve the highest possible level of health for people, taking into account how to maintain that level, so that people can work well with effective social participation. Therefore, such a strategy consists of a set of services that contribute to protecting people from diseases, and enhancing their treatment options with low costs. This strategy sought to achieve the highest possible level of health for people according to five basic principles: (a) adopting several sectoral programs; (b) preventing an outbreak of disease; (c) making decisions by community; (d) using suitable technologies; and (e) achieving equitable accessibility and spatial distribution of healthcare services [23].

Spatial equality in access to healthcare can be achieved by understanding a concept of spatial planning, and its role in providing an effective and equitable healthcare system for all [25]. However, spatial planning is a set of methods used to address the distribution of individuals and activities in different places and periods [26]. In other words, it is a set of structured actions that can be implemented in a specific period of time at one or several spatial levels (national, regional, local). A range of tools and methods are used over spatial planning to make the best sustainable use of available natural and human resources. This type of planning seeks to create the desired change in the society with the guidance, control, and follow-up of this change in different aspects of life to prevent any negative effects. At the health level, the spatial planning of the healthcare system can be defined as a detailed policy to provide healthcare services to all individuals; for example, programs and projects aimed at achieving the perfect health level of the individual and society with specific characteristics in an given period of time, by making the best use of the available materials and human resources [23].

The healthcare system consists of organizations, institutions, and resources aimed primarily at improving public health. Such a system must provide services that meet existing and future needs, that all individuals can access equitably. Nevertheless, there are a number of issues relating to healthcare systems of both developing and developed countries, the most important of which is that there are population groups with poor utilization and access to healthcare services because the equality principle is not taken into account in the planning of healthcare services. The inequality of spatial distribution of healthcare services can be overcome by practicing standards-based spatial planning for such services, thus eventually contributing to improving the spatial performance of the healthcare services system in general [23].

In light of the above, when agencies or ministries intend to adopt strategies or plans related to the allocation of healthcare services, consideration must be given for how to provide equitable access and to overcome spatial disparities. This requires taking into account spatial planning standards for the distribution of healthcare services in a specific geographical area, thus highlighting the importance of studying the spatial distribution of population densities and estimating demand for the services. Moreover, spending financial resources on healthcare services must ensure health benefits are achieved for people that equal the real value of spending. In other words, there must be a balance between the fair provision of such services and their operation at high efficiency.

3.3. Issues of Healthcare Planning and GIS Role

Several references, such as [4,27], identified the most important major issues affecting the health of societies. These issues will be reviewed, in light of the role of GIS in dealing with them, over the past three decades. In addition, the concentration will be on reviewing and discussing only empirical issues that are concerned with how to plan and organize healthcare services (spatially) within a specific geographical area.

3.3.1. Epidemiological Planning and Disease Mapping

One of the most important research areas during the past two decades is the study of spatial epidemiology by GIS [28]. However, the study of spatial epidemiology requires answering a number of important inquiries, the most important of which are: Where do these epidemics occur? What are the environmental factors that lead to outbreaks of epidemics? What is the evolution of the spatial patterns of these epidemics? [29]. These questions can be answered through the GIS tool. For instance, GIS can determine the locations of epidemics, and uses demographic, economic, and environmental data to study and analyze spatial relationships within the affected area [30].

The epidemiological planning issue has been supported by various GIS studies in the healthcare planning area [31]. Geographers and spatial planners have focused on modeling epidemic diseases in many studies [32]. The socioeconomic characteristics of the population are considered one of the most important factors on which epidemiology studies are based. Mapping the spatial distribution of epidemic diseases can be implemented by a number of methods, the most important of which is the method of choropleth GIS maps. Through these maps, disease rates are drawn on a basic map in order to determine the severity of and vulnerability to an epidemic disease. Moreover, the spatial distribution of epidemic diseases can also be implemented by modeling the prediction of disease risk using the kernel estimation method [33].

There are a number of studies that have shown that GIS is a useful tool for epidemiological planning [19]. Cliff, Haggett and Ord [34] studied and analyzed influenza outbreaks in Iceland (see Figure 7). Before 1900, there were no records of this disease in Iceland. In contrast, the outbreak of the disease over a period of three decades contributed to providing a useful mapping test related to spatial patterns of disease spread. They found that the infection moved and spread hierarchically through the air. It moved from Reykjavik (the capital) to the smaller provinces, and then to the small towns, and eventually to the rural areas. When looking at the map outputs, it became clear that the hierarchical and spatial aspects of the patterns of disease spread were useful to spatial planners. This eventually contributed to overcome the influenza disease across urban and rural areas. Gould and Wallace [35] also used a hierarchical process to observe that HIV/AIDS began to spread in the United States in the early 1980s. To remedy the situation and manage the spread of the disease, they used GIS to map the current status and potential future in terms of disease spread. Moreover, they tried to map the disease spread as clusters to contain and understand the disease.

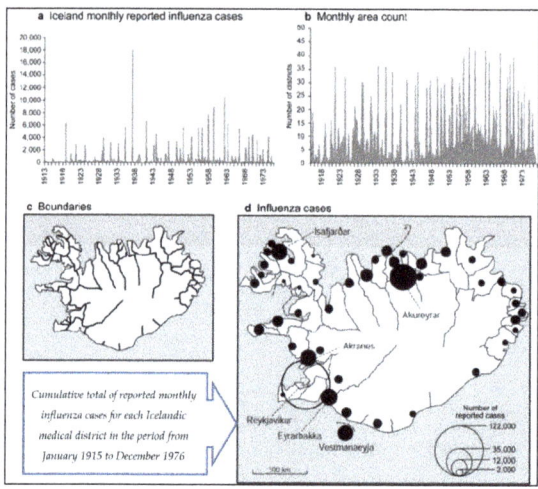

Figure 7. Reported influenza morbidity in Iceland in the period from January 1915 to December 1976. (Source: [34]).

In another work, Braga et. al [36] mapped lung cancer clusters in the cities of Viterbo and Lucca, Italy. Standard methods, such as kernel and Bayesian, were used to determine disease rates at the cluster level. Brown et al., [37] used GIS as an effective tool in investigating spatial inequality of the delivery of healthcare services in Merseyside, UK. Furthermore, Wrigley [38] used GIS to model the disease-affected areas according to the demographic characteristics and the socioeconomic variables of the population. In Johnson's work [39], prostate cancer incidence rates were modeled using GIS in New York State. In this work, infection rates (SIRs) of prostate cancer were subjected to the hierarchical modeling of Bayesian by zip code to determine the relative performance of spatial data. In this work, spatial data were linked to air quality data.

In the area of integration between GIS and epidemiological techniques, Rasam et al. [40] used an exploratory analysis approach to identify patterns of spatial distribution of cholera in the Sabah area of Malaysia. In this study, cholera cases were mapped using spatial statistics within a GIS enviroment (see Figure 8). An epidemiological technique (i.e., a cohort technique) was also used to examine the disease's spread. As a result, it became clear that the disease was easily transferred from person to person, especially in the area within 1500 meters from the patient location and with contaminated water. Hence, this study showed that GIS is considered an effective epidemiological technique for mapping patterns of the spatial distribution and directions of disease.

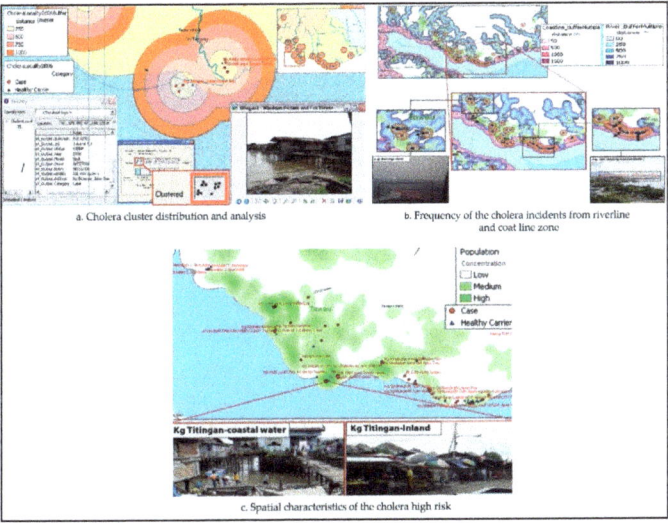

Figure 8. Spatial mapping and analysis of cholera in the Sabah area, Malaysia. (Source: [40]).

Recently, the management of outbreaks of diseases such as Ebola and measles has become one of the most advanced practices in the epidemiological planning area. For example, during a measles outbreak in Disneyland in December of 2014, GIS maps played a large role in developing a general perception of the locations where children with the disease live, and the potential spatial directions for the spread of this disease. In addition, these maps have been recently used in the field of vaccination in various countries and throughout the United States to identify the locations that need higher rates of vaccination, as well as to identify the locations that seriously suffer from outbreaks of this type of disease [41].

According to Sones [42], GIS can map outbreak of diseases. In the USA, measles was thought to be eradicated in 2000. However, measles returned in 2019, with the CDC reporting at least 764 cases in 23 states. GIS maps related to the spread of measles were used by the Washington Post newspaper, where it appeared that most cases did not receive a vaccination, while 10% of those who were infected were vaccinated. However, it became clear through GIS maps that the incidence of measles has risen in geographical areas that contained children who had not received vaccination for the disease, and particularly of parents in 17 US states who were free to choose whether to vaccinate their children. Therefore, public health officials considered such areas as sources for the spread of measles. On the other hand, it became clear that measles may be transferred from one area to another through airborne hosts, especially in unvaccinated areas. Hence, decision-makers used GIS as a tool to compute measles cases and track the directions of disease outbreaks by mapping the disease. These maps helped decision-makers to reduce gaps in health services by identifying a number of factors (e.g., locations of patients, number of disease cases, and time period of the disease spread). Analysis of such data contributed to detecting areas of population suffering from a deficit of health services, and to identify optimal locations for these services in the future.

To sum up, many references were reviewed here to reveal what was written about the issue of epidemiological planning and disease mapping. A total of 12 studies were used to investigate the role of GIS in dealing with such issues. The studies focused on the United States, England, Italy, Saudi Arabia, India, and Malaysia. In addition, they included a total of 33 authors (range: from one author to seven authors), with half of the studies conducted by one author. Moreover, they were published by a total of seven core journals in the period from 1991 to 2019.

3.3.2. Accessibility and Utilization of Healthcare Services

GIS is an effective tool for dealing with issues of healthcare services, espicially those related to service location [43]. The WHO and the World Bank [44] emphasized that nearly half the world's population faces difficulty in accessing healthcare. Thus, it is essential that easy and equitable access to healthcare services be available to all areas of the population, including those without private transportation [45]. However, there are many areas related to this issue, with the most important of them being: (1) identifying the optimal location for health care services; (2) understanding the relationship between the current locations of services and actual healthcare needs; and (3) evaluating spatial accessibility to healthcare services. There is also another very important question, namely, what are the healthcare needs for population, as well as how should authorities allocate healthcare resources to serve the population? Hence, GIS has the answer to this question [30]. For example, Jonhs and Bentham [46] used GIS to examine the relationship between healthcare and accessibility. Furthermore, Forbes and Todd [47] proposed the possible locations of new centers to treat cancer patients in England using GIS. Therefore, finding the optimum location of healthcare service is one of the resource optimization tasks for the health authority. However, there are a number of GIS models that help determine the best location for healthcare services, such as the models of location allocation that modern GIS software provides. Through these models, spatial planners can evaluate accessibility to healthcare service after identifying areas with poor accessibility to services locations. Then, they can provide planning proposals and interventions that contribute to improving poor accessibility to healthcare service locations [30].

Any study on accessibility and utilization of healthcare should be aware of a number of important factors, such as socioeconomic variables, need, equity, supply, and demand [48]. Many researchers and spatial planners have used these factors to enhance their spatial data for modeling accessibility and utilization of healthcare services [49]. For example, supply can be represented by the number of healthcare services provided in a specific geographical area or catchment area, as well as the spatial distribution patterns of service locations and their relevant operational capacity [50]. In the study of Khan and Bardwaj [51], socioeconomic variables were entered into their spatial data for developing a comprehensive understanding of accessibility. For example, they took into account the income, education, social class, insurance, and other variables that affect how people access and use healthcare services. Practically, to reach an integrated spatial model, the variables were linked to the spatial aspects of the location, supply, demand, time, and distance.

Before the advent of GIS, researchers and spatial planners used the traditional approach based on the Euclidean distance to model accessibility to healthcare services. Due to GIS, modeling accessibility to healthcare services has become more efficient and effective through using a new set of analytical approaches based on distance and travel time [49]. This modeling is based on the following spatial data layers: (1) the layer of healthcare service locations and their spatial distribution (supply) [52]; (2) the layer of population distribution and their demographic data (demand/need); and (3) layer of the transportation network linking potential patients and healthcare services [53–55]. These three preceding layers have become the most important basic spatial data that can be merged and overlapped in a GIS environment to model accessibility for the planning of healthcare services [4]. For instance, Brabyn and Skelly [56] merged the preceding layers in a vector (linear) GIS for modeling accessibility to public hospitals by distance and travel time across New Zealand. The accessibility scores were determined per area and population. As a result, they found that there are some locations with low accessibility to hospitals in New Zealand, particularly in northern and southern areas with high average travel times to hospitals (Figure 9). In addition, via GIS, Murad [57] created a geo-database including health center locations, population distribution, and road network to identify accessibility to healthcare centers in the city of Jeddah, Saudi Arabia. By the drive-time analysis technique, the study revealed that there are areas of Jeddah with low accessibility to healthcare centers since they fall outside the 30 min drive-time service area.

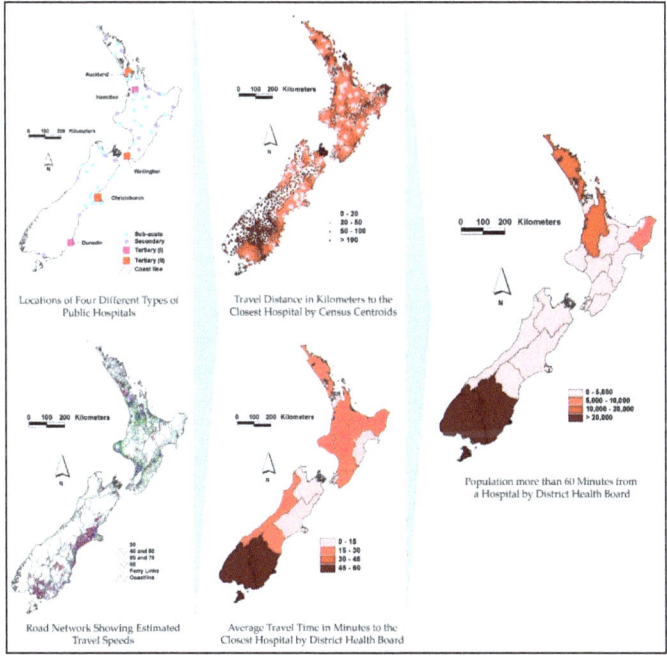

Figure 9. Modeling population access to New Zealand public hospitals. (Source: [56]).

Furthermore, in a comprehensive study, Christie and Fone [58] used GIS for modeling accessibility to hospital services in Wales. They identified the travel time per social group (weighted by deprivation score). The study found inequality in the provision of hospital services, where there were many parts (disadvantaged areas) with poor accessibility and utilization of services, in contrast to the rich population areas. However, when looking at the preceding studies, we find that they focused on using distance and travel time as techniques to model accessibility to healthcare services. In other words, with the advent of GIS, most studies have moved on from focusing on using Euclidean distance, which had been used to model accessibility, to using distance and travel time techniques, thus increasing the effectiveness and precision of accessibility modeling.

With recent developments in GIS techniques, many researchers have developed models of accessibility to healthcare services. Luo and Wang [50] developed a model of accessibility to primary care in the Chicago area. They adopted the raster travel friction approach for modeling accessibility. In the area of GIS-based accessibility analysis, Mokgalaka [59] measured accessibility to primary healthcare services to assist in spatial planning. To do this, facility utilization rates in the form of headcounts were combined with GIS-based accessibility analysis. In this study, GIS was used to define three different scenarios to identify the level of demand for primary healthcare services, where it became clear that databases and patient records are not available. These GIS-based scenarios were tested to model catchment areas. As a result, the levels of demand for primary healthcare services varied across the three scenarios, where it appeared that the number of headcounts in the facility contributed to this difference in demand; that is, the higher the number of headcounts in the facility, the higher the demand for it. Hence, spatial distribution plans for primary healthcare services can be developed by incorporating GIS-based accessibility analysis and facility utilization rates.

In addition, Luo and Wang [50] developed a gravity model approach using GIS, where they adopted the floating catchment area (FCA) weighted by location and population. In a similar study on the accessibility of primary healthcare in Washington DC, the gravity model approach was developed by Guagliardo [60] via incorporating a kernel density element. The last decade has witnessed a new wave of progress in location-based accessibility theory, especially through developing the method of the two-step floating catchment area (2SFCA), which is considered an FCA method. This method can help spatial planners to evaluate spatial inequality of providing healthcare services. For example, Kanugantia, Sarkarb and Singh [61] studied the spatial performance of the healthcare system in the Alwar district of Rajasthan. Through GIS, a two-step floating catchment area (2SFCA) was used to measure accessibility to healthcare facilities in rural areas that mainly suffer from spatial isolation from the facilities. This study contributed to recognizing areas that have low accessibility to healthcare facilities. Hence, this study helped to improve the road network and propose new healthcare facility locations in order to enhance the spatial performance of healthcare system in the region.

Another example is the work of Tao and Cheng [62], who studied accessibility to healthcare services by elderly people in Beijing (see Figure 10). A multimode and variable-demand two-step floating catchment area (2SFCA) model based on travel time technique was developed to measure the elderly's accessibility to healthcare services in Beijing, taking into account that the challenge was competition among elderly and nonelderly people for accessing services. As a result, it appeared that there is a high demand on healthcare services by the elderly, who are considered deprived of private mobility, and rely on public transportation to access services, unlike the nonelderly, who have private mobility with low demand on services. Hence, new health resources should be allocated to improving accessibility to services via public mobility, especially in areas that have low accessibility to services. In addition, Ni et al. [63] benefited from the 2SFCA method in effectively identifying more realistic details of accessibility to healthcare services. They used an improved method to integrate all modes of transportation with the 2SFCA in order to estimate accessibility to services of healthcare in Nanjing City. They used the travel-mode technique depending on distance to define the complicated multi-mode travel behavior of the population. Door-to-door approaches were proposed to define each aspect of the primary transportation. Moreover, open data was processed to compute the origin–destination time cost. In a last step, the improved method was applied to estimate the population's accessibility to healthcare services by comparing it with three single-mode 2SFCA methods.

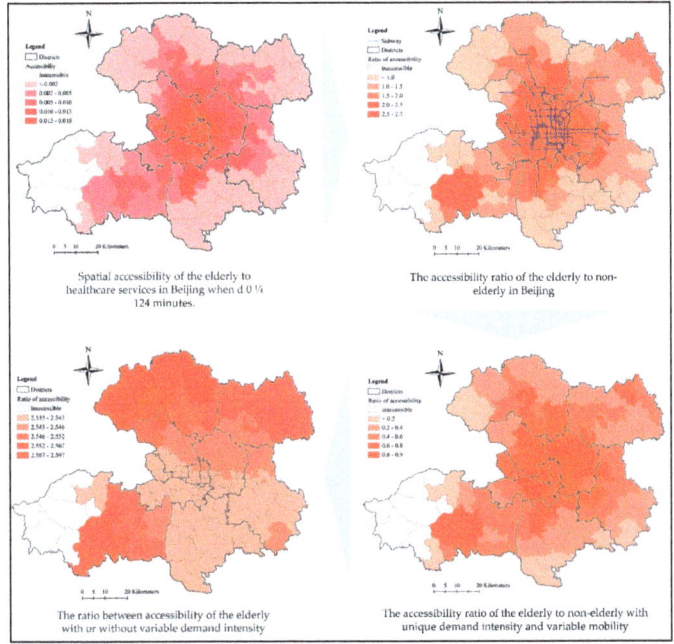

Figure 10. Modeling the spatial accessibility of the elderly to healthcare services in Beijing, China using a multimode and variable-demand two-step floating catchment area (2SFCA) model. (Source: [62]).

To summarize, many references were reviewed here to reveal what was written about the issue of accessibility and utilization of healthcare services. A total of 21 studies were used to investigate the role of GIS in dealing with such issues. The studies focused on the United States, England, Ireland, Scotland, Saudi Arabia, South Africa, China, Moldova, and India. In addition, they included a total of 42 authors (range: from one author to five authors), and half of studies were conducted with two authors. Moreover, the studies were published by a total of 17 core journals in the period from 1984 to 2018.

3.3.3. Public Health and Information Management

GIS is considered a useful tool in the Health Management Information System (HMIS); furthermore, it can make a healthcare delivery system more effective and efficient. GIS includes health planning, mapping of the risk service area, database management, and location identification [64]. During the 1980s in the UK, technical staff in the Local Health Units (LHU) looked for methods and techniques to help plan healthcare services and resources. They used GIS to develop information systems to link data attributes to each other, such as services, population, health outcomes, and socioeconomic data. This process was activated by GIS at the country level, and particularly in Italian provinces [4]. With the development of Internet platforms, healthcare information is presented and easily accessible [65]. For example, the WHO and the CDC in the US contributed to publishing several types of data and information relating to spatial healthcare during the last decade. In contrast, there is a lack of interactive information that enables the public to make spatial inquiries or analyses, since, at present, most spatial information relating to healthcare is in the form of traditional flat maps [66].

GIS has the ability to disseminate and manage the tools and base data via Internet platforms [67]. For instance, the health maps produced by the WHO are a model for addressing public health issues, and managing growing infectious diseases [66]. Moreover, the work of Singhasivanon et al. [68] is an example of the ability of GIS in sharing data and monitoring disease. They provided a spatial model and management analysis of drug-resistant malaria in the Mekong Delta. In addition, one effective and successful example is the Health Atlas produced by the Health Observatories in the UK and Ireland, which is considered a new online product [69]. In 2003, the SARS information system was managed via the development of a Web-based interactive GIS, which enabled the public to participate in preventing relevant activities (see Figure 11) [70]. In another work related to GIS on the Internet, Abdullahi, Lawal and Agushaka [71] designed a Web-based GIS for the health system. This allowed workers in the health sector to share and manage data, and access information that enables them to find the nearest hospitals that provide improved healthcare services in Zaria, Nigeria.

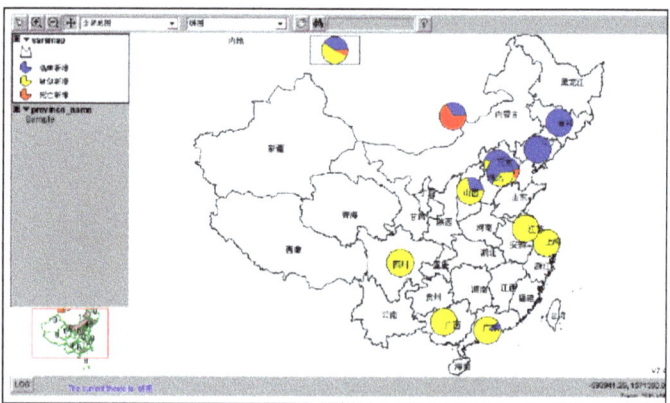

Figure 11. Web-based Geographic Information Systems (GIS) for public health information visualization: distribution map with pie chart to express public health information. (Source: [70]).

In addition, there is a relationship between epidemiological mapping and healthcare information management. For example, Masimalai [72] used GIS in analyzing the spatial directions associated with the spread of filariasis in India, taking advantage of the potential of GIS in managing health information related to the disease. As a result, it appeared that GIS is an effective tool in mapping epidemiological information of filariasis, and therefore, management and surveillance of the disease is easier for decision-makers in India. In the area of linking management of patient information and GIS, according to Moore et al. [73], the Ministry of Health coordinated with stroke centers in Kentucky to implement a project to improve the quality of stroke encounters. From 2008 to 2018, there were 23 hospitals that inserted 76,222 records of stroke patients using the Patient Management Tool (PMT). The aim of this project was to link stroke patient records with GIS to improve patient care management. As a result, the use of GIS maps has helped public health officials and hospital stroke coordinators to develop possible interventions to improve stroke care.

To sum up, many references were reviewed here to reveal what was written about the issue of public health and information management. A total of nine studies were used to investigate the role of GIS in dealing with such an issue. The studies focused on the United States, England, Ireland, Nigeria, and India. In addition, they included a total of 34 authors (range: from one author to 12 authors), and nearly half of studies were written by three authors. Moreover, they were published by a total of seven core journals in the period from 1999 to 2019.

3.3.4. Public Health Surveillance

This area is closely related to public health by collecting, analyzing, and interpreting health data to plan and evaluate public health practices. Public health surveillance helps in: (1) following up progress in achieving public health goals; (2) detecting the impact of interventions aimed at upgrading public health; (3) monitoring epidemic diseases and identifying associated problems; (4) identifying public health priorities, policies, and strategies; and (5) predicting sudden emergency cases [74]. However, in recent years, outbreaks of disease have increased in terms of number and complexity, and the threat of such diseases to the public health of societies has reached dangerous levels [75]. According to Wiafe and Davenhall [76], new diseases such as Severe Acute Respiratory Syndrome SARS have emerged, while other diseases, such as tuberculosis, have returned. These diseases have appeared for a number of reasons, the most important of which is the large increase in travel and international trade in recent years, which has led to the spread of diseases across geopolitical and international borders at large rates (for example, the outbreaks of SARS and bird flu). These diseases threaten societies, which leads to the need to establish an effective system for disease surveillance. Through this system, the information necessary will be available for public health officials to identify and manage outbreaks of disease. Successful disease surveillance requires a standardized methodology, as well as appropriate tools for collecting data rapidly and accurately, with timely dissemination. Hence, the best current system that can monitor disease is GIS, which is the preferred technology for collecting, analyzing, displaying, and sharing specific spatial data at the right time [43].

Public health surveillance is mainly based on a number of important elements, the most important of which are: (1) tracking epidemics; (2) evaluating potential infection; and (3) designing health interventions [77]. GIS is an effective tool in managing and analyzing data in health surveillance. For example, GIS has been used to successfully monitor and analyze reproductive outcomes for mothers who live near hazardous waste locations [78]. Moreover, GIS can monitor infectious diseases that basically spread by disease vectors because it has the ability to identify the environmental factors of disease vectors. GIS has contributed to the monitoring and spread limitation of a number of diseases, the most important of which are: (1) malaria; (2) onchocerciasis; and (3) Lyme disease [4].

There are many successful instances of disease surveillance using GIS. One study was the work of the WHO and UNICEF in 1993. They developed the Public Health Mapping Program to overcome Guinea worm disease, which has spread in the rural poor. They used GIS as tool to monitor the spread of disease infection and eradication efforts, and to identify populations at risk. This work is considered an effective example of how GIS could be used to control Guinea worm disease [79]. In addition, and with more advanced work, DC Health in 2016 responded to the outbreak of Zika disease. It used ArcGIS Online to accurately map mosquito trap locations and breeding grounds, leading to a more thorough understanding of mosquito populations, as well as potential health risks in the area [80].

Disease surveillance with GIS and remote sensing functions can be effective via risks maps that include areas suffering from environmental conditions that contribute to the spread of diseases [81]. According to Pam et al. [82], combining GIS and remote sensing techniques is considered an exciting development in epidemiological studies, particularly in the surveillance of vector-borne diseases. For example, Kalluri et al. [83] used GIS and remote sensing as a tool for surveillance of vector-borne diseases. In this study, remote sensing techniques were discussed for studying mosquitoes (see Figure 12), ticks, flies, and sandflies. GIS maps were used to track the climate change that may affect the abundance of vectors. As a result, the combination of GIS and remote sensing was an effective method in the surveillance of potential vector-borne diseases, and evaluating the human environmental damage. In addition, the study discovered that one of the most important contributors to vector-borne diseases is wildlife environment. Moreover, in another study related to eliminating malaria in the Solomon Islands, the government implemented a program for surveillance of the spread of the disease, and its elimination, by integrating GIS and remote sensing functions. As a result, this program significantly contributed to decreasing the incidence of malaria cases in Solomon Islands; consequently, the malaria disease-based death rate also decreased [84].

In addition, many countries have made significant progress in using infectious disease surveillance systems through GIS. These systems could somewhat control disease outbreaks. However, countries face a number of challenges that affect the operation of these systems effectively and efficiently. The most important of these challenges are: (1) weak infrastructure and coordination between relevant health organizations; (2) weak technical systems of health organizations and facilities; (3) weak financial resources for systems development; and (4) untrained human resources to use such systems. Consequently, the number of diseases and deaths may not decrease over time. These challenges will negatively contribute to the decision-making process and interventions aimed at eliminating and controlling infectious diseases effectively and efficiently [85].

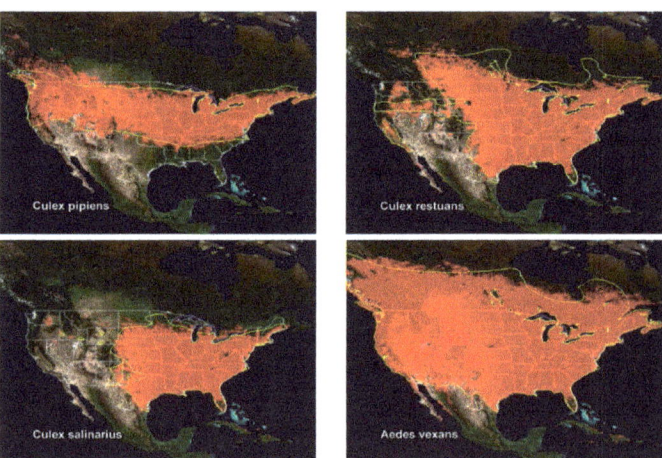

Figure 12. Maps showing the potential distribution of four species of mosquito in the United States. (Source: [83]).

To sum up, many references were reviewed here to reveal what was written about the issue of public health surveillance. A total of 11 studies were used to investigate the role of GIS in dealing with such an issue. The studies focused on the United States, Canada, Japan, Solomon Islands, India, and Zambia. In addition, they included a total of 36 authors (range: from two authors to nine authors), and nearly half of studies were written by two authors. Moreover, they were published by a total of eight core journals in the period from 1992 to 2019.

3.3.5. Location Allocation and Optimal Location Modelling

One of the important issues associated with healthcare planning is modeling the optimal allocation of healthcare service locations [86]. Therefore, this issue has been a theoretical problem facing spatial planners for some time, especially in the predigital period, when the focus was on planning the location of healthcare services efficiently, ensuring the spatial performance of healthcare systems was improved within urban and rural areas [87]. Location–allocation models are used to select optimal locations for new services, including healthcare services; for example, selecting a new location for a primary healthcare center or diabetes center taking into account existing locations for available healthcare, as well as the basic demand for services. Location–allocation models are represented in mathematical programming approaches that can be described as a set of numerical methods that contribute to solving optimization problems associated with public health scenarios. In addition to planning new locations for services, location–allocation models can contribute to evaluating service delivery in a specific geographic area [88].

The spatial decision-making associated with allocating healthcare service locations depends on a set of various scenarios, such as: (1) planning a new service location; (2) adding a new service into existing services; and (3) removing existing services. Due to the emergence of GIS in the digital period, and the discovery of geographic computational methods, analysis of spatial data for health care service locations has been enhanced, assessment of various scenarios can be undertaken more quickly, and the optimum allocation of services is much simpler [66]. Historically, several studies addressed the location–allocation models of healthcare using GIS. One of the successful examples of the location–allocation problem is the work of Forbes and Todd [47], which used GIS to assess possible locations for allocating new units to treat disease of cancer in England. This study estimated travel time for a number of potential locations by assuming specific speeds within the road network, combined with population areas to determine travel time zones. Population and patient numbers were calculated for different periods by recording population and cancer case data. The best location was the one that had the maximum population for the desired maximum travel times.

It is also possible to investigate the use of health services, and to improve or propose new services, by combining accessibility models and location–allocation models within the GIS environment [86]. For example, Abdelkarim [89] also integrated accessibility and location–allocation models into GIS to improve spatial planning and environmental sustainability of healthcare services in Al-Madinah Al-Munawwarah, Saudi Arabia. The study aimed to support the spatial allocation of health services in Al-Madinah Al-Munawwarah. The study also included many types of health services, the most important of which were hospitals and healthcare centers. The researcher used the network analysis method to measure the accessibility to health services through different time periods (i.e., 5 min, 10 min, and 15 min). Moreover, the maximum coverage model was used during a response period of no more than 15 min. As a result, the study's findings revealed that residents suffer from poor accessibility to healthcare service coverage areas due to poor spatial distribution of healthcare services. The study also proposed providing 24 new healthcare service locations to cover a lack in some areas of the city. In another work, Polo et al. [90] combined location-allocation models and accessibility models within a GIS environment in order to support health service planning (i.e., dog and cat sterilization services) in Bogota, Colombia (Figure 13). Moreover, they modified the 2SFCA method based on a set of considerations to measure the spatial accessibility to health services without modifying location–allocation models. As a result, they discovered that there were disadvantaged areas in accessing health services, especially those in central, western, and northern Bogota. Consequently, the spatial accessibility to health services was increased by moving the locations proposed by the maximum coverage model.

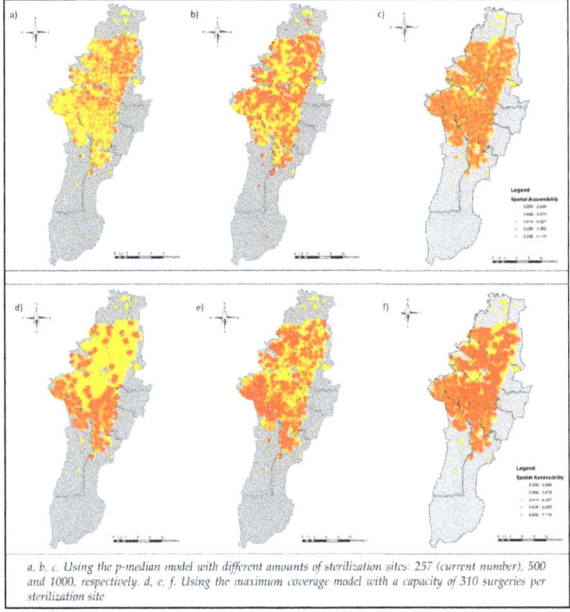

Figure 13. Spatial accessibility to sterilization sites arising from the location–allocation models in Bogota, Colombia. (Source: [90]).

To sum up, many references were reviewed here to reveal what was written about the issue of location–allocation and optimal location modelling. A total of seven studies were used to investigate the role of GIS in dealing with such an issue. The studies focused on the United States, England, Finland, Saudi Arabia, and Colombia. In addition, they included a total of 18 authors (range: from one author to four authors), and nearly half of studies were written by two authors. Moreover, they were published by a total of five core journals in the period from 1995 to 2019.

4. Discussion

In this paper, our literature review briefly surveyed the literature related to a number of key issues that fall under the field of healthcare planning. In other words, the previous research and studies related to healthcare planning were summarized and presented from the perspective of a number of key issues with examining the role of GIS in dealing with such issues. This literature contains a rich context of theoretical, analytical, and quantitative aspects that can be recognized by reviewing them fully. It was clear from the literature survey that the relationship between GIS and healthcare planning issues is constantly evolving at the global level. The tremendous and vital development of GIS technologies has contributed to understanding such issues, and its relationship with different geographical areas. Consequently, this development of GIS technologies has been efficiently supporting health professionals in studying and analyzing issues of healthcare planning by a number of applications based on analytical approaches.

Before the emergence of GIS, the spatial relationship between place and health was an important issue for scientists and researchers. This relationship was explained by simple spatial analysis based on paper maps that described the spread of epidemic diseases and were used to support spatial decisions for dealing with diseases. Ever since Dr. Snow's work aimed at overcoming cholera in London in 1854, monitoring diseases has depended on maps-based spatial analysis, including features such as disease outbreak locations, road networks, and property boundaries. Thus, making spatial decisions to address epidemic diseases was more effective and accurate, and the spatial relationship between place and health was better understood and more obvious. Over time, Dr. Snow's work has promoted the continued development of GIS, especially in the field of epidemiology, which has contributed to enhancing health officials' capabilities in terms of spatial planning, analysis, and monitoring epidemic diseases and their spread. Identifying factors of environmental risk and their role in emerging diseases has been enhanced, especially with the development of statistical and spatial analysis methods within the GIS environment. The emergence of computer systems in the 1960s led to the birth of a growth era for GIS, specifically with regard to producing digital maps, applying spatial analysis methods, and managing spatial databases. This contributed to supporting healthcare planning and responding to epidemic diseases by allocating health resources, assessing environmental risks, and managing, analyzing, and modeling spatial data.

It was clear from the literature review that there are many healthcare planning issues that have gradually emerged with the development and understanding of the relationship between health and place, which are considered the main two factors in the planning of healthcare. Based on the review and its findings regarding the recent trends in this subject, the most important issues were found to be epidemiological modeling and disease mapping, the evaluation of the accessibility and utilization of healthcare, disease surveillance, and health information management, as well as location-allocation modeling for healthcare services. These issues must be taken into consideration before working on any study of healthcare planning. Scientists and researchers have investigated these issues during the past three decades in order to develop analytical approaches that support the field of human public health. However, based on the literature examined in this paper, it appears that the analytical approaches of spatial studies associated with healthcare planning have reached an acceptable level of maturity and rationality, and it is possible to apply these approaches to more complex issues related to healthcare planning, particularly with the recent development of GIS technologies. But in contrast, the literature review confirmed that geographic researchers and spatial planners have been highly focusing on developing and applying analytical approaches to support two important issues of healthcare planning: first, modeling epidemics in order to monitor and prevent their spread, and, second, to assess inequalities in access to healthcare in order to determine the optimal allocation of health resources. Achieving these two aspects depends on robust analysis, which mainly depends on the availability of a valuable base of spatial and attribute data. Moreover, analytical statistics processes within GIS environments require a high quality and accuracy of data that facilitates comparison between scenarios and outputs of the analysis. In contrast, the development of models and analytical approaches has contributed to improving the accuracy and quality of spatial data that are processed and analyzed within the GIS environment.

Studies reviewed in this paper emphasized that GIS has a positive role in addressing a reasonable area of healthcare planning issues. It has contributed to creating an appropriate environment for utilizing analytical approaches to address healthcare planning issues, especially in terms of issues related to optimal allocation of health resources based on set spatial behaviors between supply and demand. Thus, GIS can be an effective tool for dealing with healthcare planning issues, especially with (1) the continued significant development of GIS technologies worldwide, and (2) the cognitive development of planners and health professionals in practicing applications based on analytical approaches that have been supported by advanced technologies of GIS. GIS is now used in epidemiology, specifically relating to environmental epidemics, where GIS can assist in understanding and analyzing patterns of disease spread, and modeling relevant environmental exposure factors, effects, and risks, provided that an effective system is available to manage health data and information. GIS can also help achieve equality of access to healthcare by examining and evaluating use patterns of demand for healthcare, and allocating optimal locations for healthcare facilities based on population distribution, locations of health facilities, transportation and road networks, and other factors.

Although GIS has been contributing to supporting healthcare planning using analytical approaches and statistical methods, the application of these approaches and methods to GIS-based healthcare planning faces a number of key challenges. The most important of these are, first, the lack of availability and weak management of health information, and, second, the lack of maps of spatial behaviors observed between supply and demand. Third, and most importantly, the lack of spatial data is one of the most important key challenges facing the healthcare planning process based on GIS. GIS deals with healthcare planning issues through a set of analytical approaches and statistical methods that require availability of several types of spatial data. For example, good modeling and planning of epidemics requires data on environmental risk areas and their descriptive characteristics, and this is difficult to acquire in many countries. This is particularly true of developing countries, which may also have fertile environments for the spread of epidemics and diseases, thus complicating the issue. In addition, a successful health information management system requires the availability of spatial data that allows accurate inquiries and analyses of the public and workers in the health sector. These challenges are considered as obstacles for any practical task in healthcare planning to ensure theoretical and quantitative work is logical in a real world environment.

5. Conclusions

GIS is an effective tool to support spatial decision-making in public health through applying the evolving analytical approaches to dealing with healthcare planning issues. This requires a literature review before preparing relevant studies, particularly because of the continuous development of GIS technologies. However, it is clear from the literature reviewed that there are aspects that need further investigation to be considered as future directions that health organizations and officials should deal with using GIS-based analytical approaches and statistical methods. First, the GIS-based analytical approaches used for modeling epidemics depend highly on the availability of census data to give a more realistic representation of the disease spread and prediction of locations of populations at risk. In addition, the census data used for the modeling epidemics should be of high quality and accuracy in order to be in line with the requirements of recent GIS techniques, and this is a major challenge, especially in developing countries. Second, the GIS-based analytical approaches used for modeling of accessibility to healthcare services depend on the availability of a set of spatial data (e.g., distance from origin to healthcare service) and nonspatial data (e.g., estimation of demand based on demographic characteristics of the population). Nevertheless, the biggest challenge consisted in how to estimate the demand for healthcare services in light of the low quality and accuracy of the demographic and socioeconomic data of population that can describe patients' behavior in seeking the appropriate service. Third, the GIS-based analytical approaches used for developing health information systems including epidemiology management, disease surveillance and health risk analysis require the availability of precise enviromental risk data. Nevertheless, health organizations and specialized researchers face a difficulty in using these approaches to develop their health information systems due to the lack of enviromental risk data entered into interactive information systems for disease management and surveillance. This represents a major challenge, especially at the level of conducting inquiries and spatial analyses by specialists and the public. Fourth, many health organizations and specialized researchers have been using the GIS-based analytical approaches to monitor outbreak of epidemic diseases, assess potential infections, map disease risks, and predict sudden emergencies. Public health surveillance systems need the accurate data about the surrounding environment of the population at risk. Consequently, the application of analytical approaches to improve public health surveillance facing difficulty due to the poor organization, collection, analysis and interpretation of such data. Hence, that requires the development of health information systems in general.

Author Contributions: Conceptualization, Abdulkader Murad; methodology, Abdulkader Murad; formal analysis, Bandar Fuad Khashoggi; writing—original draft preparation, Bandar Fuad Khashoggi; writing—review and editing, Abdulkader Murad; visualization, Bandar Fuad Khashoggi; supervision, Abdulkader Murad; All authors have read and agreed to the published version of the manuscript.

Funding: This research received no external funding.

Conflicts of Interest: The authors declare no conflict of interest.

References

1. Geraghty, E. Why Health is so Spatial. Available online: https://www.youtube.com/watch?v=3p7OFICg9Ak (accessed on 30 January 2020).
2. Krieger, N. Place, Space, and Health: GIS and Epidemiology. *Epidemiology* **2003**, *14*, 384–385. [CrossRef]
3. Pickle, L.W. Spatial Analysis of Disease. *Cancer Treat. Res.* **2002**, *113*, 113–150. [CrossRef] [PubMed]
4. Gatrell, A.C.; Masser, I.; Salgé, F. *GIS and Health*; Informa UK Limited: London, UK, 1998; pp. 179–187.
5. Curtis, S. *Health and Inequality*; SAGE Publications: Thousand Oaks, CA, USA, 2004.
6. Yuan, M. Adding Time into Geographic Information System Databases. In *The Handbook of Geographic Information Science*; Wiley: Hoboken, NJ, USA, 2008; pp. 169–184.
7. Koch, T. Mapping the Miasma: Air, Health, and Place in Early Medical Mapping. *Cartogr. Perspect.* **2005**, 4–27, 4–27. [CrossRef]
8. GisGeography. The Remarkable History of GIS. Available online: https://gisgeography.com/history-of-gis/ (accessed on 3 February 2020).
9. ESRI. GIS for Public Health Today and Tomorrow. Available online: https://www.esri.com/news/arcuser/0499/umbrella.html (accessed on 3 February 2020).
10. Koch, T. *Disease Maps*; The University of Chicago Press: Chicago, IL, USA, 2011; p. 247.
11. D'Onofrio, A.; Mazzetta, C.; Robertson, C.; Smans, M.; Boyle, P.; Boniol, M. Maps and atlases of cancer mortality: A review of a useful tool to trigger new questions. *Ecancermedicalscience* **2016**, *10*, 670. [CrossRef] [PubMed]
12. Yomralioglu, T.; Colak, E.H.; Aydinoglu, A.C. Geo-Relationship between Cancer Cases and the Environment by GIS: A Case Study of Trabzon in Turkey. *Int. J. Environ. Res. Public Health* **2009**, *6*, 3190–3204. [CrossRef]
13. Altonen, B. Alfred Haviland—1875 (2ed. 1893)—Cancer in Great Britain. Public Health, Medicine and History. 2019. Available online: https://brianaltonenmph.com/gis/historical-disease-maps/alfred-haviland-1875-2ed-1893-disease-in-great-britain/ (accessed on 3 February 2020).

14. Clarke, K.; McLafferty, S.L.; Tempalski, B. On epidemiology and geographic information systems: A review and discussion of future directions. *Emerg. Infect. Dis.* **1996**, *2*, 85–92. [CrossRef]
15. Croner, C. Public Health Geographic Information Systems (Gis) News and Information; 1994–1997. Center of Disease Control and Prevention. Available online: https://stacks.cdc.gov/view/cdc/13298 (accessed on 6 February 2020).
16. CDC. Our History—Our Story. Available online: https://www.cdc.gov/about/history/index.html (accessed on 6 February 2020).
17. World Health Organization. The Atlas of Heart Disease and Stroke. Available online: https://www.who.int/cardiovascular_diseases/resources/atlas/en/ (accessed on 17 February 2020).
18. CDC. Heart Disease Death Rates, Total Population Ages 35+. Available online: https://www.cdc.gov/dhdsp/maps/national_maps/hd_all.htm (accessed on 8 February 2020).
19. Musa, G.J.; Chiang, P.-H.; Sylk, T.; Bavley, R.; Keating, W.; Lakew, B.; Tsou, H.-C.; Hoven, C. Use of GIS Mapping as a Public Health Tool—From Cholera to Cancer. *Health Serv. Insights* **2013**, *6*, 111–116. [CrossRef]
20. Farnia, P.; Aghajani, J.; Velayati, A. Impact of geographical information system on public health sciences. *Biomed. Biotechnol. Res. J.* **2017**, *1*, 94. [CrossRef]
21. Briney, A. Overview of Public Health and GIS. Gislounge. Available online: https://www.gislounge.com/overview-public-health-gis/ (accessed on 8 February 2020).
22. CESCR—Committee on Economic, Social and Cultural Rights. The Right to the Highest Attainable Standard of Health. United Nations Human Rights. Available online: https://www.refworld.org/pdfid/4538838d0.pdf (accessed on 26 May 2020).
23. Sherif, A. Towards Spatial Justice in Urban Health Services Planning. Ph.D. Thesis, University of Utrecht, Utrecht, The Netherlands, 2007.
24. Drissy, A. The Evolution of Health Expenditure in Algeria and its Effectiveness in the Reform of the Health System During the Period (2013–2004). *Algerian J. Glob. Econ. Policies.* **2015**, *6*, 137–145.
25. Mokgalaka, H. Measuring Access to Primary Health Care: Use of a GIS-Based Accessibility Analysis. Semantic Scholar. Available online: https://pdfs.semanticscholar.org/5a16/14e0c2db094958a992a2b8a30c335b55d22b.pdf?_ga=2.240499466.883523912.1577652254-1188223766.1576187194 (accessed on 29 December 2019).
26. Dallhammer, E.; Gaugitsch, R.; Neugebauer, W. *Spatial Planning and Governance within EU Policies and Legislation and Their Relevance to the New Urban Agenda (p. 2)*; European Committee of the Regions: Bruxelles, Belgium, 2018; Available online: https://cor.europa.eu/en/engage/studies/Documents/Spatial-planning-new-urban-agenda.pdf (accessed on 26 May 2020).
27. McLafferty, S.L. GIS and Health Care. *Annu. Rev. Public Health* **2003**, *24*, 25–42. [CrossRef]
28. Kirby, R.S.; Delmelle, E.; Eberth, J.M. Advances in spatial epidemiology and geographic information systems. *Ann. Epidemiol.* **2016**, *27*, 1–9. [CrossRef] [PubMed]
29. Nicol, J. Geographic information systems within the national health service: The scope for implementation. *Plan. Outlook* **1991**, *34*, 37–42. [CrossRef]
30. Murad, A. Using GIS for Planning Public General Hospitals at Jeddah City. *J. King Abdulaziz Univ. Des. Sci.* **2005**, *3*, 3–22. [CrossRef]
31. Datta, D.; S G, R.K.; Mb, A.N.; Bapilus, L.; Anandan, S. Spatial Epidemiology: Geostatistical Tool for Disease Mapping. *World J. Pharm. Res.* **2017**, *6523*, 1771–1780. [CrossRef]
32. Little, M.; Meade, M.; Florin, J.; Gesler, W. Medical Geography. *Geogr. Rev.* **1989**, *79*, 247. [CrossRef]
33. Gatrell, A.; Senior, M. *Health and health care application in Longley P, Goodchild M, Maguire D and Rhind D, Geographical Information System Principles and Application*; John Wiley & Sons: Hoboken, NJ, USA; pp. 925–938.
34. Cliff, A.D.; Haggett, P.; Ord, J.K. *Spatial Aspects of Influenza Epidemics*; Pion: London, UK, 1986.
35. Gould, P.; Wallace, R. Spatial Structures and Scientific Paradoxes in the AIDS Pandemic. *Geografiska Annaler* **1994**, *76*, 105–116. [CrossRef]
36. Braga, M.; Cislaghi, C.; Luppi, G.; Tasco, C. A Multipurpose. Interactive Mortality Atlas of Italy. In *GIS and Health*; Gatrell, A.C., Löytönen, M., Eds.; Taylor and Francis: London, UK, 1998; pp. 125–138.
37. Brown, P.J.B.; Hirschfield, A.; Batey, P.W.J. Applications of geodemographic methods in the analysis of health condition incidence data. *Pap. Reg. Sci.* **1991**, *70*, 329–344. [CrossRef]
38. Wrigley, N. Market-based systems of health-care provision, the NHS Bill, and geographical information systems. *Environ. Plan. A.* **1991**, *23*, 5–8.

39. Johnson, G.D. Small area mapping of prostate cancer incidence in New York State (USA) using fully Bayesian hierarchical modelling. *Int. J. Health Geogr.* **2004**, *3*, 29. [CrossRef]
40. Rasam, A.A.R.; Ghazali, R.; Noor, A.M.M.; Naim, W.M.; Hamid, J.R.A.; Bazlan, M.J.; Ahmad, N. Spatial epidemiological techniques in cholera mapping and analysis towards a local scale predictive modelling. In *Proceedings of the IOP Conference Series: Earth and Environmental Science*; IOP Publishing: Bristol, UK, 2014; Volume 18, p. 12095.
41. Brown, B. 5 Benefits of Geographic Information Systems in Healthcare. Hitconsultant. Available online: https://hitconsultant.net/2015/10/29/5-benefits-of-geographic-information-systems-in-healthcare/#.Xe0UX-jXJPY (accessed on 8 December 2019).
42. Sones, M. Reveal: Mapping and Tracking the Spread of Deadly Diseases. Available online: https://www.esri.com/about/newsroom/blog/reveal-mapping-and-tracking-the-spread-of-deadly-diseases/ (accessed on 18 December 2019).
43. Fradelos, E.C.; Papathanasiou, I.V.; Mitsi, D.; Tsaras, K.; Kleisiaris, C.F.; Kourkouta, L. Health Based Geographic Information Systems (GIS) and their Applications. *Acta Inform. Medica* **2014**, *22*, 402–405. [CrossRef]
44. WHO. World Bank and WHO: Half the World Lacks Access to Essential Health Services, 100 Million Still Pushed Into Extreme Poverty Because of Health Expenses. Available online: https://www.who.int/news-room/detail/13-12-2017-world-bank-and-who-half-the-world-lacks-access-to-essential-health-services-100-million-still-pushed-into-extreme-poverty-because-of-health-expenses (accessed on 21 December 2019).
45. Bhatt, J.; Bathija, P. Ensuring Access to Quality Health Care in Vulnerable Communities. *Acad. Med.* **2018**, *93*, 1271–1275. [CrossRef] [PubMed]
46. Jones, A.P.; Bentham, G. Emergency medical service accessibility and outcome from road traffic accidents. *Public Health* **1995**, *109*, 169–177. [CrossRef]
47. Forbers, H.; Todd, P. Review of Cancer Services, Northwest Regional Health Authority, Urban Research and Policy Evaluation Regional Research Laboratory. University of Liverpool: Liverpool, UK, 1995.
48. World Health Organization. *Barriers and Facilitating Factors in Access to Health Services in the Republic of Moldova. Health Policy Paper*; WHO: Moldova, 2012; pp. 4–22. Available online: http://www.euro.who.int/__data/assets/pdf_file/0018/183510/e96775-final.pdf (accessed on 21 December 2019).
49. Mohan, J.; Joseph, A.E.; Phillips, D.R. Accessibility and Utilization: Geographical Perspectives on Health Care Delivery. *Trans. Inst. Br. Geogr.* **1986**, *11*, 121. [CrossRef]
50. Luo, W.; Wang, F. Measures of Spatial Accessibility to Health Care in a GIS Environment: Synthesis and a Case Study in the Chicago Region. *Environ. Plan. B Plan. Des.* **2003**, *30*, 865–884. [CrossRef]
51. Khan, A.A.; Bhardwaj, S.M. Access to Healthcare: A Conceptual framework and its relevance to Health Care Planning. *Eval. Health Prof.* **1994**, *17*, 60–76. [CrossRef]
52. Foley, R. Assessing the applicability of GIS in a health and social care setting: Planning services for informal carers in East Sussex, England. *Soc. Sci. Med.* **2002**, *55*, 79–96. [CrossRef]
53. Teljeur, C.; Barry, J.; Kelly, A. The potential impact on travel times of closure and redistribution of A&E units in Ireland. *Ir. Med J.* **2004**, *97*, 6.
54. Kumar, N. Changing geographic access to and locational efficiency of health services in two Indian districts between 1981 and 1996. *Soc. Sci. Med.* **2004**, *58*, 2045–2067. [CrossRef]
55. Parker, E.B.; Campbell, J.L. Measuring access to primary medical care: Some examples of the use of geographical information systems. *Health Place* **1998**, *4*, 183–193. [CrossRef]
56. Brabyn, L.; Skelly, C. Modeling population access to New Zealand public hospitals. *Int. J. Health Geogr.* **2002**, *1*, 3. [CrossRef]
57. Murad, A. Using GIS for Determining Variations in Health Access in Jeddah City, Saudi Arabia. *ISPRS Int. J. Geo-Inf.* **2018**, *7*, 254. [CrossRef]
58. Christie, S.; Fone, D. Equity of access to tertiary hospitals in Wales: A travel time analysis. *J. Public Health Med.* **2003**, *25*, 344–350. [CrossRef] [PubMed]
59. Mokgalaka, H. GIS-Based Analysis of Spatial Accessibility: An Approach to Determine Public Primary Healthcare Demand in Metropolitan Areas. Master's Thesis, University of Cape Town, Cape Town, South Africa, 2015.

60. Guagliardo, M.F. Spatial accessibility of primary care: Concepts, methods and challenges. *Int. J. Health Geogr.* **2004**, *3*, 3. [CrossRef] [PubMed]
61. Kanuganti, S.; Sarkar, A.; Singh, A.P. Quantifying Accessibility to Health Care Using Two-step Floating Catchment Area Method (2SFCA): A Case Study in Rajasthan. *Transp. Res. Procedia* **2016**, *17*, 391–399. [CrossRef]
62. Tao, Z.; Cheng, Y. Modelling the spatial accessibility of the elderly to healthcare services in Beijing, China. *Environ. Plan. B: Urban Anal. City Sci.* **2018**, *46*, 1132–1147. [CrossRef]
63. Ni, J.; Liang, M.; Lin, Y.; Wu, Y.; Wang, C. Multi-Mode Two-Step Floating Catchment Area (2SFCA) Method to Measure the Potential Spatial Accessibility of Healthcare Services. *ISPRS Int. J. Geo-Inf.* **2019**, *8*, 236. [CrossRef]
64. Sharma, A.K. Role of GIS in Health Management Information System and Medical Plan: A Case Study of Gangtok area, Sikkim, India. *Int. J. Environ. Geoinform.* **2015**, *2*, 16–24. [CrossRef]
65. Cockerham, W. *International Encyclopedia of Public Health*, 2nd ed.; Elsevier: Birmingham, UK, 2017; p. 414.
66. Foley, R.; Charlton, M.; Fotheringham, S. GIS in Health and Social Care Planning. Available online: https://www.semanticscholar.org/ (accessed on 12 December 2019).
67. Gong, H.; Simwanda, M.; Murayama, Y. An Internet-Based, IS Platform Providing Data for Visualization and Spatial Analysis of Urbanization in Major Asian and African Cities. *ISPRS Int. J. Geo-Inf.* **2017**, *6*, 257. [CrossRef]
68. Singhasivanon, P.; Kidson, C.; Supavej, S. Mekong Malaria. Malaria, multi-drug resistance and economic development in the Greater Mekong sub-region of South-East Asia, incorporating geographical information systems databases. *Southeast Asian J. Trop. Med. Public Health* **1999**, *30*, 4.
69. Pringle, D.; Johnson, H.; Cullen, C.; Boyle, E.; Doyle, D.; Brazil, J.; McKeown, P.; Staines, A.; Beaton, D.; McIntyre, M.; et al. *Health Atlas Ireland: An Open-Source Mapping, Database and Statistical System*; GeoComputation 2007; National University of Ireland: Maynooth, Ireland, 2008.
70. Lu, X. A Framework of Web GIS Based Unified Public Health Information Visualization Platform. In *Applications of Evolutionary Computation*; Springer Science and Business Media LLC: Berlin, Germany, 2005; Volume 3482, pp. 256–265.
71. Abdullahi, F.; Lawal, M.; Agushaka, J. Design and Implementation of A Web-Based Gis for Public Healthcare Decision Support System in Zaria Metropolis. Ijrras, 4(4), p. 1. Available online: https://core.ac.uk/download/pdf/25731372.pdf (accessed on 21 December 2019).
72. Masimalai, P. GIS for rapid epidemiological mapping and health-care management with special reference to filariasis in India. *Int. J. Med. Sci. Public Health* **2015**, *4*, 1. [CrossRef]
73. Moore, K.; Merritt, A.; Bobo, B.; Graham, A.; Kuhn, A. Kentucky Stroke Encounter Quality Improvement Project (SEQIP) Abstract 141: Using Geographic Information Systems (GIS) to Analyze Statewide Regional Data—A Feasibility Project from the Kentucky Stroke Encounter Quality Improvement Project (SEQIP). *Circ. Cardiovasc. Qual. Outcomes* **2019**, *12*, 1. [CrossRef]
74. World Health Organization. Public Health Surveillance. Available online: https://www.who.int/topics/public_health_surveillance/en/ (accessed on 24 December 2019).
75. Morens, D.M.; Fauci, A.S. Emerging Infectious Diseases: Threats to Human Health and Global Stability. *PLoS Pathog.* **2013**, *9*, e1003467. [CrossRef] [PubMed]
76. Wiafe, S.; Davenhall, B. Extending Disease Surveillance with GIS. ESRI. Available online: https://www.esri.com/news/arcuser/0405/disease_surveil1of2.html (accessed on 13 December 2019).
77. Lee, L.M.; Teutsch, S.M.; Thacker, S.B.; Louis, M.E.S. *Principles & Practice of Public Health Surveillance*; Oxford University Press (OUP): Oxford, UK, 2010.
78. Stallones, L.; Nuckols, J.R.; Berry, J.K. Surveillance around hazardous waste sites: GIS and reproductive outcomes. *Environ. Res.* **1992**, *59*, 81–92. [CrossRef]
79. Law, D.; Wilfert, R. Infectious Disease Surveillance and Outbreak Investigation using GIS. Focus, Volume 5, p. 3. Available online: https://nciph.sph.unc.edu/focus/vol5/issue2/5-2Mapping_issue.pdf (accessed on 13 December 2019).
80. ASTHO Organization Technologies for Vector-Borne Disease Surveillance. p. 3. Available online: https://astho.org/Programs/Environmental-Health/Natural-Environment/VBD-Tech-Surveillance-Scan/ (accessed on 13 December 2019).

81. Kazmi, S.J.H.; Usery, E.L. Application of remote sensing and gis for the monitoring of diseases: A unique research agenda for geographers. *Remote Sens. Rev.* **2001**, *20*, 45–70. [CrossRef]
82. Pam, D.D.; Omalu, I.C.J.; Akintola, A.A.; Dan, A.Y.; Kalesanwo, A.O.; Babagana, M.; Muhammad, S.A.; Ocha, I.M.; Adeniyi, K.A. The Role of GIS And Remote Sensing in the Control of Malaria. *Online J Health Allied Scs.* **2017**, *16*, 7. Available online: http://www.ojhas.org/issue63/2017-3-7.html (accessed on 26 May 2020).
83. Kalluri, S.; Gilruth, P.; Rogers, D.; Szczur, M. Surveillance of Arthropod Vector-Borne Infectious Diseases Using Remote Sensing Techniques: A Review. *PLoS Pathog.* **2007**, *3*, e116. [CrossRef]
84. Jeanne, I.; Chambers, L.E.; Kazazic, A.; Russell, T.L.; Bobogare, A.; Bugoro, H.; Otto, F.; Fafale, G.; Amjadali, A. Mapping a Plasmodium transmission spatial suitability index in Solomon Islands: A malaria monitoring and control tool. *Malar. J.* **2018**, *17*, 381. [CrossRef] [PubMed]
85. Mandyata, C.B.; Olowski, L.K.; Mutale, W. Challenges of implementing the integrated disease surveillance and response strategy in Zambia: A health worker perspective. *BMC Public Health* **2017**, *17*, 746. [CrossRef]
86. Rahman, S.-U.; Smith, D.K. Use of location-allocation models in health service development planning in developing nations. *Eur. J. Oper. Res.* **2000**, *123*, 437–452. [CrossRef]
87. Afshari, Q.P.H.; Peng, H.A.A.Q. Challenges and Solutions for Location of Healthcare Facilities. *Ind. Eng. Manag.* **2014**, *3*. [CrossRef]
88. Kotavaara, O.; Pohjosenperä, T.; Juga, J.; Rusanen, J. Accessibility in designing centralised warehousing: Case of health care logistics in Northern Finland. *Appl. Geogr.* **2017**, *84*, 83–92. [CrossRef]
89. Abdelkarim, A. Integration of Location-Allocation and Accessibility Models in GIS to Improve Urban Planning for Health Services in Al-Madinah Al-Munawwarah, Saudi Arabia. *J. Geogr. Inf. Syst.* **2019**, *11*, 633–662. [CrossRef]
90. Polo, G.; Acosta, C.M.; Ferreira, F.; Dias, R.A. Location-Allocation and Accessibility Models for Improving the Spatial Planning of Public Health Services. *PLoS ONE* **2015**, *10*, e0119190. [CrossRef] [PubMed]

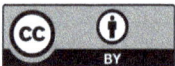

© 2020 by the authors. Licensee MDPI, Basel, Switzerland. This article is an open access article distributed under the terms and conditions of the Creative Commons Attribution (CC BY) license (http://creativecommons.org/licenses/by/4.0/).

MDPI
St. Alban-Anlage 66
4052 Basel
Switzerland
Tel. +41 61 683 77 34
Fax +41 61 302 89 18
www.mdpi.com

ISPRS International Journal of Geo-Information Editorial Office
E-mail: ijgi@mdpi.com
www.mdpi.com/journal/ijgi

www.ingramcontent.com/pod-product-compliance
Lightning Source LLC
LaVergne TN
LVHW070423100526
838202LV00014B/1514